AHMAD ASSALIA   MICHEL GAGNER   MOSHE SCHEIN (EDS.)

Controversies in Laparoscopic Surgery

Ahmad Assalia   Michel Gagner
Moshe Schein (Eds.)

Controversies in
Laparoscopic Surgery

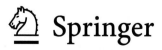 Springer

Ahmad Assalia, MD
Deputy Director and Chief of Laparoscopic Service,
Department of Surgery B, Rambam Health Care Campus,
Lecturer in Surgery,
The Bruce Rappaport Faculty of Medicine, Technion,
Israel Institute of Technology,
Haifa 31906, Israel
(e-mail: Assaliaa@aol.com)

Michel Gagner, MD, FRCSC, FACS
Professor of Surgery, Chief,
Division of Laparoscopic and Bariatric Surgery, Department of Surgery,
Joan and Standford I. Weill Medical College of Cornell University,
New York Presbyterian Hospital-Weill Cornell Medical Center,
525 East 68th Street, Mailbox 294, New York, NY 10021, USA
(e-mail: gagnerm@aol.com)

Moshe Schein, MD, FACS, FCS (SA)
Surgical Specialties of Keokuk
1425 Morgan Street ,
Keokuk, IA 52632 , USA
Professor of Surgery, Weill College of Medicine,
Cornell University, New York
(e-mail: mschein1@mindspring.com)

ISBN-10   3-540-21158-6 Springer-Verlag Berlin Heidelberg New York
ISBN-13   978-3-540-21158-6 Springer-Verlag Berlin Heidelberg New York

Library of Congress Control Number: 2004111360

Springer-Verlag is a part of Springer Science+Business Media

springeronline.com

© Springer-Verlag Berlin Heidelberg 2006
Printed in Germany

Editor: Gabriele Schröder, Heidelberg
Desk Editor: Stephanie Benko, Heidelberg
Production: PRO EDIT GmbH, 69126 Heidelberg, Germany
Cover design: E-Studio Calamar, Spain
Typesetting: SDS, Leimen, Germany
Printed on acid-free paper   24/3151Re – 5 4 3 2 1 0

Preface

"If you are too fond of new remedies, first you will not cure your patients; secondly, you will have no patients to cure."
(Astley Paston Cooper, 1768–1841)

Today Dr. Cooper would have to modify his aphorism to:
"If you are *not* too fond of new remedies you will have no patients to cure..."

That controversy exists implies that evidence supporting an unequivocally "correct" position is lacking. *Laparoscopy, however, was born into controversy*. Some would even say that the majority of laparoscopy is still controversial. By challenging established concepts in surgery, laparoscopy was very often met with skepticism and even fierce objection. Beginning in the early days of laparoscopic cholecystectomy, opinions were divided as to the role of laparoscopic surgery as an acceptable, viable or a better substitute to the open surgical counterparts. In addition to the feasibility and applicability, the controversy involved the various ways to best perform the laparoscopic approach and to achieve at least a similar outcome to that with open surgery.

After a decade and a half of vast experience and progress, except of a few instances (e.g., cholecystectomy, adrenalectomy, esophageal myotomy, splenectomy for normal-sized spleens and possibly Nissen's fundoplication), debate still surrounds most of the laparoscopic procedures. Many of them, in fact, are still considered experimental or immature. Growing experience, daring and technological advances made most of operations to be feasible laparoscopically resulting in the well-known advantages of minimal access surgery. But beyond feasibility, laparoscopy has struggled to prove itself comparable to, or even better, than traditional techniques. The learning curves and specific inherent problems associated with laparoscopy created additional dimensions of complications. Issues of operating times and cost further complicated the continuing debate.

Very few randomized controlled trials were conducted to scientifically evaluate the role of laparoscopy. Nevertheless, several procedures practically replaced open surgery even without high levels of evidence. The success was determined most often by the patients rather than the well established and often conservative medical community. Therefore, and mainly because of patient demand, large scale randomized controlled trials will most probably not be performed for many procedures.

Even so, laparoscopy is now commonplace in every hospital and almost in every country around the world, mainly because patients tend to seek comfort and "easier" procedures. Hospitals are striving to expand their laparoscopic services and new generation of young surgeons are being born into this minimally invasive era or this new "state of mind". New territories in surgery are being conquered by laparoscopy and, as experience is accumulating, it is becoming clear that the opponents or "laparo-skeptics" are tempering their criticism. It seems that the laparoscopic momentum will not be stopped. Even though the industry seems to have an important role in the development and promotion of laparoscopy, often for its own gain, we will do better if we know where to draw the line between fruitful cooperation (while keeping in mind standards of care) and personal profits. At the same time, while striving to improve and innovate, we, as balanced surgeons, need to moderate and curb our over-enthusiasm for the sake of our integrity and, most importantly, for the sake of our patients.

That was the rationale behind this book: to critically evaluate the current status of laparoscopy and provide a balanced, evidence-based opinion. The inclusion of one editor who is not an advanced laparoscopic surgeon (MS) reflects our intentions. For each topic, a known laparoscopic pioneer in the field has critically evaluated the available evidence "flavored" with his personal experience, which was then balanced or "counter-balanced", in most cases, by a known non-laparoscopic surgical authority.

Unlike other available texts in laparoscopy, this book is not intended to be a substitute for or "just another" textbook. Rather, the authors assume that the reader has a fundamental grasp of relevant basic knowledge and thus focus on sharp points of dispute. Even though it sheds a different light on the field of laparoscopy, it should serve not only the dedicated laparoscopic surgeon but also general surgeons with the quest for evidence-based practice and interest in laparoscopy, as well as surgical trainees.

Could this book have been written a decade ago? Yes, but in the absence of experience and sufficient data it would have been a futile non-scientific debate between the conservative surgeon trying to protect his well-established practice, and avoiding the learning of the "new trick", and the open-minded enthusiastic pioneer trying to accomplish his dream. The main and almost only controversy was the mere justification of laparoscopic surgery. Today, after almost 15 years of experience, when some of the laparoscopic procedures are considered as the new "gold standard", considerable data exist to afford a more educated debate.

In the preface to the first surgical text addressing controversies (RL Varco, JP Delaney, Controversy in Surgery, W.B. Saunders, Philadelphia, 1976), James P. Shannon, wrote:

"One mark of an educated man is his ability to differ without becoming angry, sarcastic or discourteous. Such a man recognizes that in contingent matters there will always be a place for legitimate difference of opinion ... he respects the honesty and the intellectual integrity of others and ... if his be a disciplined mind, he does not lightly forsake the intellectual ground he has won at great cost. He yields only to evidence, proof or demonstration."

Let us hope that this spirit of intellectual debate will continue to lead us in our future endeavors.

The Editors
New York, 2005

Contents

Chapter 22
Cystic Parasitic and Non-parasitic Liver Disease. . . . 273
SELÇUK MERCAN

Chapter 23
Liver Surgery for Solid Tumors 287
W.R. JARNAGIN, YUMAN FONG

List of Contributors

Michel B. Aboutanos, MD, MPH
(e-mail: mbaboutanos@vcu.edu)
Assistant Professor of Surgery, Director of Injury
Prevention Program, Division of Trauma/Critical Care,
Department of Surgery, West Hospital, 15th Floor,
1200 East Broad St., PO Box 980454, Richmond,
VA 23298-0454, USA

Ahmad Assalia, MD
(e-mail: Assaliaa@aol.com)
Deputy Director and Chief of Laparoscopic Service,
Department of Surgery B, Rambam Health Care Campus,
Lecturer in Surgery,
The Bruce Rappaport Faculty of Medicine, Technion,
Israel Institute of Technology, Haifa 31906, Israel

Laurent Biertho, MD
(e-mail: laurentbiertho@hotmail.com)
Surgical resident, Department of Abdominal Surgery,
Les Cliniques Saint Joseph, Rue de Hesbaye, 75, 4000 Liege,
Belgium

Molly Buzdon, MD
(e-mail: mbuzdon@smail.umaryland.edu)
Assistant Chief of Surgery, Director of Laparoscopic Surgery,
Union Memorial Hospital, 201 East University Parkway,
Baltimore, MD 21218, USA

Marco Catarci, MD
(e-mail: m.catarci@sanfilipponeri.roma.it)
Staff Surgeon, General & Oncologic Surgery Unit,
San Filippo Neri Hospital, Via G. Martinotti, 20, 00135 Rome,
Italy

Bipan Chand, MD
(e-mail: Larsons@ccf.org)
Associate Staff, Department of General Surgery,
Cleveland Clinic Foundation, 9500 Euclid Avenue,
Cleveland, OH 44195,
USA

Eugene Cho, MD, FACS
(e-mail: Escho@mail.com)
Program Director -- Advance Laparoscopy Fellowship Program,
Franciscan Health System, 233 St Helens #505, Tacoma,
WA 98402,
USA

Paul T. Cirangle, MD, FACS
(e-mail: pcirangle@lapsf.com)
Assistant Professor of Surgery,
Uniformed Services University of the Health Sciences,
California Pacific Medical Center, San Francisco, California,
USA

Federico Cuenca-Abente, MD
(e-mail: federicoca@hotmail.com)
Fellow, Center for Videoendoscopic Surgery,
Department of Surgery,
University of Washington Medical Center Seattle,
WA 98195-6410,
USA

Myriam J. Curet, MD, FACS
(e-mail: mcuret@stanford.edu)
Associate Professor of Surgery, Department of Surgery,
Stanford University, 701B Welch Road, Stanford, CA 94305,
USA

Donald R.Czerniach, MD
(e-mail: drczern@laparoendoscopy.com)
Assistant Professor of Surgery, Department of Surgery,
University of Massachusetts Medical School, 55 Lake Avenue
North, Worcester, MA 01655,
USA

Bernard Dallemagne, MD
(e-mail: BernardDallemagne@lescliniquesstjoseph.be)
Head, Department of Abdominal Surgery,
Les Cliniques Saint Joseph, Rue de Hesbaye, 75, 4000 Liege,
Belgium

Salvadora Delgado, MD, PhD
Consultant, Gastrointestinal Surgery, Hospital Clinic,
University of Barcelona, Villarroel 170, 08036 Barcelona,
Spain

Eric J. DeMaria, MD
(e-mail: edemaria@hsc.vcu.edu)
Professor of Surgery, Chief, General Surgery Section, Director,
Minimally Invasive Surgery Center, Department of Surgery,
Virginia Commonwealth University, 1200 East Broad Street,
West Building, 16th Floor, Richmond, VA 23298,
USA

Claude Deschamps, MD
(e-mail: deschamps.claude@mayo.edu)
Professor of Surgery, Division of Thoracic Surgery,
Mayo Clinic College of Medicine, 200 First Street, SW, Rochester,
MN 55905,
USA

Adolfo Z. Fernandez Jr., MD
Assistant Professor of Surgery, Department of Surgery,
Wake Forest University School of Medicine,
Medical Center Boulevard, Winston-Salem, NC 27157,
USA

Yuman Fong, MD
(e-mail: dimarioa@MSKCC.ORG)
Murray F. Brennan Chair in Surgery,
Memorial Sloan-Kettering Cancer Center, Professor of Surgery,
Weill Medical College of Cornell University,
Memorial Sloan-Kettering Cancer Center, 1275 York Avenue,
New York, NY 10021,
USA

Dennis L. Fowler, MD
(e-mail: dlf91@columbia.edu)
U.S. Surgical Professor of Clinical Surgery,
Columbia College of Physicians and Surgeons,
Professor of Clinical Surgery,
Weill Medical College of Cornell University, Director,
Minimal Access Surgery Center, New York Presbyterian Hospital,
622 W. 168th St., PH 12, Room 126, New York, NY 10032,
USA

Michel Gagner, MD, FRCSC, FACS
(e-mail: mig2016@med.cornell.edu)
Professor of Surgery, Division of Laparoscopy, Chief,
Bariatric Surgery, Department of Surgery,
Weill-Cornell College of Medicine,
New York-Presbyterian Hospital, New York, NY 10032,
USA

Gian Mattia del Genio, MD
(e-mail: gdg@doctor.com)
Resident in Surgery, Ospedale Molinette, University of Turin,
Corso AM Dogliotti 14, 10126 Turin,
Italy

Paolo Gentileschi, MD
(e-mail: gentilp@yahoo.com)
Assistant Professor of Surgery, Department of Surgery,
University of Rome Tor Vergata, Via A. Bosio, 13, 00161 Rome,
Italy

Jacques M. Himpens, MD
(e-mail: Jaques_himpens@hotmail.com)
Chief, Department of Laparoscopic Bariatric Surgery,
St Blasius General Hospital, 50 Kroonveldlaan,
Dendermonde 9200,
Belgium

Alberto de Hoyos, MD
(e-mail: dehoyosa@upmc.edu)
Director, Minimally Invasive Thoracic Surgery,
Northwestern Memorial Hospital, Chicago, IL,
USA

John G. Hunter, MD
(e-mail: hunterj@ohsu.edu)
Mackenzie Professor and Chair, Department of Surgery,
Oregon Health & Science University,
3181 SW Sam Jackson Park Road, Portland, OR 97239-3098,
USA

William B. Inabnet, MD, FACS
(e-mail: wbi2102@columbia.edu)
Chief, Section of Endocrine Surgery,
College of Physicians and Surgeons of Columbia University,
161 Fort Washington Ave, New York, NY 10032,
USA

J. Andrew Isch, MD
Senior Fellow & Acting Instructor,
Center for Video Endoscopic Surgery,
University of Washington Medical Center,
Department of Surgery,
1959 NE Pacific Street, Box 356410, Seattle, WA 98195-6410,
USA

Rao Ivatury MD, FACS
(e-mail: rivatury@hsc.vcu.edu)
Professor of Surgery, Emergency Medicine & Physiology,
Virginia Commonwealth University, Chief,
Division of Trauma, Critical Care & Emergency Surgery,
VCU Medical Center, Richmond, Virginia,
USA

Glyn G. Jamieson, MD, FRACS, FACS
(e-mail: Chris.batesbrownsword@adelaide.edu.au)
Professor and Chairman, Department of Surgery,
Royal Adelaide Hospital, The University of Adelaide,
Adelaide SA 5000,
Australia

William R. Jarnagin
(e-mail: jarnagiw@mskcc.org)
Assistant Attending Surgeon,
Memorial Sloan-Kettering Cancer Center,
Assistant Professor of Surgery,
Weill Medical College of Cornell University,
Department of Surgery,
Memorial Sloan-Kettering Cancer Center,
1275 York Avenue, New York, NY 10021,
USA

Gregg H. Jossart, MD, FACS
(e-mail: gjossart@lapsf.com)
Director of Minimally Invasive Surgery,
Advanced Laparoscopic and Endocrine Surgery,
Surgery for Morbid Obesity, California Pacific Medical Center,
2100 Webster Street, Suite 518, San Francisco, CA 94115,
USA

Gordie K. Kaban, MD, FRCSC
(e-mail: kabang@ummhc.org)
Fellow in Minimally Invasive Surgery, Department of Surgery,
University of Massachusetts Medical School,
55 Lake Avenue North, Worcester, MA 01655,
USA

Seigo Kitano, MD, FACS
(e-mail: kitano@oita-med.ac.jp)
Professor and Chairman, Department of Surgery I,
Oita Medical University, 1-1 Idaigaoka,
Hasama-machi, Oita 879-5593,
Japan

Antonio M. Lacy, MD, PhD
(e-mail: alacy@clinic.ub.es)
Professor of Surgery, Gastrointestinal Surgery, Hospital Clinic,
University of Barcelona, Villarroel 170, 08036 Barcelona,
Spain

Karl A. LeBlanc, MD, MBA, FACS
(e-mail: DOCMBA2@aol.com)
Minimally Invasive Surgery Institute, Inc.,
1111 Hennessy Blvd. Suite 612,
Baton Rouge, Louisiana, USA,
and Clinical Associate Professor of Surgery,
Louisiana State University, New Orleans, Louisiana,
USA

Demetrius E.M. Litwin, MD, FRCSC
(e-mail: litwind@ummhc.org)
Professor of Surgery, Vice-Chairman, Department of Surgery,
University of Massachusetts Medical School,
55 Lake Avenue North, Worcester, MA 01655,
USA

James D. Luketich, MD
(e-mail: luketichjd@upmc.edu)
Associate Professor and Chief,
Division of Thoracic and Foregut Surgery,
Co-Director, The Minimally Invasive Surgery Center,
University of Pittsburgh Medical Center Health System,
Pittsburgh, Pennsylvania, USA,
and Division of Thoracic and Foregut Surgery,
UPMC Presbyterian, Suite 800, 200 Lothrop Street,
Pittsburgh, PA 15213,
USA

Joe Mamazza MD, FRCSC
(e-mail: mamazzaj@smh.toronto.on.ca)
Medical Director, Minimal Access Therapeutics Program,
St. Michael's Hospital, University of Toronto, 30 Bond Street,
M5B 1W8, Toronto, Ontario,
Canada

Payam Massaband, MD
(e-mail: payam@stanford.edu)
Resident in surgery, Stanford University, 701B Welch Road,
Stanford, CA 94305,
USA

Ronald Matteotti, MD
(e-mail: rom203@med.cornell.edu)
Fellow, Division of Laparoscopy and Bariatric Surgery,
Department of Surgery, Weill-Cornell College of Medicine,
New York-Presbyterian Hospital, New York, NY 10021,
USA

Selcuk Mercan, MD
(e-mail: smercan2000@yahoo.com)
Professor of Surgery, Department of General Surgery,
Faculty of Medicine, University of Istanbul,Capa, Topkapý,
Ýstanbul, Turkey

Mario Morino, MD
(e-mail: mario.morino@unito.it)
Professor of Surgery, General and Minimally Invasive Surgery,
Ospedale Molinette, University of Turin, Italy,
Corso AM Dogliotti 14, 10126 Turin, Italy

Brant K. Oelschlager, MD
(e-mail: brant@u.washington.edu)
Director, Laparoscopic Fellowship,
Co-director of Swallowing Center, Assistant Professor,
University of Washington Medical Center,
Department of Surgery, 1959 NE Pacific Street, Box 356410,
Seattle, WA 98195-6410,
USA

Masayuki Ohta, MD
Assistant Professor, Department of Surgery I,
Oita University Faculty of Medicine, 1-1 Idaigaoka,
Hasama-machi, Oita 879-5593,
Japan

Adrian Park, MD, FRCSC, FACS
(e-mail: apark@smail.umaryland.edu)
Campbell and Jeanette Plugge Professor of Surgery,
Chief, Division of General Surgery, Department of Surgery,
University of Maryland Medical Center, University of Maryland,
22 South Greene Street, S4B14, Baltimore, MD 21201-1595,
USA

Carlos A. Pellegrini, MD
(e-mail: pellegri@u.washington.edu)
Henry Harkins Professor and Chairman, Department of Surgery,
University of Washington Medical Center,
Department of Surgery, 1959 NE Pacific Street, Box 356410,
Seattle, WA 98195-6410,
USA

Alfons Pomp, MD, FRCSC, FACS
(e-mail: alp2014@med.cornell.edu)
Associate professor of Surgery, Division of Laparoscopy
and Bariartic Surgery, Department of Surgery,
Weill-Cornell College of Medicine,
New York-Presbyterian Hospital,
New York, NY 10021, USA

Jeffrey Ponsky, MD
(e-mail: ponskyj@ccf.org)
Professor of Surgery, Department of General Surgery,
Center of Minimally Invasive Surgery,
Cleveland Clinic Lerner College of Medicine of CWRU,
The Cleveland Clinic Foundation,
9500 Euclid Ave, Cleveland, OH 44195,
USA

Eric C. Poulin, MD, FRCSC
(e-mail: eric.poulin@utoronto.ca)
Wilbert J. Keon Chair of Surgery,
University of Ottawa Surgeon-in-Chief, University of Ottawa,
Ottawa,
Canada

E. Matt Ritter, MD
Fellow, Advanced Laparoscopic and GI Surgery,
Emory Endosurgery Unit, Department of Surgery,
Emory University School of Medicine,
1364 Clifton Road, NE, Suite H-122, Atlanta, GA 30322,
USA

Homero Rivas, MD
(e-mail: homerorivas@msn.com)
Fellow of Gastrointestinal Surgery, Gastrointestinal Surgery,
Hospital Clínic, University of Barcelona, Villarroel 170, 08036
Barcelona,
Spain

Addi Z. Rizvi
General Surgery Resident, Department of Surgery,
Oregon Health & Science University,
3181 SW Sam Jackson Park Road,
Portland,OR 97239-3098, USA

Christopher M. Schlachta, MD, FRCSC
(e-mail: christopher.schlachta@utoronto.ca)
Chief Division of General Surgery, St. Michael's Hospital,
University of Toronto, 30 Bond Street, M5B 1W8, Toronto,
Ontario, Canada

Carol E.H. Scott-Conner, MD, PhD
(e-mail: Scott-ConnerC@mail.medicine.uiowa.edu)
Professor and Head, Department of Surgery,
Roy J and Lucille A Carver College of Medicine,
University of Iowa, 200 Hawkins Drive, 1516 JCP, Iowa City,
IA 52242-1086, USA

Norio Shiraishi, MD
Associate Professor, Department of Surgery I,
Oita University Faculty of Medicine, 1-1 Idaigaoka,
Hasama-machi, Oita 879-5593,
Japan

C. Daniel Smith, MD, FACS
(e-mail: csmit27@emory.edu)
Associate Professor of Surgery and Surgical Anatomy,
Chief, General and Gastrointestinal Surgery, Director,
Emory Endosurgery Unit, Department of Surgery,
Emory University School of Medicine, 1364 Clifton Road, NE,
Suite H-122, Atlanta, GA 30322,
USA

Mark A. Talamini, MD
(e-mail: talamini@jhmi.edu)
Professor of Surgery, Director of Minimally Invasive Surgery,
Department of Surgery, Johns Hopkins Hospital,
Johns Hopkins University School of Medicine,
600 North Wolfe Street, block 665, Baltimore, MD 21287-4665,
USA

David S. Tichansky, MD
(e-mail: Newsky15@aol.com)
Assistant Professor of Surgery,
Minimally Invasive Surgery Section, Department of Surgery,
University of Tennessee, Memphis, 956 Court Ave, E232,
Memphis, TN 38103-2822,
USA

Mauro Toppino, MD
Associate professor of Surgery, General Surgery
and Minimally Invasive Surgery, Ospedale Molinette,
University of Turin, Corso AM Dogliotti 14, 10126 Turin,
Italy

David R. Urbach, MD, MSc
(e-mail: david.urbach@ices.on.ca)
Assistant Professor, Departments of Surgery and Health Policy,
Management and Evaluation, Staff Surgeon,
Division of General Surgery, University Health Network,
University of Toronto, Toronto, Ontario,
Canada

Tom P. Vleugels
(e-mail: TomVleugels@hotmail.com)
Department of abdominal surgery, Heilig Hart general hospital,
105 Naamse Straat, Leuven 3000,
Belgium

John Wayman, MD, FRCS
Upper GI Fellow, Department of Surgery, University of Adelaide,
Royal Adelaide Hospital, Adelaide, SA 5000,
Australia

Kaare Weber, MD
(e-mail: kaareweber@hotmail.com)
Assistant Professor of Surgery,
Divisions of General and Laparoscopic Surgery,
Department of Surgery,
Mount Sinai Medical Center, New York, NY,
USA

Donald B. Witzke, PhD
(e-mail: Don.Witzke@uky.edu)
Research Associate Professor,
Department of Pathology & Laboratory Medicine, Suite MS 117,
College of Medicine, University of Kentucky, Lexington,
KY 40536-0298,
USA

List of Commentators

Göran Åkerström, MD, PhD
(e-mail: iva.kulhanek@kirurgi.uu.se)
Professor, Department of Surgical Sciences,
University Hospital, SE-751 85 Uppsala,
Sweden

Nick Alexakis, MD
(e-mail: nalexakis@yahoo.co.uk)
Clinical Fellow, Department of Surgery, University of Liverpool,
Royal Liverpool University Hospital, Daulby Street, Liverpool,
L69 3GA,
UK

Carmen Balagué, MD, PhD
(e-mail: cbp64@yahoo.com)
Staff Surgeon, Service of Surgery, Hospital de Sant Pau,
P Claret 167, 08025 Barcelona,
Spain

Philip S. Barie, MD, MBA, FCCM, FACS
(e-mail: pbarie@med.cornell.edu)
Professor of Surgery and Public Health,
Weill Medical College of Cornell University,
NewYork-Presbyterian Hospital, New York,
NY 10021, USA

Willem A Bemelman
(e-mail: w.a.bemelman@amc.nl)
Laparoscopic Surgery/Colorectal Surgery,
Academic Medical Center, Department of Surgery,
Meibergdreef 9, 1105 AZ Amsterdam,
The Netherlands

Markus W. Büchler, MD
(e-mail: markus_buechler@med.uni-heidelberg.de)
Professor and Chairman, Department of General Surgery,
University of Heidelberg, Im Neuenheimer Feld 110,
69120 Heidelberg,
Germany

Andres Castellanos MD
(e-mail: Andres.E.Castellanos@drexel.edu)
Assistant professor of surgery,
Drexel University College of Medicine,
245 N. 15th St., Philadelphia, PA 9102,
USA

Wim P. Ceelen, MD
(e-mail: wim.ceelen@ugent.be)
Department of Surgery, Gent University Hospital 2K12 IC,
University Hospital De Pintelaan 185, 9000 Gent,
Belgium

Nicolas V. Christou, MD, PhD
(e-mail: Nicolas.Christou@MUHC.McGill.ca)
Head, Division of General Surgery, MUHC and McGill University,
Director, Section of Bariatric Surgery,
Division of General Surgery,
Room s9.30, Royal Victoria Hospital Site, 687 Pine Avenue West,
Montreal, QC H3A 1A1,
Canada

Pierre-Alain Clavien, MD, PhD, FACS, FRCS
(e-mail: clavien@chir.unizh.ch)
Professor and Chairman,
Division of Visceral and Transplantation Surgery,
University Hospital of Zürich, Rämistrasse 100, 8091 Zürich,
Switzerland

Robert E. Condon, MD, MSc, FACS
(e-mail: rec@wolfenet.com)
Professor and Chairman, Emeritus, Department of Surgery,
The Medical college of Wisconsin, Clinical Professor of Surgery,
The University of Washington, 2722 86th Ave. NE, Clyde Hill,
WA 98004-1653, USA

Ibrahim Dagher, MD, PhD
Attending Surgeon, Department of Digestive Surgery,
Paris-Sud University, Hôpital Antoine-Béclère,
157 rue de la Porte de Trivaux, 92141 Clamart Cédex,
France

Ara Darzi, KBE MD FRCS FRCSI FACS FRCPSG FMedSci
(e-mail: a.darzi@imperial.ac.uk)
Professor and Head, Department of Surgical Oncology
and Technology, Imperial College London, St Mary's Hospital,
Praed Street, London W2 1NY,
UK

Demetrios Demetriades, MD, PhD, FACS
(e-mail: demetria@usc.edu)
Professor of Surgery, Director,
Division of Trauma and Surgical Critical Care,
Department of Surgery,
University of Southern California Keck School of Medicine,
LAC and USC Medical Center, 1200 N State Street, Los Angeles,
CA 90033,
USA

David M. Dent
(e-mail: dmdent@UCTGSH1.UCT.AC.ZA)
Professor and Head, Department of Surgery,
University of Cape Town Faculty of Health Sciences
and Groote Schuur Hospital, Cape Town,
South Africa

Quan-Yang Duh MD
(e-mail: quan-yang.duh@med.va.gov)
Professor of Surgery, Department of Surgery,
University of California,
San Francisco, Surgical Service 112,
Veterans Affairs Medical Center,
4150 Clement Street, San Francisco, CA 94121,
USA

Jean Emond, MD
(e-mail: je111@columbia.edu)
Zimmer Professor of Surgery,
Vice-chair and Chief of Transplantation,
Columbia College of Physicians and Surgeons,
Center for Liver Diseases, New York Presbyterian Hospital,
622 W. 168th St. 14th floor, New York,
NY 10032, USA

Abe Fingerhut, MD, FACS, FRCSG
(e-mail: AbeFinger@aol.com)
Associate Professor, Louisiana State University,
New Orleans, Louisiana, USA, and Chief of Surgery,
Centre Hospitalier Intercommunal,
78303 Poissy,
France

Dominique Franco, MD
(e-mail: dominique.franco@abc.ap-hop-paris.fr)
Professor of Digestive Surgery,
Chief of Department of Digestive Surgery,
Paris-Sud University, Hôpital Antoine-Béclère,
157 rue de la Porte de Trivaux, 92141 Clamart cédex,
France

Gary Gecelter, MD, FACS
(e-mail: GGecelter@lij.edu)
Associate Professor of Clinical Surgery,
Albert Einstein College of Medicine, Department of Surgery,
Long Island Jewish Medical Center, 270-05 76th Avenue,
New Hyde Park, New York,
USA

Dirk J. Gouma, MD
(e-mail: d.j.gouma@amc.nl)
Professor of Surgery, General Surgery/G.I. Surgery,
Academic Medical Center,
Department of Surgery, Meibergdreef 9,
1105 AZ Amsterdam,
The Netherlands

Adam Griesemer, MD
Resident, Department of Surgery,
Columbia University Medical Center,
622 W 168th Street, New York, NY 10032,
USA

Harrith M. Hasson, MD
(e-mail: drhasson@aol.com)
Clincial Professor, Department of OB/GYN,
Weiss Hospital University of Chicago,
4646 N. Marine Drive, Suite Chicago, IL 60640
USA

Peter Kienle, MD
(e-mail: Peter.Kienle@med.uni-heidelberg.de)
Department of General Surgery, University of Heidelberg,
Im Neuenheimer Feld 110, 69120 Heidelberg,
Germany

Zygmunt H. Krukowski. PhD, FRCS, FRCP
(e-mail: suro13@abdn.ac.uk)
Consultant Surgeon, Aberdeen Royal Infirmary,
Professor of Surgery,
University of Aberdeen, Polwarth Building,
Aberdeen AB25 2ZN, Scotland,
UK

Picard Marceau, MD, PhD, FRCSC FACS
(e-mail: picard.marceau@chg.ulaval.ca)
Professor of Surgery, Department of Surgery, Laval University,
2725 chemin Sainte-Foy, Quebec G1V 4G5,
Canada

Edward E. Mason MD, PhD
(e-mail: edward-mason@uiowa.edu)
Emeritus Professor, University of Iowa College of Medicine,
Iowa City, Iowa,
USA

William Clark Meyers, MD, MBA
(e-mail: wcm23@drexel.edu)
Assistant Dean for Interdisciplinary Studies
and Chair of Surgery, Senior Associate Dean for Clinical Affairs,
Chairman -- Department of Surgery,
Drexel University College of Medicine,
245 N. 15th Street, MS 413, Philadelphia, PA 19102,
USA

John P. Neoptolemos, MA, MB, BChir, MD, FRCS
(e-mail: J.P.Neoptolemos@liverpool.ac.uk)
Professor of Surgery, Head -- Department of Surgery,
Royal Liverpool University Hospital, UCD Building,
Daulby Street,
Liverpool, L69 3GA, UK

Per-Olof Nyström, MD, PhD
(e-mail: p-o.nystrom@lio.se)
Associate Professor of Surgery, Consultant Colorectal Surgeon,
Department of Surgery, Linkoping University Hospital,
581 85 Linkoping,
Sweden

Mark B. Orringer, MD
(e-mail: morrin@med.umich.edu)
Professor and Head, Section of Thoracic Surgery,
University of Michigan Medical School, Ann Arbor, MI 48109,
USA

E. Patchen Dellinger, MD
(e-mail: patch@u.washington.edu)
Professor and Vice-chairman, Department of Surgery, Chief,
Division of General Surgery, University of Washington,
Box 356410, Room BB 428, 1959 NE Pacific Street, Seattle,
WA 98195-6410,
USA

J. David Richardson, MD, FACS
(e-mail: jdrich01@louisville.edu)
Professor and Vice-chairman, Department of Surgery,
University of Louisville, 530 S. Jackson Street, Louisville, KY
40292, USA

Raul J. Rosenthal, MD, FACS
(e-mail: rosentr@ccf.org)
Director, The Bariatric Institute, Head,
Section of Minimally Invasive Surgery, Cleveland Clinic Florida,
2950 Cleveland Clinic Blvd., Weston, FL 33331,
USA

Michael G. Sarr, MD
(e-mail: sarr.michael@mayo.edu)
James C. Masson Professor of Surgery, Department of Surgery,
Division of Gastroenterologic and General Surgery,
Mayo Clinic and Mayo Clinic College of Medicine,
200 First Street S.W., Rochester, MN 55905,
USA

Markus Schäfer, MD
Senior Staff Surgeon,
Division of Visceral and Transplantation Surgery,
University Hospital of Zürich, Rämistrasse 100, 8091 Zürich,
Switzerland

Ulrich Schöffel, MD
(e-mail: Ulrich.Schoeffel@swmbrk.de)
Associate Professor of Surgery,
University of Freiburg Medical School,
Chief of General and Visceral Surgery, Department of Surgery,
University of Freiburg, Germany,
and Red-Cross Hospital Lindenberg,
Jägerstr.41, 88161 Lindenberg,
Germany

Seymour I. Schwartz, MD
(e-mail: Seymour_Schwartz@URMC.Rochester.edu)
Distinguished Alumni Professor of Surgery,
University of Rochester School of Medicine and Dentistry,
Rochester, NY 14642,
USA

Eduardo M. Targarona, MD, PhD
(e-mail: etargarona@hsp.santpau.es)
Chief of Section of Endoscopic Surgery,
Associate Professor of Surgery, Service of Surgery,
Hospital de Sant Pau,
Medical School of the Autonomous University of Barcelona,
P Claret 167, 08025 Barcelona,
Spain

Manuel Trias, MD, PhD
Director of the Service of Surgery, Associate Professor of Surgery,
Hospital de Sant Pau,
Medical School of the University of Barcelona,
P Claret 167, 08025 Barcelona,
Spain

J. Stuart Wolf, Jr., MD
(e-mail: wolfs@umich.edu)
Associate Professor of Urology, Director,
Division of Minimally Invasive Urology, University of Michigan,
Department of Urology, 1500 E. Medical Center Dr.,
Ann Arbor, MI 48109-0330,
USA

Sen-Chang Yu MD, PhD
(e-mail: senchang@ha.mc.ntu.edu.tw)
Associate Professor, Department of Surgery,
National Taiwan University Hospital, President,
Minimally Invasive Surgery Medical Foundation,
7, Chung-Shan S. Rd., Taipei 100,
Taiwan

Abdalla E. Zarroug, MD
Resident in Surgery, Department of Surgery,
Mayo Clinic and Mayo Clinic College of Medicine,
200 1st Street SW, Rochester, MN 55905,
USA

Education and Training

ADRIAN PARK, DONALD WITZKE

▶ **Key Controversy**

– Who should be trained and how should we train them?

1.1
Introduction

Two major controversial issues dominate minimally invasive surgery (MIS) training: who should be trained and how should we train them? Although we focus on these two issues, it will become apparent that they are interconnected and that a large number of "smaller" issues are nested within each of them. We suggest that these issues reveal that the surgical training system is not working; nor is it currently taking a path that will lead to its healthy rebuilding.

MIS, compared to its open surgery (OS) counterpart, has generally been shown to reduce patient hospital-stays and complications, to speed patient recovery, return patients to work more quickly, and to improve cosmesis. Historically, the public demand for MIS procedures has caused surgical centers to increasingly offer this approach to their patient population. This patient demand has also challenged medical centers' ability to provide service – the number of trained laparoscopic surgeons has often been insufficient to meet the demand for surgery. Along with the supply–demand gap is a history of complications associated with early experience with different procedures. Thus the birth of a unique surgical methodology began in controversy, which continues today with training issues.

1.1.1
Minimally Invasive Surgery: Born in Controversy

The first procedure to be at the center of controversy was laparoscopic cholecystectomy (LC), which set the modern era of MIS in motion in 1987 [1]. In addition to the limitations posed by rather primitive instruments, there were a number of questionable solutions and outcomes related to training.

— Medical education seminars and workshops began to be offered, folowing traditional training designs, as a weekend solution to training surgeons in LC.
— Surgeons who had undergone this training began to perform LC without the benefit of preceptorship or performance certification of their competence.
— LC began to be the treatment of choice for gall bladder problems, without first undergoing the scientific rigor of clinical trials research to determine its benefits.
— Complication rates for LCs were far greater than the corresponding rates for the open surgery counterpart.

Research reports began to shed light on the reasons why these complication rates were so high, concluding that there was a steep curve associated with learning how to perform LC [2–8]. One study suggested that, using time as a criterion, a performance plateau was only reached after 200 patients [7]. Other procedures studied also provided evidence of steep learning curves [9–19].

1.2
Discussion

1.2.1
Training Issues

1.2.1.1
New and Evolving Laparoscopic Procedures

As "expert" laparoscopic surgeons become more comfortable with MIS by honing their skills in one procedure, there is a natural propensity to want to extend their repertoire to other procedures. To date, this expansion has resulted in more than 100 different MIS procedures being explored in the general surgical literature. The Society of American Gastrointestinal Endoscopic Surgeons (SAGES) has classified three laparoscopic procedures as core (cholecystectomy, appendectomy, and exploratory laparoscopy), calling the rest advanced [20, 21]. While there is evidence in the literature that trials of many of these new laparoscopic procedures are increasingly being reported, many procedures have been accepted without the benefit of randomized, prospective clinical trails (e.g., laparoscopic adrenalectomy, splenectomy, donor nephrectomy, fundoplication) [22]. Further, we have evidence, vis-à-vis the learning curve data reported, that surgeons with inadequate training and/

or experience are still performing MIS in their practices. This has led some authors to conclude that perhaps all training in MIS be done in residency [23]. At the very least, it is argued, any sanctioned post-residency laparoscopy training with a focus on developing clinical and cognitive skills should include a preceptorship with sufficient non-patient (i.e., simulator) practice time so that requisite perceptual motor skills can be mastered as well [24, 25]. Still, others have proposed that advanced training in laparoscopy should only be done through fellowships [26], or is already being done by fellows [27].

While this is a partial solution to giving surgeons extended experience in their craft, the number of programs offering MIS fellowships, although limited, is growing rapidly. The critical element in establishing a productive MIS training program is having a full-time director of MIS – an experienced laparoscopic surgeon [28]. Given the large and increasing need for highly trained laparoscopists, however, this path will only prolong the discrepancy between the number of skilled laparoscopists needed and the number produced. As a result, it appears that other training methods such as Continuing Medical Education conferences and courses will still play some role in the education of minimally invasive surgeons.

1.2.1.2
Continuing Medical Education

Surgeons in practice would seem to be in the best position to benefit from workshops and seminars focused on learning laparoscopy. It is, however, now well documented that attending this type of training does not necessarily result in enabling surgeons to safely perform laparoscopic procedures [29, 30]. There is a learning curve that not only requires a mature surgeon's learned clinical judgment but his or her learning and practice of perceptual motor skills as well. There is some evidence to suggest that even once the perceptual motor skills are mastered there is only minimal transfer of surgical skill and judgment from one laparoscopic procedure to the next. There appears to be a reasonable learning curve for each new procedure [8]. Providers of Continuing Medical Education (CME) for MIS are limited in terms of what they can promise surgeons who attend their courses. It seems that the most that can be offered is "an appreciation for" the requirements of the procedure, a series of stepwise progressions through the procedure and an introduction to the skill development required [31, 32].

Since there appears to be only limited transfer of training from one procedure to another, it is still questionable whether a surgeon well trained in LC can attend a weekend seminar and learn how to safely perform a laparoscopic fundoplication. Thus, those classically trained surgeons without MIS experience who are seeking to *learn* afresh the skills of laparoscopic surgery in a limited time-frame are likely to be disappointed by the results. Further, it should not surprise anyone familiar with the literature of MIS training that, if these surgeons choose to return to their practices to perform the newly learned procedures, a high incidence of poor patient outcomes is likely to occur. In considering which training methods *should* be used to provide surgeons with the necessary skills to ensure that their patients receive high quality care, traditional CME is probably not the answer. Coupling CME with an extensive preceptorship will more likely satisfy the requirement for learning and practicing any newly learned procedure [33].

1.2.1.3
Resident Training

A brief review of the training data compiled by the US Accreditation Council for Graduate Medical Education (ACGME) reveals another training controversy – the apparent focus on providing residents with abundant experience in LC (63% of all laparoscopic procedures reported for residents) with an attendant dearth of experience in other laparoscopic procedures (9% for the second highest procedure – laparoscopic appendectomy, LA). For the top three procedures, these percentages work out to an average of 90% LCs per resident, 13% LAs per resident, and 10% inguinal herniorrhaphies per resident. Residents are possibly being "over-trained" in LC, perhaps at the cost of learning and practicing other laparoscopic procedures [34].

The number of abdominal and alimentary tract procedures reported for residents' total laparoscopic experience compares unfavorably with their open surgery experience at an MIS:OS ratio of 1:4. Clearly, opportunities for residents to gain MIS skills are being minimized in training programs; this is especially problematic for a method of surgery that one author claims to be the future of general surgery [35]. Change in surgical training curricula is slow to occur. While resistance to change is not unexpected, a part of the controversy that might be difficult to resolve is the need to train all surgeons in open procedures so that when indicated, conversions from a laparoscopic to an open method is possible in a safe and timely manner. Further complicating the problem is the concurrent demand for programs to limit the number of hours of training each week to 80 h per resident, along with a notable pressure for academic surgeons to increase their clinical output. These changes, viewed against the backdrop of increased accountability, federal control (via Health Insurance Portability and Accountability Act [HIPAA] and Institutional Review Boards [IRB]), mounting costs for malpractice insurance (even the name sounds menacing), suggest that the current situation may only get worse. Given the mandated reduction in resident training hours, will it be possible for residents to assimilate the increased training time demanded by learning both MIS and OS techniques?

As with others, we think that dependence on the operating room (OR) to train novice residents in laparoscopy is problematic even though some have argued that insufficient evidence exists to validate the use of simulations over OR experience. The use of simulations to learn and practice MIS perceptual-motor skills has been validated to limited OR performance [36, 37]. Considering the amount of perceptual-motor skill involved in the competent manipulation of laparoscopic instruments, using the OR for such training increases the risks to patients, uses master surgeon's time wastefully, and increases the length and cost of the operation [38, 39]. In fact, some have argued that the sheer complexity of the training context (e.g., the OR) may interfere with efficient and effective learning. Coupled with studies finding no advantage in using high fidelity simulations for training novices, less expensive simulations may be optimal in many training situations [40–44].

While it is not universally supported by surgeons, many think that not only should perceptual-motor skills be learned and practiced in a training laboratory, but that successfully measuring up to specific performance criteria should also be used as a "ticket" to the OR. Further, we suggest that resident access to different segments of a laparoscopic procedure (e.g., suturing) can be tied to that individual achieving an acceptable level of performance on a mechanical or virtual reality simulator. This sounds like a straightforward suggestion; however, pitfalls abound. For example, some argue that low-cost mechanical trainers using inexpensive part-tasks (e.g., "bagging" a simulated appendix as part of a laparoscopic appendectomy) would be insufficient to train residents adequately. Others argue that it is more likely that resident training would be more effective being learned and practiced in a high fidelity computer-based simulator. However, there is evidence to suggest that while it may be important to use high-fidelity simulations to evaluate performance, it is more than likely adequate to use lower-fidelity simulations for learning and practice [45].

Added to these controversies is the emerging recognition that "master" laparoscopic surgeons are required to teach others the art and science of MIS. This suggests that until we can prepare a significant number of surgeons well-trained in MIS (e.g., when the ratio of laparoscopic to open experience changes from 1:4 to 4:1), such training will be marginalized.

One additional controversial issue related to training is that some surgical residents (as with some surgeons in practice) may not have the natural ability (i.e., perceptual-motor aptitude) to efficiently learn MIS. Indeed, if this contention is true, then it is important that either specific programs, surgical societies, or the ACGME develop and provide valid and reliable methods to make residency selection decisions or to redirect some surgical residents into subspecialties that require a different set of abilities. Although this is not necessarily a palatable direction, the recommendation has been made [46].

1.3
Summary

What is needed are residency programs that acknowledge the increasing role that MIS will play in general surgery by offering:
— A structured training program
— Priority of training over "service" at the elbow of the attending
— Validated and reliable resident selection and evaluation methods
— Institutional infrastructure support including an adequately equipped training laboratory
— A critical mass of residency-trained or preceptored MIS surgeons
— Education and research support staff

These suggestions are consistent with, and would support, the new focus on resident competence required by the ACGME and the Surgery Residency Review Committee (RRC) in the USA [34, 47]. However, we had better hurry – the next innovation of endoluminal surgery is already upon us [48]!

References

1. Litynski GS. Highlights in the history of laparoscopy. Frankfurt/Main: Barbara Bernert Verlag; 1996.
2. Dent TL. Training, credentialing, and granting of clinical privileges for laparoscopic general surgery. Am J Surg 1991;161:399–403.
3. Hawasli A, Lloyd LR. Laparoscopic cholecystectomy: the learning curve: report of 50 patients. Am Surg 1991;57:542–4.
4. Cagir B, Rangraj M, Maffuci L, Herz BL. The learning curve for laparoscopic cholecystectomy. J Laparoendosc Surg 1994;4:419–27.
5. Hunter JG, Sackier JM, Berci G. Training in laparoscopic cholecystectomy: quantifying the learning curve. Surg Endosc 1994;8:28–31.
6. Moore MJ, Bennett CL; Southern Surgeons Club. The learning curve for laparoscopic cholecystectomy. Am J Surg 1995;170:55–9.
7. Voitk AJ, Tsao SGS, Ignatius S. The tail of the learning curve for laparoscopic cholecystectomy. Am J Surg 2001;182:250–3.
8. Park AE, Witzke DB, Donnelly MB. Ongoing deficits in resident training for minimally invasive surgery. J Gastrointest Surg 2002;6:501–9.
9. Meinke AK, Kossuth T. What is the learning curve for laparoscopic appendectomy? Surg Endosc 1994;8:371–5.

10. Senagore AJ, Luchtefeld MA, MacKeigan JM. What is the learning curve for laparo-scopic colectomy?. Am Surg 1995;61:681–5.

11. Watson DI, Baigne RJ, Jamieson GG. A learning curve for laparoscopic fundoplication: definable, avoidable, or a waste of time? Ann Surg 1996;224:198–203.

12. Watson DI, Jamieson GG, Baigrie RJ, Mathew G, Devitt PG, Game PA, Britten-Jones R. Laparoscopic surgery for gastroesophageal reflux: beyond the learning curve. Br J Surg 1996;83:1284–7.

13. Reissman P, Cohen S, Weiss EG, Wexner SD. Laparoscopic colorectal surgery: ascending the learning curve. World J Surg 1996;20:277–82.

14. Ford WDA, Crameri JA, Holland AJA. The learning curve for laparoscopic pyloromy-otomy. J Pediatr Surg 199732:552–4.

15. Meehan JJ, Georgeson KE. The learning curve associated with laparoscopic antireflux surgery in infants and children. J Pediatr Surg 1997;32:426–9.

16. Poulin EC, Mamazza J. Laparoscopic splenectomy: lessons from the learning curve. Can J Surg 1998;41:28–36.

17. Querleu D, Lanvin D, Elhage A, Henry-Buisson B, Leblanc E. An objective experimen-tal assessment of the learning curve for laparoscopic surgery: the example of pelvic and para-aortic lymph node dissection. Eur J Obstet Gynecol Reprod Biol 1998;81:55–8.

18. Soot SJ, Eshraghi N, Farahmand M, Sheppard BC, Deveney CW. Transition from open to laparoscopic fundoplication: the learning curve. Arch Surg 1999134:278–81.

19. Rege RV, Joehl RJ. A learning curve for laparoscopic splenectomy at an academic insti-tution. J Surg Res 1999;81:27–32.

20. Society of American Gastrointestinal Endoscopic Surgeons (SAGES). SAGES position statement on advanced laparoscopic training. Surg Endosc 1998;12:377.

21. Society of American Gastrointestinal Endoscopic Surgeons (SAGES). Integrating ad-vanced laparoscopy into surgical residency training. Surg Endosc 1998;12:374–6.

22. Hunter JG. Clinical trials and the development of laparoscopic surgery. Surg Endosc 2001;15:1–3.

23. Nussbaum MS. Surgical endoscopy training is integral to general surgery residency and should be integrated into residency and fellowships abandoned. Semin Laparosc Surg 2002;9:212–5.

24. Society of American Gastrointestinal Endoscopic Surgeons (SAGES). SAGES Guide-lines (replaces #26): framework for post-residency surgical education and training. Surg Endosc Online 1998; 1–11.

25. Hamilton EC, Scott DJ, Fleming JR, Rege RV, Laycock R, Bergen PC, Tesfay ST, Jones DB. Comparison of video trainer and virtual reality training systems on acquisition of laparoscopic skills. Surg Endosc 2002;16:406–11.

26. Pace DE, Chiasson CM, Schlachta CM, Mamazza J, Poulin EC. Laparoscopic splenec-tomy: does the training of minimally invasive surgical fellows affect outcomes? Surg Endosc 2002;16:954–6.

27. Hunter JG. Fellowships in minimally invasive surgery: a fait accompli. Semin Laparosc Surg 2002;9:216–7.

28. Fowler DL, Hogle N. The impact of a full-time director of minimally invasive surgery: clinical practice, education, and research. Surg Endosc 2000;14:444–7.

29. Cuschieri A. Reflections on surgical training [Editorial]. Surg Endosc 1993;7:73–4.

30. Rogers DA, Elstein AS, Bordage G. Improving continuing medical education for surgical techniques: applying the lessons learned in the first decade of minimal access surgery. Ann Surg 2001;233:159–66.

31. See WA, Cooper CS, Fisher RJ. Predictors of laparoscopic complications after formal training in laparoscopic surgery. JAMA 1993;270:2689–92

32. Morino M, Festa V, Garrone C. Survey on Torino courses. The impact of a two-day practical course on appendiceship and diffusion of laparoscopic cholecystectomy in Italy. Surg Laparosc Endosc 19959:46–8.

33. Rogers DA. Ethical and educational considerations in minimally invasive surgery training for practicing surgeons. Semin Laparosc Surg 2002;9:206–11.

34. Residency Review Committee for Surgery. Accreditation Council for Graduate Medical Education (ACGME) web site. Surgery resident statistics summary. Available from http://www.acgme.org/RRC/reports/GSReportCo102.pdf

35. Himal HS. Minimally invasive (laparoscopic) surgery: the future of general surgery. Surg Endosc 2002;16:1647–52.

36. Hyltander A, Liljegren E, Rhodin PH, Lönroth H. The transfer of basic skills learned in a laparoscopic simulator to the operating room. Surg Endosc 2002;16:1324–8.

37. Seymour NE, Gallagher AG, Roman SA, O'Brien MK, Bansal VK, Andersen DK, Satava RM. Virtual reality training improves operating room performance: results of a randomized, double-blinded study. Ann Surg 2002;236:458–64.

38. Bridges M, Diamond DL. The financial impact of teaching surgical residents in the operating room. Am J Surg 1999;177:28–32.

39. Scott DJ, Bergen PC, Rege RV, Laycock R, Tesfay ST, Valentine RJ, Euhus DD, Jeyarajah DR, Thompson WM. Jones DB. Laparoscopic training on bench models: better and more cost effective than operating room experience? J Am Coll Surg 2000;191:272–83.

40. Prophet WW, Boyd HA. Device-task fidelity and transfer of training: aircraft cockpit procedures training. Technical Report 70-10, Fort Rucker AL: Human Resources Research Organization; 1970. p. 1–26.

41. Alessi SM. Fidelity in the design of instructional simulations. J Comput Based Instr 1998;15:40–7.

42. Longridge T, Bürki-Cohen J, Go TH, Kendra AJ. Simulation fidelity considerations for training and evaluation of today's airline pilots. In: Proceedings of the 11th International Symposium on Aviation Psychology, Columbus OH, 9–11 March 2001.p. 1–7.

43. Matsumoto ED, Hamstra SJ, Radomski SB, Cusimano MD. The effect of bench model fidelity on endourological skills: a randomized controlled study. J Urol 2002;167:1243–7.

44. Noble CE. The relationship between fidelity and learning in aviation training and assessment. J Air Transp 2002;7:33–54.

45. Park A, Witzke DB. Training and educational approaches to minimally invasive surgery: state of the art. Semin Laparosc Surg 2002;9:198–205.

46. Cuschieri A, Francis N, Crosby J, Hanna GB. What do master surgeons think of surgical competence and revalidation? Am J Surg 2001;182:110–6.

47. Dunnington GL, Williams RG. Addressing the new competencies for residents' surgical training. Acad Med 2003;78:14–21.

48. Spivak H, Hunter JG. Endoluminal surgery. Surg Endosc 1997;11:321–5.

Commentary

ROBERT E. CONDON

Laparoscopy has a long history among general surgeons. I remember using an old Wolf laparoscope in the 1950s as a diagnostic tool, most frequently in patients with abdominal pain of obscure cause. But, it was our colleagues in gynecology who recognized in the 1970s that the laparoscope could be used therapeutically. Therapeutic laparoscopy, now termed minimally invasive surgery, began among general surgeons in the 1980s with the introduction of laparoscopic cholecystectomy. The range of laparoscopic procedures has rapidly expanded, not only in general surgery but in many other specialties as well.

Unlike many technical innovations in modern surgery, MIS did not begin in a traditional surgical education center. Laparoscopic cholecystectomy was introduced and promoted by a surgical entrepreneur who had no philosophical commitment to the usual condition of surgical education – the sharing of new knowledge without personal profit to surgical teachers or their institutions. Thus, instead of this technical development taking place in a environment of critical appraisal, careful evaluation, and freely shared new knowledge, it occurred in an environment that required payment of fees by surgeons for access to the operating room to view the new procedure. High fees were charged for weekend "courses" providing minimal instruction, and no requirements or standards were set to objectively define the accomplishment of expertise.

Industry quickly saw the potential in MIS of new disposable instrumentation – disposable and thus profitable – and promoted MIS to both physicians and the public. Additionally, the media touted the virtues, assumed but unproved, of the new technique. Patients clamored for "laser surgery." There was a rush by a portion of the surgical community to quickly adopt, and for their hospitals to advertise the availability of laparoscopic cholecystectomy.

The result in the early 1990s was that many surgeons in academic teaching centers, and some of their community clinical allies, found themselves in a unique and unwonted position. They were unable at that time to provide residents completing their programs with the skills needed to perform MIS because the teachers, for the most part, did not possess the skills and therefore could not teach them.

So, the academics paid up, attending the same inadequate weekend "courses" as their community-practicing colleagues, and then scrambled to educate their residents in the new and rapidly evolving field of MIS. They tried their best to overcome the twin problems of the dearth of technical training available to academic surgeons that would meet reasonable standards and the clearly inadequate numbers of patients having MIS procedures in their institutions with whom to educate their residents.

Initially, the results fell short of the desired mark. Graduating residents in the early to mid 1990s often did not have the desired level of expertise to independently perform MIS. But, they were no worse off than most community surgeons then already practicing MIS. Both groups really learned their skills on their initial patients having MIS, with the predictable outcome of sometimes higher-than-desirable complication rates.

MIS requires a fundamentally different skill set than does open surgery. While three-dimensional understanding of human anatomy carries over, the eye–hand motor skills of open surgery do not serve. MIS requires a new set of eye–hand coordinated motor skills that cannot easily be learned in the same manner as were the skills of traditional open operations.

The skills needed for MIS are not as easily practiced informally and without supervision as are, for example, the skill involved in tying the surgical knots used in open surgery. Rather, the learning of MIS technical skills – if it is not to be done in patients – requires the use of complex simulator models and expensive equipment. And, once acquired, the initial application of MIS skills cannot be practiced in groups but requires one-on-one guidance of the resident by the teaching staff.

The patient substrate needed for teaching MIS is much larger than that needed for learning the skills of open surgery. Many of the skills used in open surgery can be acquired over time by observing and participating in a number of open procedures whose primary educational focus is learning by another. Several trainees at differing levels of experience can be involved with a single open operation, thus enriching their knowledge base of each of them. Such exposure is more difficult to achieve in MIS procedures, in which the ability to handle instruments and to dissect is limited pretty much to a preceptor-trainee pair. Thus, many more patients and procedures are needed to fully educate the graduating general surgery resident in technical MIS surgery. And, the cadre of teachers likewise needs to larger since the MIS educational process is so much less susceptible to sharing among multiple learners, and requires more dedicated one-on-one teaching time.

Much has been made of the early high complication rates of MIS as being due to an effect of "the learning curve," as if such complications were inevitable. I disagree. My personal observations of a successful, novel MIS teaching program in an academic medical center indicates that the "learning curve" is primarily a matter of poor judgment by novice surgeons. Complication rates can be kept low, even early in MIS experience, if the surgeon avoids blind maneuvers, positively identifying and completely dissecting structures before cutting or clamping, and maintains a low threshold for conversion to an open procedure. Many complications comprising the "learning curve" are, in reality, failure by an unwilling surgeon to follow these precepts.

Doctors Park and Witzke correctly point out that deficiencies in MIS educational programs persist. In my view, these deficiencies are rooted in the legacy generated by the adverse educational environment surrounding the introduction of therapeutic laparoscopy into general surgery, and the lingering effects today are due to the failure of the academic surgical educational system to catch up. But, the reality that MIS requires the acquisition of an entirely new set of eye-hand motor skills that cannot easily be learned in the same manner as traditional open operations also plays an important role.

The authors identify a number of problems: (1) insufficient numbers of well-trained MIS surgeons in academic centers; (2) resident MIS experience skewed to cholecystectomy; (3) overall marginalization of MIS within the residency experience; (4) failure to identify whether or not prospective residents possess the natural ability to learn MIS; (5) the need for training laboratories to overcome the inefficiency of teaching MIS in the operating room; (6) the continuing need to train residents in open procedures, and (7) the as yet unmeasured but probably deleterious effects of the 80-h work week limitation on the education of residents.

As a response to these problems, the authors suggest a number of items that are listed in their Summary paragraph. But, they fail to specify the mechanisms or the means by which these elements are to be included in programs of surgical education.

I have some suggestions about how to get the job done within the limitations of the 80-h resident work week. My proposals require the Residency Review Committee for Surgery (RRC), with the support of the American Board of Surgery (ABS), to step up to the plate, to take some courage, and to specify to hospitals conducting surgical residencies that they must immediately stop abusing surgical residents. If hospitals do not act, the RRC should threaten withdrawal of approval of the residency program, and must be prepared do so if a hospital proves recalcitrant.

There are two major abuses of surgical residents perpetrated today by nearly all teaching hospitals. First, hospitals fail to provide sufficient infrastructure and staffing so that residents have to perform many tasks that are unrelated to their education. If residents did not have to spend so much time doing these service chores for hospitals, 80 h a week would be more than enough time in which to receive their professional education, including education-related patient care. Second, hospitals divert income received for residency support from Federal and State health care programs – such as Medicare, Crippled Children and many others – to other uses within the institution. A surgical residency is a profit center for most hospitals. That is an egregious abuse of residents and their educational programs.

The RRC must insist that institutions conducting surgical residencies provide adequate infrastructure and support, and that dollars received by hospitals to cover the costs of surgical education are, in fact, spent on education. The financial records of such funding should be audited by independent accountants chosen by and answerable to the RRC. The hospitals will plead that they cannot afford these reforms, but if the RRC insists, they will find a way to do the right thing.

With these work and financing abuses corrected, there will then be resources available to help build the needed structured educational experiences in MIS. Skills laboratories, with both basic and advanced simulation devices, need to be a organized and directed by surgeons skilled in MIS and committed to the education of residents. The experience to be gained in these laboratories needs to be specified for each residency year, and acquisition of the required skills needs to be certified by an objective testing process.

The skills laboratory also can be part of a program of structured education in MIS for practicing surgeons, including certification of skill acquisition, that can be conducted in 2-week increments (so that the practitioner-students need not close their practice). Both residents and practicing surgeons should move on to supervised experience in the operating room only after they demonstrate that they have acquired the eye-hand motor skills needed for MIS.

The basic simulation level of the skills laboratory should also be available, perhaps even required, for medical students on their general surgery rotation. Such experience, paralleling their experience gained with the basic skills used in open operations, will help students to identify whether they have the natural eye-hand motor skills required for MIS, and will enhance the self-selection process that students use to identify that a surgical career is appropriate for them.

All general surgery residency programs should be required by the RRC to have a skills laboratory, and educators should be required by both the RRC and the ABS to have demonstrated MIS competence in their area of practice. Such a requirement will stimulate the training of the additional MIS-competent faculty that general surgery residency programs need. These faculty can use the resources, and the objective tests of accomplishment, provided by their institutional skills laboratory for part of their own education. They then should take the time necessary, either in their own institution or in another having appropriate numbers of patients available for education, to acquire clinical MIS competence.

Further, the RRC should broaden its requirements for MIS experience by residents, and consider increasing the number of procedures required. If necessary, the number of residents in some programs may need to be reduced to conform to the numbers of MIS procedures done in their affiliated hospitals. Further, post-residency MIS fellowships of any type should be interdicted in those programs and their institutions in which patient numbers are not sufficiently generous to serve the needs of all general surgery residents.

Getting the RRC and the ABS, the bodies responsible for standards in the education of general surgeons, to put in place reforms such as those outlined above will not be easily accomplished. Opposition is predictable. But, unless and until something of the nature of my proposals is actually done, the lingering educational deficits of MIS will not be overcome. These deficits have a negative impact on the quality of patient care, and we have an obligation to see that they are corrected. But, the deficits will not go away spontaneously. They need to be driven away by those dedicated surgeon-educators who sit on the RRC and ABS.

Access to the Abdomen

PAOLO GENTILESCHI, MARCO CATARCI

▶ **Key Controversy**

A. Type of access
  – Open versus Veress needle/trocar access
  – Direct Trocar versus Veress needle/trocar access
  – Umbilical versus other site and new devices access
B. Choice of access

2.1
Introduction

The great majority of specific complications associated with laparoscopic surgery occur during access and the creation of pneumoperitoneum [1–5]. The umbilical area is the thinnest portion of the abdominal wall and is therefore often the preferred access site. However, immediately below this point is the aortic bifurcation, the bowel and omentum. Access-related injuries have been well documented at each of these sites, as well as at the colon, stomach, inferior vena cava and iliac veins, ureter, bladder, iliac and epigastric arteries [6, 7]. Major vascular injuries are rare but, once inflicted, between 9% and 13% of patients will die [7–9]. Access-related bowel or visceral injuries are relatively more common. Reports indicate that between 50–66% of bowel or visceral injuries are undiagnosed at the time of primary surgery and can lead to major complications such as sepsis or peritonitis [7]. As a result of these injuries, this initial phase of any laparoscopic procedure has a mortality rate varying from 0.05 to 0.2% [2].

There are two basic forms of access – open and closed. Open laparoscopy is usually undertaken via a Hasson-type approach. This access method allows direct visualization through the use of an initial incision and dissection down to the peritoneum, followed by insertion of the blunt Hasson trocar, secured with stay or purse-string sutures, and then insufflation with carbon dioxide [10, 11]. Closed laparoscopy is performed using a blind approach, with either pre-insufflation before laparoscope insertion (Veress needle/trocar method) or insufflation after laparoscope insertion (direct trocar method) [12, 13].

One other hybrid form of closed laparoscopy involves limited visual access through the use of an optical needle or trocar [14, 15]. As every method of entering the abdominal cavity is associated with risks, many controversies in this crucial step of every laparoscopic procedure exist and are discussed in this chapter.

2.2
Discussion

2.2.1
Type of Access

2.2.1.1
Open versus Veress Needle/Trocar Access

Closed laparoscopy has been used for decades in gynecology [16]. With the introduction of laparoscopy into general surgery, the closed access technique was preferred initially [17], although this appears to be changing. Recent figures show an increased trend towards the use of open and/or optical access techniques [18, 19] and commercial data show that the sales of disposable Hasson and optical trocars in Italy have nearly doubled during the last 5 years (Ethicon Endo-Surgery, Rome, Italy; personal communication, 2003). Actually, some authors suggested that routine use of the open approach can effectively lower the operative time needed to achieve pneumoperitoneum while protecting from major vascular injuries [2, 20, 21]. However, two cases of major vascular injury occurring during an open approach were recently reported [22], confirming that there is no "foolproof" technique for the creation of the pneumoperitoneum. A search for evidence is therefore strongly needed.

Four systematic reviews recently addressed the methods used to establish laparoscopic pneumoperitoneum [23–26]. In addition, several population-based studies evaluated the incidence of adverse events related to the laparoscopic access [19, 27–29]. The following discussion is based on the analysis of their results. Outcome measures are related to safety of the access [mortality rate, major complications (major vessel and/or hollow viscus injuries) rate, minor complications (wound infection, omental injury, extraperitoneal insufflation) rate] and to efficacy of the access [failure rate and mean time to obtain pneumoperitoneum].

A total of four randomized controlled trials (RCTs), all from general surgery centers, compared open versus Veress needle/trocar access [30–33] (Table 2.1). According to the data available from these RCTs, the only significant conclusion is that open access is faster than the closed one. There were no

Table 2.1. Randomized controlled trials comparing open versus Veress needle/trocar techniques (NR not reported)

Authors [ref]	Technique	No. of patients	No. of mortalities	No. with major morbidity (%)	No. with minor morbidity (%)	No. of failures (%)	Mean insertion time ±SD (min)
Peitgen et al. [30]	Open	26	0	0 (–)	0 (–)	9 (34.6)	1.8±0.5
	Closed	24	0	0 (–)	0 (–)	6 (25.0)	3.8±1.5
Cogliandolo et al. [31]	Open	75	0	1 (1.3)	5 (6.7)	NR	3.2±0.2
	Closed	75	0	3 (4.0)	5 (6.7)	NR	4.5±0.4
Bemelman et al. [32]	Open	20	0	0 (–)	0 (–)	5 (25.0)	5.8±1.7
	Closed	20	0	0 (–)	0 (–)	0 (–)	4.0±0.9
Bernik et al. [33]	Open	34	0	0 (–)	1 (2.9)	2 (5.9)	4.3±1.0
	Closed	28	0	0 (–)	3 (10.7)	3 (10.7)	5.2±0.9
Total	Open	155	0	1 (0.6)	6 (3.9)	16 (20.0)	3.7±1.7
	Closed	147	0	3 (2.0)	8 (5.4)	9 (12.5)	4.4±0.6free

deaths reported as a consequence of primary access complications in either the open or closed laparoscopy groups. Three out of four RCTs [30, 32, 33] showed no major complication, and only two [31, 33] reported minor complications, without significant differences between the two groups. Unfortunately, the number of patients enrolled in these RCTs is largely undersized and insufficient to avoid a type-II error, a significant bias present in many reports from negative RCTs published in the surgical literature [34].

Given the relatively low rate of adverse events, definitive evidence regarding the safety of either open or closed access would only be reached through a multicenter RCT with over 10,000 cases in each study arm. Although difficult to perform, such a trial might be the only way to find a final answer to this ongoing debate.

Concerning the results of lower-level evidence studies, one systematic review [24] pooled the results of comparative non-randomized studies dividing prospective from retrospective ones. Analyzing retrospective studies only, it seems that the risk of major complications is 2.7 times higher with open, as opposed to Veress needle/trocar access (risk ratio, RR, 2.70; 95% confidence interval, CI, 1.57–4.63), mainly due to overlooked small bowel injuries. When only prospective studies were analyzed, the reverse was true, the risk of major injuries with open access being 0.3 times that of Veress needle/trocar access (RR 0.30, 95% CI 0.09–1.03). Actually, retrospective studies did not report the proportion of patients in each group with a history of prior abdominal surgery. It is therefore possible that their results were biased by the surgical preference of operating those patients with adhesions caused by previous abdominal surgery with an open access. Population-based studies confirm a significant reduction of major complications with the open access compared to the Veress needle/trocar one [19, 27].

Major retroperitoneal vascular injuries occurred most often, if not exclusively, with the Veress needle/trocar technique varying from 0.02 to 0.24% [19, 23–27, 29]. The most common major complication associated with access was bowel injury, with a reported incidence ranging from 0 to 4% [19, 23–27, 29]. The main risk factor for bowel injury during laparoscopic access was obviously previous abdominal surgery. In non-randomized trials, the risk of bowel injury was higher with the open technique compared with that of the closed technique, although again a selection bias probably affected the results of these studies. On the other hand, herniation of the primary access site and extraperitoneal insufflation were less frequently reported during the open access technique.

2.2.1.2
Direct Trocar versus Veress Needle/Trocar Access

Three RCTs, all from gynecological centers, compared direct trocar insertion with Veress needle/trocar access [35–37] (Table 2.2). As with previous comparisons, here again the absence of mortality, the rarity of major adverse events and the undersized patient sample make any conclusion about the safety impossible. The only significant conclusion deriving from data pooling is a reduced minor morbidity rate with the direct trocar technique. As for the efficacy, it was not possible to establish a comparison between the two techniques due to inconclusive information.

The direct insertion technique has a number of very eminent gynecological laparoscopists as proponents and it is undisputedly the most rapid method for gaining access to the abdomen [23]. Actually, the diffusion of this technique among general surgery centers is quite modest, probably due to its low reproducibility in inexperienced hands.

2.2.1.3
Umbilical versus Other Site and New Devices Access

Depending upon the suspected presence of periumbilical adhesions and the surgical procedure to be performed, alternative entry sites include the left upper quadrant, the suprapubic area, the transfundal site and through the posterior vaginal fornices, the latter being preferred by gynecologists. In the average patient, the area of the left hypochondrium shows the lowest rate of intra-abdominal adhesions. Only one RCT comparing periumbilical versus transfundal Veress needle insufflation was available [38], but its results were inconclusive.

Concerning new devices for laparoscopic access (optical trocars), no comparison to date has been presented with the open access technique, whereas a paucity of useful information in comparison with the Veress needle/trocar technique was available [39–41]. Conclusions regarding their comparative safety and efficacy cannot therefore be drawn to date, even though a recent three-armed RCT found it easier to establish the pneumoperitoneum with a new access device (TrocDoc) than with the open technique or the Veress needle [32]. However, commercial data shows a 140% increase in the sales of disposable optical trocars in Italy during the last 5 years (Ethicon Endo-Surgery, Rome, Italy; personal communication 2003) and, therefore, more investigational trials about their safety and efficacy can be anticipated.

Table 2.2. Randomized controlled trials comparing direct trocar insertion versus Veress needle/trocar techniques (VNT)

Author [ref.]	Technique	No. of patients	No. of mortalities	No. with major morbidity (%)	No. with minor morbidity (%)	No. of failures (%)
Borgatta et al. [35	Direct	103	0	1 (1.0)	4 (3.9)	0 (–)
	VNT	110	0	1 (0.9)	15 (13.6)	6 (5.5)
Nezhat et al. [36	Direct	100	0	0 (–)	3 (3.0)	6 (6.0)
	VNT	100	0	0 (–)	22 (22.0)	3 (3.0)
Byron et al. [37]	Direct	111	0	0 (–)	1 (0.9)	2 (1.8)
	VNT	141	0	0 (–)	7 (5.0)	4 (2.8)
Total	Direct	314	0	1 (0.3)	8 (2.5)	8 (2.5)
	VNT	351	0	1 (0.3)	44 (12.5)	13 (3.7)

2.2.2
Choice of Access

The need to perforate the abdominal wall in order to perform a laparoscopic procedure will probably always be associated with the risk of damaging structures beneath. This risk is so low that no individual surgeon's personal experience can provide enough data to evaluate the relative risks of alternative approaches. It is also so low that it would be at least very difficult if not impossible to perform a properly designed and sized RCT. The choice of the access to the abdomen, therefore, cannot be based upon data deriving from top-evidence studies, and should be based also on other considerations.

Patient and public expectations are growing higher every day and major surgical accidents, although rare, are no longer tolerated, and frequently if not always lead to litigation in order to gain financial compensation [42]. A recent injury-based study [28] showed a large aggregate of such injuries, suggesting that they are probably under reported in procedure-based studies. In our recent enquiry about iatrogenic injuries during the creation of pneumoperitoneum in the area of Rome, it appeared that one-third of surgical centers reported at least one major retroperitoneal vessels injury [19]. Open laparoscopy with good visualization seems to have theoretical advantages in terms of prevention of major vascular injuries. Even if only to prevent one major vascular injury in one surgeon's life, we favor open laparoscopy as the routine method of gaining abdominal access. Concerning small bowel injuries, open laparoscopy is not safer than other types of access, even though it can help immediate injury recognition and management.

At our Institutions, we were exposed early in our experience (namely, during our residencies) to laparoscopic surgery. After a short period of few months in which a Veress needle/trocar access technique was used, we both moved to the routine use of an open access method, feeling confident that open laparoscopy was a wise alternative to the closed access, especially because it was totally under the visual control of the surgeon. Our experience with this technique together with the collected access methods of other centers in the area of Rome have been previously published [19, 20]. We strongly believe that, when routinely used, the open technique has to be preferred to the closed one because it's faster, safer and equally effective, even in the absence of clear recommendations in current guidelines [24, 26].

2.3
Summary

No single method of abdominal access in laparoscopic surgery has been clearly proved to be superior. There is insufficient data to prove the safety and efficacy of one abdominal access technique over another, and probably there will never be due to the large number of patients to be enrolled in randomized trials.

The mortality rate due to injuries occurring during this obligatory phase of any laparoscopic procedure varies from 0.05 to 0.2%, and is strongly related to either major vascular injuries or unrecognized bowel injuries.

Open laparoscopy can virtually eliminate the risk of major vascular injuries. For this reason, it is and will remain our preferred method of access to the abdomen.

References

1. Karam KS, Hajj SN. Mesenteric hematoma – Meckel's diverticulum: a rare laparoscopic complication. Fertil Steril 1977;28:1003–5.
2. Nuzzo G, Giuliante F, Tebala GD, et al. Routine use of open technique in laparoscopic operations. J Am Coll Surg 1997;184:58–62.
3. Lacey CG. Laparoscopy. A clinical sign for intraperitoneal needle placement. Obstet Gynecol 1976;47:625–7.
4. Leron E, Piura B, Ohana E, et al. Delayed recognition of major vascular injury during laparoscopy. Eur J Obstet Gynecol Reprod Biol 1998;79:91–3.
5. Riedel HH, Lehmann WE, Mecke H, et al. The frequency distribution of various laparoscopic operations, including complication rates – statistics of the Federal Republic of Germany in the years 1983–1985. Zentralbl Gynakol 1989;111:78–91.
6. Airan MC. Basic techniques. In: McFayden BV, Ponsky JL, editors. Operative laparoscopy and thoracoscopy. Philadelphia: Lippincott-Raven; 1996. p. 93–123.
7. Rosen DM, Lam AM, Chapman M, Carlton M, Cario GM. Methods of creating pneumoperitoneum: a review of techniques and complications. Obstet Gynecol Surv 1998;53:167–74.
8. Chapron CM, Pierre F, Lacroix S, et al. Major vascular injuries during gynecologic laparoscopy. J Am Coll Surg 1997;185:461–5.
9. Deziel DJ, Millikan KW, Economou SG, et al. Complications of laparoscopic cholecystectomy: a national survey of 4,292 hospitals and analysis of 77,604 cases. Am J Surg 1993;165:9–14.
10. Hasson HM. Modified instrument and method for laparoscopy. Am J Obstet Gynecol 1971;110:886.
11. Hasson HM. Open laparoscopy vs. closed laparoscopy: a comparison of complication rates. Adv Plan Parent 1978;13:41–50.

12. Dingfender JR. Direct laparoscope trocar insertion without prior pneumoperitoneum. J Reprod Med 1978;21:45–7.
13. Woolcott R. The safety of laparoscopy performed by direct trocar insertion and carbon dioxide insufflation under vision. Aust N Z J Obstet Gynaecol 1997;37:216–9.
14. Schaller G, Kuenkel M, Manegold BC. The optical „Veress-needle" – initial puncture with a minioptic. Endosc Surg Allied Technol 1995;3:55–7.
15. Hallfeldt KKJ, Trupka A, Kalteis T, et al. Safe creation of pneumoperitoneum using an optical trocar. Surg Endosc 1999;13:306–7.
16. Phillips JM, Hulka JF, Peterson HB; American Association of Gynecologic Laparoscopists. 1982 Membership survey. J Reprod Med 1984;29:592–4.
17. Bonjer HJ, Hazebroek EJ, Kazemier G, et al. Open versus closed establishment of pneumoperitoneum in laparoscopic surgery. Br J Surg 1997;84:599–602.
18. Wherry DC, Marohn MR, Malanoski MP, et al. An external audit of laparoscopic cholecystectomy in the steady state performed in medical treatment facilities of the department of defense. Ann Surg 1996;224:145–54.
19. Catarci M, Carlini M, Gentileschi P, et al. Major and minor injuries during the creation of pneumoperitoneum. A multicenter study on 12,919 cases. Surg Endosc 2001;15:566–9.
20. Zaraca F, Catarci M, Gossetti F, et al. Routine use of open laparoscopy: 1,006 consecutive cases. J Laparoendosc Adv Surg Tech 1999;9:75–80.
21. Thomas WEG. Section C. Minimal access surgery. In: Basic surgical skills: a participants' handbook. London: Royal College of Surgeons of England; 1996. p. 43–65.
22. Hanney RM, Carmalt HL, Merret N, et al. Use of the Hasson cannula producing major vascular injury at laparoscopy. Surg Endosc 1999;13:1238–40.
23. Garry R. Towards evidence-based laparoscopic entry techniques: clinical problems and dilemmas. Gynaecol Endosc 1999;8:315–26.
24. Merlin T, Maddern G, Jamieson G, et al. A systematic review of the methods used to establish laparoscopic pneumoperitoneum. ASERNIP-S Report No. 13. Adelaide, South Australia: ASERNIP-S. October 2001. Available from http://www.surgeons.org/asernip-s/systematic_review/MELPreview1001.pdf (cited 30 March 2003).
25. Centre for Clinical Effectiveness. What is the safety of open versus closed technique for laparoscopy? Melbourne: Southern Health/Monash Instuitute of Public Health; 2001. Available from http://www.med.monash.edu.au/healthservices/cce/evidence/pdf/c/512.pdf (cited 30 March 2003).
26. Neudecker J, Sauerland S, Neugebauer E, et al. The European Association for Endoscopic Surgery clinical practice guideline on the pneumoperitoneum for laparoscopic surgery. Surg Endosc 2002;16:1121–43.
27. Hashizume M, Sugimachi K; Study Group of Endoscopic Surgery in Kyushu, Japan. Needle and trocar injury during laparoscopic surgery in Japan. Surg Endosc 1997;11:1198–1201.
28. Chandler JG, Corson SL, Way LW. Three spectra of laparoscopic entry access injuries. J Am Coll Surg 2001;192:478–91.
29. Bhoyrul S, Vierra MA, Nezhat CR, et al. Trocar injuries in laparoscopic surgery. J Am Coll Surg 2001;192:677–83.
30. Peitgen K, Nimtz K, Hellinger A, et al. Offener zugang oder Veress-nadel bei laparoskopischen eingriffen? Ergebnisse einer prospektiv randomisierten studie. Chirurg 1997;68:910–3.

31. Cogliandolo A, Manganaro T, Saitta FP, et al. Blind versus open approach to laparoscopic cholecystectomy: a randomized study. Surg Laparosc Endosc 1998;8:353–5.

32. Bemelman WA, Dunker MS, Busch OR, et al. Efficacy of establishment of pneumoperitoneum with the Veress needle, Hasson trocar, and modified blunt trocar (TrocDoc): a randomized study. J Laparoendosc Adv Surg Tech A 2000;10:325–30

33. Bernik TR, Trocciola SR, Mayer DA, et al. Balloon blunt-tip trocar for laparoscopic cholecystectomy: improvement over the traditional Hasson and Veress needle methods. J Laparoendosc Adv Surg Tech A 2001;11:73–8.

34. Dimick JB, Diener-West M, Lipsett PA. Negative results of randomized clinical trials published in the surgical literature. Equivalency or error? Arch Surg 2001;136:796–800.

35. Borgatta L, Gruss L, Barad D, et al. Direct trocar insertion vs Veress needle use for laparoscopic sterilization. J Reprod Med 1990;35:891–4.

36. Nezhat FR, Silfen SL, Evans D, et al. Comparison of direct insertion of disposable and standard reusable laparoscopic trocars and previous pneumoperitoneum with Veress needle. Obstet Gynecol 1991;78:148–150.

37. Byron JW, Markenson G, Miyazawa K. A randomized comparison of Veress needle and direct trocar insertion for laparoscopy. Surg Gynecol Obstet 1993;177:259–62.

38. Santala M, Jarvela I, Kauppila A. Transfundal insertion of a Veress needle in laparoscopy of obese subjects: a practical alternative. Hum Reprod 1999;14:2277–8.

39. Mettler L, Ibrahim M, Vinh VQ, et al. Clinical experience with an optical access trocar in gynecological laparoscopy-pelviscopy. J Soc Laparoendosc Surg 1997;1:315–8.

40. Marcovich R, Del Terzo MA, Wolf JS. Comparison of transperitoneal laparoscopic access techniques: Optiview visualizing trocar and Veress needle. J Endourol 2000;14:175–179.

41. String A, Berber E, Foroutani A, et al. Use of the optical access trocar for safe and rapid entry in various laparoscopic procedures. Surg Endosc 2001;15:570–3.

42. Natali J. Implications médico-légales des traumatismes vasculaires au cours de la chirurgie vidéo-endoscopique. J Mal Vasc 1996;21:223–6.

Commentary

Harrith M. Hasson

The authors present a concise and balanced treatment of the subject to which I should like to add a few comments. When I introduced the instruments and technique of open laparoscopy in 1971, it seemed intuitive that entering the abdomen under visual control through a carefully dissected minilaparotomy incision using a blunt trocar would eliminate most of the risks associated with blind abdominal access using needles and sharp trocars. However, as with any new procedure, I had to go through a learning phase associated with prolonged operative time and increased risk of complications, before mastering the technique and realizing its safety potential. This was demonstrated in my group's recently published experience involving 5284 patients in whom access to the abdominal cavity was with open laparoscopy [1]. In our first 50 cases the incidence of wound infection was 6% that of bowel injury was 2%. These rates dropped to 0.3% and 0%, respectively, in the next 1436 cases. In the last 3798 cases, the wound infection rate remained stable at 0.3%, there were no instances of bowel injury, but we had one case of postoperative hernia due to slippage of the approximating suture knot. We did not experience any cases of failed laparoscopy attempt, inappropriate insufflation, gas embolism, organ injury or major vessel injury. Other investigators [2, 3] made similar observations.

Variations in open laparoscopy complication rates are probably related to one or more of the following factors:
— Employment of appropriate instruments and techniques
— Existing expertise relative to case selection
— Knowledge of abdominal wall anatomy

Proper technique is based on four points: (1) the minilaparotomy incision is dissected in layers. The fascial and, if necessary, the peritoneal layers, are elevated during incision to protect the abdominal structures, (2) after abdominal entry is visually confirmed, the blunt-tipped cannula is introduced with guidance into the abdomen and gas is insufflated through it to establish the pneumoperitoneum, (3) a system is devised to hold the cannula in place and maintain the pneumoperitoneum during the operation, and (4) at the end of the procedure, the fascial defect is closed with sutures.

Entering the abdomen with a knife (or scissors) without elevation of the fascia is in fact closed laparoscopy using a knife rather than a sharp trocar. Introducing a bare cannula into the abdomen without a protective blunt obturator may cause damage to internal structures by the sharp edge of the bare cannula. Failure to guide the blunt-tipped cannula into the abdomen, confirm successful access to the abdominal cavity by visual means, or stabilize the cannula on the abdominal wall while attaching the stay sutures may cause the cannula to be displaced in the pre-peritoneal space with subsequent pre-peritoneal insufflation. Failure to use adequate means to seal the incision and block escape of the gas may cause gas leaks and increase the risk of intraoperative injury due to poor visualization. Finally, failure to close the fascial defect adequately may result in postoperative herniation [4].

Open and closed laparoscopies were utilized on equal basis in four studies [5–8]. One was prospective [5], the others retrospective. Three were general surgery studies [5, 6, 8] and one involved gynecologic oncology patients [7]. In each case outcome data favored the open method. Cumulatively, there were 866 open laparoscopy and 2,286 closed laparoscopy cases. The rate of failed laparoscopy attempts in the open method was 0.1% and there were no cases of inappropriate insufflation, vascular or visceral injury. The rate of failed attempts in the closed method was 0.6%, inappropriate insufflation 1%, vascular injury 0.2% and visceral injury 0.5%. On the other hand, when open laparoscopy was used only in high-risk patients, it did not prevent bowel injury (0.4% of 258 patients) as opposed to 0.2% of 2,066 low-risk patients in whom closed method access was used [9].

Published data confirm the safety and efficacy of open laparoscopy in low-risk patients and suggest that surgeons who perform it routinely experience few problems even in high-risk patients. On the other hand, surgeons who perform closed laparoscopy routinely and reserve the open method of access to the most difficult patients may lack the expertise needed to handle the associated anatomic alterations. However, it must be recognized that high-risk patients such as those with dense bowel adhesions, cancer or Crohn's disease will continue to be at risk for bowel injury with open laparoscopy as they do with open surgery.

References

1. Hasson HM, Rotman C, Rana N, Kumari, NA. Open laparoscopy: 29 year experience. Obstet Gynecol. 2000;96:763–6.
2. Zaraca F, Catarci M, Gossetti F, Mulieri G, Carboni M. Routine use of open laparoscopy: 1006 consecutive cases. J Laparosc Endosc Adv Surg Tech 1999;9:75–80.
3. Schnepper FW. Sterilization by open laparoscopy in a private office. J Am Assoc Gynecol Laparosc 1999;4:469–72.
4. Hasson HM. Open laparoscopy: In: J.J. Sciarra, editors. Gynecology and obstetrics, vol. 1. Philadelphia: Lippincott Williams and Wilkins; 2003. Chap. 122.
5. Sigman HH, Fried GM, Garzon J, Hinchey EJ, Wexler MJ, Meakins JL, et al. Risks of blind versus open approach to celiotomy for laparoscopic surgery. Surg Laparosc Endosc 1993;3:296–9.
6. Ballem RV, Rudomanski J. Techniques of pneumopertioneum. Surg Laparosc Endosc 1993;3:42–3.
7. Casey AC, Farias-Eisner R, Pisani,AC, Cirisano FD, Kim YB, Muderspach L, et al. What is the role of reassessment laparoscopy in the management of gynecologic cancers in 1995? Gynecol Oncol 1996;60:454–61.
8. Bonjer HJ, Haxebroek EJ, Kazemier G, Guiffrida MC, Meijer WS, Lange JF. Open versus closed establishment of pneumoperitoneum in laparoscopic surgery. Br J Surg 1997;84:599–602.
9. Bateman BG, Kolp LA, Hoeger K. Complications of laparoscopy: operative and diagnostic. Fertil Steril 1996;66:30–5.

Establishing Pneumoperitoneum:
The Ideal Gas
and Physiological Consequences

► **Key Controversy**

― What is the ideal gas for pneumoperitoneum?

3.1
Introduction

In 1901, Georg Kelling first described the technique of creating pneumo-peritoneum and performing celioscopy, now known as laparoscopy. His intent for creating "lufttamponade" or pneumoperitoneum, in a dog model, was to develop methods for controlling intra-abdominal blood loss. In 1924 Zollikofer described the use of carbon dioxide to create pneumoperitoneum. Over the past 20 years the field of laparoscopic surgery has grown tremendously. There are now longer, more technically difficult procedures being performed on older, less healthy patients. The physiological effects of pneumoperitoneum have been studied extensively, but controversy regarding the ideal gas for pneumoperitoneum still exists.

3.1.1
Physiology of the Pneumoperitoneum

3.1.1.1
Cardiovascular

The effects of increased intra-abdominal pressure (IAP) on cardiovascular physiology have been well studied. In euvolemic patients there is an observed decrease in venous return, increase in peripheral resistance, and increase in intrathoracic/pleural pressure. Most clinical studies show that these changes result in little change or a decrease in cardiac output at an IAP of 15 mmHg [1–6]. At an IAP of 15 mmHg heart rate generally remains unchanged [7, 8]. Kashtan et al. showed in a canine model that compensatory changes in cardiac function maintained blood pressure and cardiac output (CO) until IAP reached 40 mmHg [7]. The decrease in cardiac function was thought to be related to an increase in afterload.

Mean arterial pressure increases with increased IAP. Systemic hypertension observed with increased IAP is a result of elevated intracranial pressures. In turn, elevated intracranial pressure is a result of decreased venous drainage resulting from high right atrial pressures. Elevated intracranial pressure triggers the medulla oblongata to release catecholamines and vasopressin, which causes systemic vasoconstriction [9]. Systemic hypertension is an autoregulatory response to maintain cerebral perfusion pressures.

During pneumoperitoneum, intra-abdominal venous return is altered by elevated right atrial pressures and mechanical constriction at the level of the diaphragm. In the abdominal vascular compartment, flow through the inferior vena cava is related to the pressure difference between the upstream IAP and the downstream right atrial pressure. Thus, intra-abdominal venous return to the heart increases when right atrial pressure is <IAP, but decreases when right atrial pressure is >IAP [8, 10]. Cardiac output changes during pneumoperitoneum may reflect intravascular volume status. In hypovolemic patients, the vena cava is easily compressible, and there is diminished venous return to the heart. In hypervolemic patients, the increase in IAP slightly augments venous return and CO [7]. Venous return may be diminished by narrowing of the suprahepatic inferior vena cava at the level of the diaphragm during elevated IAP, but this effect is rarely a problem in the euvolemic patient [11, 12]. In an animal study, Ridings et al. showed that crystalloid volume resuscitation at IAP of 25 mmHg returned cardiac index to normal baseline without significantly worsening cardiopulmonary function or further elevating IAP [13].

Most studies addressing the hemodynamic effects of pneumoperitoneum have used carbon dioxide as the insufflation gas. There is controversy as to whether the cardiac depressive affects of pneumoperitoneum are due to increased IAP or the hypercapnea and acidemia created by the pharmacological effects of carbon dioxide. Ho et al. concluded that 15 mmHg of carbon dioxide pneumoperitoneum alone does not account for the reduction of stroke volume, and this reduction of stroke volume persisted as long as there was an excess of carbon dioxide body buffers [14].

Thus, increased IAP causes a net decrease in cardiac output, an increase in systemic blood pressure and minimal effects on the heart rate independent of insufflating agent. In patients with underlying cardiac disease, the physiology of elevated IAP – particularly prolonged pneumoperitoneum – may cause significant cardiac stress.

3.1.1.2
Pulmonary

Increased IAP raises the diaphragm causing marked changes in respiratory function. The underlying cause of these respiratory alterations is decreased respiratory excursion of the diaphragm, resulting in restriction of lung expansion. This decrease in pulmonary compliance results in reductions of total lung capacity, functional residual capacity and residual volume [15]. Pulmonary compliance decreases by 50% as IAP is increased from 10 to 16 mmHg [16]. As IAP rises from 10 to 40 mmHg, there is a gradual increase in peak airway pressures from 15 to 35 mmHg. Significant hypoxemia and hypercapnia also ensues as IAP is increased to these levels resulting in a slight acidemia [13, 17]. Patient positioning also has an effect on pulmonary compliance. There is a greater decrease in compliance in the Trendelenberg position than there is in the reverse Trendelenberg position [16]. A combination of diminished diaphragmatic compliance as well as the weight of the abdominal viscera against the diaphragm adds to the decrease in pulmonary compliance in the Trendelenberg position. It is important to closely monitor ventilatory parameters as well as serial arterial blood gases in patients undergoing laparoscopic procedures who have baseline pulmonary compromise. When pulmonary dysfunction proceeds to the state of hyperventilation, carbon dioxide elimination is impossible and respiratory acidosis results. Management of this situation requires a reduction in IAP and/or choosing an alternative insufflating gas that is more metabolically inert.

3.1.1.3
Renal

There is a complex interplay between increased IAP and renal function. Harman initially suggested that the decrease in renal function from increased IAP is a result of direct renal parenchymal compression, rather than a decrease in cardiac output (CO) [18]. However, decrease in blood flow to all intraabdominal organs except the adrenal gland has been demonstrated at IAP of 20 and 40 mmHg [19]. There is decreased renal cortical blood flow and increased medullary blood flow with increasing IAP [20]. Of the three factors, compression of the renal parenchyma, decreased CO, and impaired venous return- local compressive effects appears to have the greatest effect on renal function. IAP greater than 15 mmHg results in elevated plasma renin and aldosterone levels, which may contribute to further local vasoconstriction and diminished renal blood flow [21, 22]. The exact mechanism for elevated plasma renin activity and aldosterone levels is unclear. It is most likely a combination of decreased CO, diminished renal perfusion, and increased renal venous pressures.

Studies have shown some improvement in renal function with intravascular volume expansion and use of vasoactive drugs. With the use of either isotonic or hypertonic saline, the adverse affects of IAP on urine output and renal blood flow were reversed, but creatinine clearance remained diminished [23]. The use of "renal dose" dopamine (2 µg/kg per min) may have some beneficial effect in limiting the renal dysfunction during prolonged pneumoperitoneum [24]. In a clinical study, clonidine was shown to suppress the renin-angiotensin-aldosternone system by decreasing plasma renin activity. This resulted in decreased catecholamine levels, more stable hemodynamics and possible renal protection from vasoconstriction [24, 25]. In patients with normal preoperative renal function, elevated IAP from pneumoperitoneum causes observable physiological changes but limited clinical detriment. However, in patients with baseline renal insufficiency, care should be made in monitoring fluid status closely, and using pharmacological agents as needed.

3.1.1.4
Endocrine

The body's neuroendocrine response to surgical stress and trauma has been well studied. Elevated IAP also results in a complex neuroendocrine response. An increase in IAP from baseline to 20 mmHg, causes an increase in plasma epinephrine and norepinephrine levels regardless of the type of gas used to obtain pneumoperitoneum [26]. Most clinical studies that have documented the neuroendocrine response to pneumoperitoneum have compared conventional open cholecystectomy (OC) to laparoscopic cholecystectomy (LC). Both OC and LC show similar intraoperative elevation in plasma adrenocorticotrophic hormone (ACTH), cortisol, norepinephrine, epinephrine, insulin and glucose concentrations [27–29]. In the OC patients, plasma epinephrine, norepinephrine, and glucose levels remain elevated in the first 24-h postoperative period [27, 29]. Plasma thyroid markers are also elevated at a similar magnitude for OC and LC [28]. Elevation of vasopressin or antidiuretic hormone (ADH) is seen early in LC but not OC, in concert with changes in systemic vascular resistance [25]. The proposed mechanism for rise in vasopressin/ADH levels has been previously mentioned. Another proposed mechanism may be the activation of periteoneal nerve endings, which are stimulated by intra-abdominal pH changes secondary to carbon dioxide pneumoperitoneum. The neurohypophysis is stimulated to release vasopressin via a vagal neurogenic pathway [30]. Alternatively, decreased venous return may stimulate right atrial volume receptors which trigger the pituitary to release vasopressin/ADH [28]. Regardless, the elevated levels of vasopressin/ADH results in decreased urine output in LC compared with that in OC, but this physiological effect reverses within an hour after pneumoperitoneum is terminated. Clinically, increased IAP and increased vasopressin/ADH lead to profound intraoperative oliguria in many patients despite adequate intravascular volume. Attempts to correct intraoperative oliguria with fluid and sodium replacement may lead to significant volume overload.

The systemic stress response during both LC and OC is similar to that observed with the neuroendocrine markers mentioned above. However stress hormone levels remain elevated in the immediate postoperative period in OC patients, while these levels return to baseline quickly in LC patients. This may contribute to the quicker recovery seen in patients undergoing LC as compared to OC.

3.1.1.5
Immunology

Operative procedures under general anesthesia result in significant immune suppression, and the severity of immune suppression is directly related to the magnitude of the operation. Laparoscopic surgery does not suppress the immune system to the same degree as open procedures, and this may contribute to the diminished postoperative pain and quick recovery after LC [31]. The physiological response to surgery or trauma is an immediate elevation of the stress hormones and a decrease in overall cellular immune response. Acute phase response and cytokine levels do not directly correlate with the body's immune status but they are well studied markers for the activation of the immune system. C-reactive protein (CRP) has been shown to rise 4–12 h after surgery and peak at 24–72 h [32]. Clinical studies have shown a lower elevation of CRP during LC and in the postoperative period as compared to OC [33–35]. Interleukin-6 (IL-6) is another cytokine that is elevated in postsurgical states, and its elevation correlates with the degree of surgical injury [36]. Most studies have shown that serum levels of IL-6, like CRP, is less affected by LC than by OC [27, 37, 38]. Initial studies comparing open and laparoscopic assisted colon resection were unable to demonstrate a difference in CRP levels, but this may be due to small patient numbers, a non-randomized population, and a heterogeneous group of operations for both malignant and benign diseases. Recent studies of colorectal resection are more consistent with the cholecystectomy data that demonstrates a smaller elevation in immune markers with a laparoscopic approach than with the open procedure [38–42]. This benefit of laparoscopic surgery may be most valuable in immuno-compromised patient populations.

In addition to the cytokine and acute phase response studies, there have been numerous studies evaluating the effect of laparoscopy on the cellular components of the immune system. Comparing OC to LC there was a greater increase in overall peripheral leukocyte count with OC [34]. Cell-mediated immunity (CMI), as measured by T-cell proliferation, was more depressed in patients undergoing OC than in LC patients [43]. Brune et al. showed less suppression of CMI following LC by comparing levels of interferon-γ, tumor necrosis factor-α, and interleukin-2 with those in a control group undergoing OC [44]. CMI was suppressed on postoperative day 1 in both groups, but the effect was more profound in OC patients than in LC patients. T-cell function has also been examined by studying animal models of delayed type hypersensitivity. Allendorf et al. showed a greater reduction in delayed-type hypersensitivity in a rat model following open cecectomy versus laparoscopic cecectomy [45]. Similarly, Trokel et al. showed that delayed-type hypersensitivity is better preserved after laparoscopy than after laparotomy in a rat model [46]. Thus, most studies to date support improved postoperative immune system preservation in laparoscopic surgery compared to open surgery (Table 3.1). Whether these animal studies and limited clinical studies have any impact on clinical outcomes is yet to be decided, and further research is necessary.

3.2
Discussion

3.2.1
In Search of the Ideal Gas

Today, advanced laporoscopic surgery involves technically difficult cases, long operative times, and old patients with significant comorbidities. Under these circumstances, the ideal gas for pneumoperitoneum should be readily available, relatively inexpensive and should be chemically, physiologically and pharmacologically inert. The gas should also be colorless, odorless, highly soluble in plasma, and noncombustible when used with electrocautery or laser coagulation.

3.2.1.1
Carbon Dioxide

Carbon dioxide is currently the gas of choice for pneumoperitoneum. It is a very soluble gas in plasma (solubility coefficient of 0.570), its cost is relatively low and it suppresses combustion. However, carbon dioxide is not physiologically inert. Carbon dioxide is readily absorbed across the peritoneum into the blood stream. The majority of carbon dioxide is transported as bicarbonate ion. The precursor to this is carbonic acid, which rapidly dissoci-

Table 3.1. Summary of comparative systemic immunological changes following open surgery and laparoscopy (*CRP* C-reactive protein, *HLA* human leukocyte antigen, *IL* interleukin, *PMN* polymorphonuclear neutrophil, *NK* natural killer, *Th* T helper cell, *TNF* tumor necrosis factor). From: Gupta and Watson, Br J Surg 2001;88:1296–1306

Marker of systemic immune response	Changes following open surgery	Changes following laparoscopy
CRP	↑↑↑	↑
IL-1	↑↑	↑
IL-6	↑↑↑	↑
IL-8	↑↑	↑
IL-10	Data unclear	Data unclear
TNF	Data unclear	Data unclear
Fibrinogen, transferrin	Data unclear	Data unclear
Elastase	↑	↑ (Returns to preop. levels early)
Albumin	Data unclear	Data unclear
PMN number	↑↑	↑
PMN function	↓↓	↓
Delayed hypersensitivity	↓↓↓	↓
Th1, Th2	↓↓	↓
CD4$^+$/CD8$^+$	↓↓	↓
Monocyte HLA-DR expression	↓↓↓	↓
Monocyte-mediated cytotoxicity	↓↓	↓
Kupffer cell activity	Data unclear	Data unclear
NK cell number and function	↓	↓

ates to form bicarbonate and hydrogen ions. The net effect is plasma acidemia and hypercarbia. Acidemia causes myocardial depression and lowers the arrhythmia threshold, while hypercarbia causes indirect sympathetic stimulation and release of catecholamines [47]. Total body stores of carbon dioxide remain elevated even after the pneumoperitoneum is ceased. Thus, there may be prolonged hypercarbia in the postoperative state.

As suggested earlier, some of the effects of laparoscopy on cardiac physiology may be more related to the pharmacological effects of hypercarbia and acidemia rather than the effects of increased IAP. In young, healthy patients, slight acidemia and hypercarbia are clinically tolerated. In the elderly patient with cardiopulmonary comorbidities, the concern for the negative physiological effects of carbon dioxide on the cardiopulmonary system is significant. The use of carbon dioxide for pneumoperitoneum results in elevated intracranial pressures as compared to helium and nitrous oxide. The central nervous system autoregulatory response to elevated $PaCO_2$ is to increase cerebral perfusion resulting in elevated intracranial pressure [48]. Currently the role of carbon dioxide pneumoperitoneum for trauma laparoscopy, or laparoscopy in patients with suspected head injury may be limited by this physiological side effect. The high solubility of carbon dioxide is beneficial in the rare event of carbon dioxide gas embolism. The end result of this event is occlusion of the right ventricle with a gas bubble leading to rapid cardiac collapse. Carbon dioxide is more soluble in plasma and has a higher affinity for hemoglobin than other gases, making it less likely to create a gas embolus if inadvertently injected into the liver or a vein.

3.2.1.2
Nitrous Oxide

Nitrous oxide was used extensively as a gas for pneumoperitoneum in the 1970s and 1980s. It is inexpensive, chemically inert, readily soluble in plasma, and is quickly cleared by the body. Nitrous oxide causes few cardiovascular alterations when compared to CO_2. The effects of nitrous oxide on the cardiovascular system are related to increased IAP rather than the pharmacological effects of the gas. Nitrous oxide pneumoperitoneum does not result in hypercarbia or respiratory acidosis [49, 50]. In a pregnant ewe model, we showed that nitrous oxide pneumoperitoneum did not cause fetal respiratory acidosis, and there was less fetal tachycardia and hypertension than with carbon dioxide pneumoperitoneum [51].

An additional benefit of nitrous oxide is its analgesic properties. In several studies, nitrous oxide pneumoperitoneum resulted in less postoperative pain when than carbon dioxide pneumoperitoneum [52–54]. This may be related to the irritating effects of carbonic acid – a byproduct of carbon dioxide breakdown – on the peritoneum or the anesthetic effects of nitrous oxide on the central nervous system [54, 55].

The concern of using nitrous oxide as an insufflating gas is related to its inability suppress combustion relative to carbon dioxide or other inert gases.

Nitrous oxide itself is not combustible, but in the presence of a volatile gas (i.e., methane or hydrogen) it may support combustion similar to air (80% nitrogen, 20% oxygen). We have shown that the concentration of methane and hydrogen detected during standard laparoscopic cases was less than 1/50 of the combustion threshold [56]. There is a theoretical risk of injuring the intestinal tract during surgery and releasing colonic methane and hydrogen normally produced by the bacterial flora. The incidence of intestinal injuries is 0.2–1.28%, and colon injuries seen in less than 1 in 2,000 [54]. There is an extremely low risk of combustion, as both an injury to the colon and high intraperitoneal concentrations of methane or hydrogen would be necessary to support combustion. The "scare" created about nitrous oxide for insufflation emanated from two case reports in the 1970s [57, 58]. Neither case could prove the incident was due to the type of gas used. Since then, there has been a clinical moratorium on the use of nitrous oxide as an insufflating gas, but the lack of scientific credibility associated with these events has led us to reinstitute the use of nitrous oxide in selected patients undergoing long operations, especially those with cardiopulmonary compromise or advanced age.

3.2.1.3
Helium

In the search for an alternative gas for pneumoperitoneum, helium has been studied in both animal models and clinically. Similar to carbon dioxide and nitrous oxide, helium is chemically inert, readily available, and inexpensive. It is a gas that is absorbed quickly and is rapidly eliminated by the pulmonary system. Helium does not cause hypercarbia or respiratory acidemia like carbon dioxide, and like nitrous oxide it causes few alterations in cardiopulmonary parameters. The cardiopulmonary changes that are observed are due to elevated IAP. Similar to carbon dioxide, helium also suppresses combustion. In the setting of pregnancy, helium does not cause maternal and fetal acidosis like carbon dioxide [59]. The disadvantage of helium is its low solubility in water, making it more dangerous than other gases in the event of a gas embolism. In small clinical studies comparing helium with carbon dioxide in LC, there was no hypercarbia or respiratory acidosis with helium. Interestingly, up to 15% of the patients who underwent helium insufflation developed prolonged postoperative subcutaneous emphysema. Although alarming to the patient, this does not affect recovery [60–62].

3.2.1.4
Argon and Nitrogen

Both argon and nitrogen have been studied only in animal models. Similar to nitrous oxide and helium, there is no hypercarbia or respiratory acidosis with these two gases. Through unknown mechanisms argon causes a slight increase in systemic vascular resistance, and a reduction in cardiac index relative to carbon dioxide in a swine model [63, 64]. In another study using a swine model, there was no decrease in stroke volume, mean arterial pressure did not increase, and pulmonary artery pressure remained unchanged in the animals that underwent nitrogen pneumoperitoneum compared to carbon dioxide pneumoperitoneum [14]. The downside of these two gases is their low plasma solubility, which makes them less desirable in the event of an air embolus, and may lead to prolonged subcutaneous emphysema. Currently the use of nitrogen and argon is limited to animal studies only.

3.3
Summary

— Laparoscopic surgery represents a dramatic surgical revolution in the past two decades. The variety and complexity of operations continue to increase. Although well studied, the physiology of pneumoperitoneum is still being elucidated, and the ideal gas for insufflation has yet to be determined.
— Increased IAP causes physiological changes in each organ system. With elevated IAP, cardiac output decreases and the systemic vascular resistance increases, while heart rate remains unchanged. The decrease in CO is related to both an increase in afterload and a decrease in venous return, whereas the increase in mean arterial pressure is thought to be related to a central nervous system response to elevated intracranial pressures resulting in release of catecholamines and vasopressin/ADH. Increased IAP results in decreased pulmonary compliance, and an overall reduction in total lung capacity, functional residual capacity and residual volume. The decrease in renal function from elevated IAP is related to compression of the renal parenchyma, diminished renal blood flow and impaired venous return. There is also a neurohormonal response by the kidney from elevated IAP resulting in increased plasma renin and aldosterone levels.
— Compared to OC, LC results in a similar rise in plasma markers of systemic stress. These levels return to baseline once pneumoperitoneum is ceased, whereas they remain elevated in patients undergoing OC. The systemic immune function is better maintained in patients undergoing LC than in

OC patients. The exact role of the systemic stress and immune response in laparoscopic procedures and its effects on postoperative outcomes is unclear and still being examined.

— Carbon dioxide is currently the most common gas used in clinical practice. It is well tolerated in young healthy patients undergoing short operative procedures. However, the negative physiological impact of prolonged hypercarbia and acidemia, especially in older patients with underlying cardiopulmonary disease, has forced us to search for a more physiologically inert gas.

— Nitrous oxide and helium pnuemoperitoneum do not result in the acid-base alterations seen with carbon dioxide. The concern about nitrous oxide's inability to suppress combustion is based on anecdotal evidence and has just recently been questioned based on scientific evidence.

— Helium has also been studied clinically as an alternative to carbon dioxide. It also is more physiologically inert, but concerns for its use are because of its low plasma solubility and higher risk in cases of air embolism.

— Both argon and nitrogen have only been used in animal models.

— Laparoscopic procedures are now technically more challenging, longer in operative time and are being performed on an older population with numerous underlying comorbidities. With the known physiological alterations from increased IAP, and the acid-base disturbances from carbon dioxide insufflation a physiologically "safer" gas should be sought. Both nitrous oxide and helium are gases that are physiologically more inert and may be alternatives to carbon dioxide pneumoperitoneum.

References

1. Dorsay DA, Greene FL, Baysinger CL. Hemodynamic changes during laparoscopic cholecystectomy monitored with transesophageal echocardiography. Surg Endosc 1995;9:128–33.
2. Myre K, Buanes T, Smith G, Stokland O. Simultaneous hemodynamic and echocardiographic changes during abdominal gas insufflation. Surg Laparosc Endosc 1997;7:415–9.
3. Elliott S, Savill P, Eckersall S. Cardiovascular changes during laparoscopic cholecystectomy: a study using transoesophageal Doppler monitoring. Eur J Anaesthesiol 1998;15:50–5.
4. Harris SN, Ballantyne GH, Luther MA, Perrino AC Jr. Alterations of cardiovascular performance during laparoscopic colectomy: a combined hemodynamic and echocardiographic analysis. Anesth Analg 1996;83:482–7.
5. Joris JL, Noirot DP, Legrand MJ, Jacquet NJ, Lamy ML. Hemodynamic changes during laparoscopic cholecystectomy. Anesth Analg 1993;76:1067–71.

6. Mann C, Boccara G, Pouzeratte Y, Navarro F, Domergue J, Colson P. Hemodynamic monitoring using esophageal Doppler ultrasonography during laparoscopic cholecystectomy. Can J Anaesth 1999;46:15–20.

7. Kashtan J, Green JF, Parsons EQ, Holcroft JW. Hemodynamic effect of increased abdominal pressure. J Surg Res 1981;30:249–55.

8. Kitano Y, Takata M, Sasaki N, Zhang Q, Yamamoto S, Miyasaka K. Influence of increased abdominal pressure on steady-state cardiac performance. J Appl Physiol 1999;86:1651–6.

9. Ben-Haim M, Mandeli J, Friedman RL, Rosenthal RJ. Mechanisms of systemic hypertension during acute elevation of intraabdominal pressure. J Surg Res 2000 15;91:101–5.

10. Takata M, Wise RA, Robotham JL Effects of abdominal pressure on venous return: abdominal vascular zone conditions. J Appl Physiol 1990;69:1961–72.

11. Rosenthal RJ, Friedman RL, Kahn AM, Martz J, Thiagarajah S, Cohen D, Shi Q, Nussbaum M. Reasons for intracranial hypertension and hemodynamic instability during acute elevations of intra-abdominal pressure: observations in a large animal model. J Gastrointest Surg 1998;2:415–25.

12. Wachsberg RH. Narrowing of the upper abdominal inferior vena cava in patients with elevated intraabdominal pressure: sonographic observations. J Ultrasound Med 2000;19:217–22.

13. Ridings PC, Bloomfield GL, Blocher CR, Sugerman HJ. Cardiopulmonary effects of raised intra-abdominal pressure before and after intravascular volume expansion. J Trauma 1995;39:1071–5.

14. Ho HS, Saunders CJ, Gunther RA, Wolfe BM. Effector of hemodynamics during laparoscopy: CO_2 absorption or intra-abdominal pressure? J Surg Res 1995;59:497–503.

15. Mutoh T, Lamm WJ, Embree LJ, Hildebrandt J, Albert RK. Abdominal distension alters regional pleural pressures and chest wall mechanics in pigs in vivo. J Appl Physiol 1991;70:2611–8.

16. Obeid F, Saba A, Fath J, Guslits B, Chung R, Sorensen V, Buck J, Horst M. Increases in intra-abdominal pressure affect pulmonary compliance. Arch Surg 1995;130:544–7.

17. Richardson JD, Trinkle JK. Hemodynamic and respiratory alterations with increased intra-abdominal pressure. J Surg Res 1976;20:401–4.

18. Harman PK, Kron IL, McLachlan HD, Freedlender AE, Nolan SP. Elevated intra-abdominal pressure and renal function. Ann Surg 1982;196:594–7.

19. Caldwell CB, Ricotta JJ. Changes in visceral blood flow with elevated intraabdominal pressure. J Surg Res 1987;43:14–20.

20. Chiu AW, Chang LS, Birkett DH, Babayan RK. The impact of pneumoperitoneum, pneumoretroperitoneum, and gasless laparoscopy on the systemic and renal hemodynamics. J Am Coll Surg 1995;181:397–406.

21. Gudmundsson FF, Gislason HG, Myking OL, Viste A, Grong K, Svanes K. Hormonal changes related to reduced renal blood flow and low urine output under prolonged increased intra-abdominal pressure in pigs. Eur J Surg 2002;168:178–86.

22. Bloomfield GL, Blocher CR, Fakhry IF, Sica DA, Sugerman HJ. Elevated intra-abdominal pressure increases plasma renin activity and aldosterone levels. J Trauma 1997;42:997–1004.

23. London ET, Ho HS, Neuhaus AM, Wolfe BM, Rudich SM, Perez RV. Effect of intravascular volume expansion on renal function during prolonged CO_2 pneumoperitoneum. Ann Surg 2000;231:195–201.
24. Perez J, Taura P, Rueda J, Balust J, Anglada T, Beltran J, Lacy AM, Garcia-Valdecasas JC. Role of dopamine in renal dysfunction during laparoscopic surgery. Surg Endosc 2002;16:1297–301.
25. Joris JL, Chiche JD, Canivet JL, Jacquet NJ, Legros JJ, Lamy ML. Hemodynamic changes induced by laparoscopy and their endocrine correlates: effects of clonidine. J Am Coll Cardiol 1998;32:1389–96.
26. Mikami O, Fujise K, Matsumoto S, Shingu K, Ashida M, Matsuda T. High intra-abdominal pressure increases plasma catecholamine concentrations during pneumoperitoneum for laparoscopic procedures. Arch Surg 1998;133:39–43.
27. Karayiannakis AJ, Makri GG, Mantzioka A, Karousos D, Karatzas G. Systemic stress response after laparoscopic or open cholecystectomy: a randomized trial. Br J Surg 1997;84:467–71.
28. Ortega AE, Peters JH, Incarbone R, Estrada L, Ehsan A, Kwan Y, Spencer CJ, Moore-Jeffries E, Kuchta K, Nicoloff JT. A prospective randomized comparison of the metabolic and stress hormonal responses of laparoscopic and open cholecystectomy. J Am Coll Surg 1996;183:249–56.
29. Glaser F, Sannwald GA, Buhr HJ, Kuntz C, Mayer H, Klee F, Herfarth C. General stress response to conventional and laparoscopic cholecystectomy. Ann Surg 1995;221:372–80.
30. Mann C, Boccara G, Pouzeratte Y, Eliet J, Serradel-Le Gal C, Vergnes C, Bichet DG, Guillon G, Fabre JM, Colson P. The relationship among carbon dioxide pneumoperitoneum, vasopressin release, and hemodynamic changes. Anesth Analg 1999;89:278–83.
31. Grace PA, Quereshi A, Coleman J, Keane R, McEntee G, Broe P, Osborne H, Bouchier-Hayes D. Reduced postoperative hospitalization after laparoscopic cholecystectomy. Br J Surg 1991;78:160–2.
32. Ohzato H, Yoshizaki K, Nishimoto N, Ogata A, Tagoh H, Monden M, Gotoh M, Kishimoto T, Mori T. Interleukin-6 as a new indicator of inflammatory status: detection of serum levels of interleukin-6 and C-reactive protein after surgery. Surgery 1992;111:201–9.
33. Halevy A, Lin G, Gold-Deutsch R, Lavi R, Negri M, Evans S, Cotariu D, Sackier JM. Comparison of serum C-reactive protein concentrations for laparoscopic versus open cholecystectomy. Surg Endosc 1995;9:280–2.
34. Redmond HP, Watson RW, Houghton T, Condron C, Watson RG, Bouchier-Hayes D. Immune function in patients undergoing open vs laparoscopic cholecystectomy. Arch Surg 1994;129:1240–6.
35. Roumen RM, van Meurs PA, Kuypers HH, Kraak WA, Sauerwein RW. Serum interleukin-6 and C reactive protein responses in patients after laparoscopic or conventional cholecystectomy. Eur J Surg 1992;158:541–4.
36. Cruickshank AM, Fraser WD, Burns HJ, Van Damme J, Shenkin A. Response of serum interleukin-6 in patients undergoing elective surgery of varying severity. Clin Sci (Lond) 1990;79:161–5.
37. Grande M, Tucci GF, Adorisio O, Barini A, Rulli F, Neri A, Franchi F, Farinon AM. Systemic acute-phase response after laparoscopic and open cholecystectomy. Surg Endosc 2002;16:313–6.

38. Delgado S, Lacy AM, Filella X, Castells A, Garcia-Valdecasas JC, Pique JM, Momblan D, Visa J. Acute phase response in laparoscopic and open colectomy in colon cancer: randomized study. Dis Colon Rectum 2001;44:638–46.
39. Wu FP, Sietses C, von Blomberg BM, van Leeuwen PA, Meijer S, Cuesta MA. Systemic and peritoneal inflammatory response after laparoscopic or conventional colon resection in cancer patients: a prospective, randomized trial. Dis Colon Rectum 2003;46:147–55.
40. Leung KL, Lai PB, Ho RL, Meng WC, Yiu RY, Lee JF, Lau WY. Systemic cytokine response after laparoscopic-assisted resection of rectosigmoid carcinoma: A prospective randomized trial. Ann Surg 2000;231:506–11.
41. Schwenk W, Jacobi C, Mansmann U, Bohm B, Muller JM. Inflammatory response after laparoscopic and conventional colorectal resections – results of a prospective randomized trial. Langenbecks Arch Surg 2000;385:2–9.
42. Harmon GD, Senagore AJ, Kilbride MJ, Warzynski MJ. Interleukin-6 response to laparoscopic and open colectomy. Dis Colon Rectum 1994;37:754–9.
43. Griffith JP, Everitt NJ, Lancaster F, Boylston A, Richards SJ, Scott CS, Benson EA, Sue-Ling HM, McMahon MJ. Influence of laparoscopic and conventional cholecystectomy upon cell-mediated immunity. Br J Surg 1995;82:677–80.
44. Brune IB, Wilke W, Hensler T, Holzmann B, Siewert JR. Downregulation of T helper type 1 immune response and altered pro-inflammatory and anti-inflammatory T cell cytokine balance following conventional but not laparoscopic surgery. Am J Surg 1999;177:55–60.
45. Allendorf JD, Bessler M, Whelan RL, Trokel M, Laird DA, Terry MB, Treat MR. Better preservation of immune function after laparoscopic-assisted vs. open bowel resection in a murine model. Dis Colon Rectum 1996;39 Suppl:S67–72.
46. Trokel MJ, Bessler M, Treat MR, Whelan RL, Nowygrod R. Preservation of immune response after laparoscopy. Surg Endosc 1994;8:1385–7.
47. Rasmussen JP, Dauchot PJ, DePalma RG, Sorensen B, Regula G, Anton AH, Gravenstein JS. Cardiac function and hypercarbia. Arch Surg 1978;113:1196–200.
48. Schob OM, Allen DC, Benzel E, Curet MJ, Adams MS, Baldwin NG, Largiader F, Zucker KA. A comparison of the pathophysiologic effects of carbon dioxide, nitrous oxide, and helium pneumoperitoneum on intracranial pressure. Am J Surg 1996;172:248–53.
49. Rademaker BM, Odoom JA, de Wit LT, Kalkman CJ, ten Brink SA, Ringers J. Haemodynamic effects of pneumoperitoneum for laparoscopic surgery: a comparison of CO_2 with N_2O insufflation. Eur J Anaesthesiol 1994;11:301–6.
50. El-Minawi MF, Wahbi O, El-Bagouri IS, Sharawi M, El-Mallah SY. Physiologic changes during CO_2 and N_2O pneumoperitoneum in diagnostic laparoscopy. A comparative study. J Reprod Med 1981;26:338–46.
51. Hunter JG, Swanstrom L, Thornburg K. Carbon dioxide pneumoperitoneum induces fetal acidosis in a pregnant ewe model. Surg Endosc 1995;9:272–7.
52. Aitola P, Airo I, Kaukinen S, Ylitalo P. Comparison of N_2O and CO_2 pneumoperitoneums during laparoscopic cholecystectomy with special reference to postoperative pain. Surg Laparosc Endosc 1998;8:140–4.
53. Sharp JR, Pierson WP, Brady CE 3rd. Comparison of CO2- and N_2O-induced discomfort during peritoneoscopy under local anesthesia. Gastroenterology 1982;82:453–6.

54. Tsereteli Z, Terry ML, Bowers SP, Spivak H, Archer SB, Galloway KD, Hunter JG. Prospective randomized clinical trial comparing nitrous oxide and carbon dioxide pneumoperitoneum for laparoscopic surgery. J Am Coll Surg 2002;195:173–9.
55. Phillips RS, Goldberg RI, Watson PW, Marshall JR, Barkin JS Mechanism of improved patient tolerance to nitrous oxide in diagnostic laparoscopy. Am J Gastroenterol 1987;82:143–4.
56. Hunter JG, Staheli J, Oddsdottir M, Trus T. Nitrous oxide pneumoperitoneum revisited. Is there a risk of combustion? Surg Endosc 1995;9:501–4.
57. Gunatilake DE. Case report: fatal intraperitoneal explosion during electrocoagulation via laparoscopy. Int J Gynaecol Obstet 1978;15:353–7.
58. El-Kady AA, Abd-El-Razek M. Intraperitoneal explosion during female sterilization by laparoscopic electrocoagulation. A case report. Int J Gynaecol Obstet 1976;14:487–8.
59. Curet MJ, Weber DM, Sae A, Lopez J. Effects of helium pneumoperitoneum in pregnant ewes. Surg Endosc 2001;15:710–4.
60. McMahon AJ, Baxter JN, Murray W, Imrie CW, Kenny G, O'Dwyer PJ. Helium pneumoperitoneum for laparoscopic cholecystectomy: ventilatory and blood gas changes. Br J Surg 1994;81:1033–6.
61. Neuberger TJ, Andrus CH, Wittgen CM, Wade TP, Kaminski DL. Prospective comparison of helium versus carbon dioxide pneumoperitoneum. Gastrointest Endosc 1996;43:38–41.
62. Bongard FS, Pianim NA, Leighton TA, Dubecz S, Davis IP, Lippmann M, Klein S, Liu SY. Helium insufflation for laparoscopic operation. Surg Gynecol Obstet 1993;177:140–6.
63. Junghans T, Bohm B, Grundel K, Schwenk W. Effects of pneumoperitoneum with carbon dioxide, argon, or helium on hemodynamic and respiratory function. Arch Surg 1997;132:272–8.
64. Eisenhauer DM, Saunders CJ, Ho HS, Wolfe BM. Hemodynamic effects of argon pneumoperitoneum. Surg Endosc 1994;8:315–20.

Commentary

Raul Rosenthal

Drs. Rizvi and Hunter have done an extraordinary work in highlighting the physiological changes that occur when establishing pneumoperitoneum. An understanding of potential complications related to the use of pneumoperitoneum during laparoscopic surgery is also necessary. Most physiological changes observed during pneumoperitoneum are self limited and related to alterations produced by mechanical effects of pneumoperitoneum [1]. However, it would be appropriate to mention and describe some of the most life-threatening complications that can be associated with the establishment of a pneumoperitoneum which will not necessarily reverse after insuflation has been discontinued.

Gas embolism, though rare, represents a potentially fatal event that requires rapid intervention [2, 3]. Bradycardia, cyanosis and cardiovascular collapse are some of the most obvious but late manifestations. Early detection can be achieved if we monitor and recognize a sudden drop in the end tidal CO2 (ETCO2). The immediate decompression of the abdominal cavity followed by placement of the patient in the Durant position (left lateral decubitus that will release the gas lock in the pulmonary outflow tract), and administration of 100% oxygen are the most powerful treatment options [4].

The development of a pneumothorax may arise from various mechanisms. The incidence of 0.1/1000 is extremely low; however, early recognition and timely intervention is paramount. Intraoperative findings suggesting a pneumothorax include subcutaneous emphysema, abrupt rise in the ETCO2, increased ventilatory pressures, hypoxemia and diminished breath sounds. A bulging diaphragm will also be diagnostic of pneumothorax. Treatment options are decompression of the abdominal cavity followed by tube thoracostomy if the patient is hemodynamically unstable versus conservative treatment with serial radiographs [1].

The clinical significance of subcutaneous emphysema lies in the development of hypercarbia to a degree not seen with pneumoperitoneum alone and it is mainly due to the larger absorptive surface area. Signs that will allow us to early recognize this complication are crepitus and increase in $ETCO_2$. After a pneumothorax has been ruled out, N_2O should be discontinued as anesthetic agent and ventilation corrected to maintain acceptable $ETCO_2$ [2, 3].

Cardiac arrhythmias are generally associated with hypercarbia and acidosis, however in laparoscopy you might see them even before hypercarbia ensues during rapid insufflation of the abdominal cavity. Bradycardia is the most common arrhythmia and is mainly due to vagal tone stimulation by sudden stretching of the pneumoperitoneum. Ectopic beats and asystole have been also reported in the early phase of insufflation [5].

Finally pulmonary aspiration is another complication that surgeons should be aware of during laparoscopy. The rise in intraabdominal pressure promotes gastric regurgitation. This event may be missed by the anesthesiologist and manifest postoperatively as pneumonitis. An early sign would be rise in ventilatory pressures and drop in O_2 saturation. The best treatment is prevention by routine decompression of the stomach with orogastric tubes before insufflation [4].

An understanding of potential complications related to the use of pneumoperitoneum during laparoscopic surgery is necessary. As a general rule we can say that the lower the insufflation pressure the lower the incidence of pulmonary complications. Therefore, the insufflation pressure should be kept as low as possible without compromising exposure. Continuous monitoring of respiratory and homodynamic parameters will allow early detection, preventive and therapeutic measures that will further reduce this rare complications and improve patient outcome [4].

References

1. Lowham AS, Fillipi CJ and Tomonaga T. Pneumoperitoneum related complications: diagnosis and treatment. In: Rosenthal RJ, Friedman RL, Phillips EH, editors. The pathophysiology of pneumoperitoneum; 1998. Berlin, Heidelberg New York: Springer Verlag. p. 131–146.
2. Kent RB. Subcutaneous emphysema and hypercarbia following laparoscopic cholecystectomy. Arch Surg 1991;126:1154–6.
3. Puri GD, Singh H. Ventilatory effects of laparoscopy under general anesthesia. Br J Anesth 1992;68:211–3.
4. Azar I, Monitoring and management of physiological changes caused by pneumoperitoneum. In: Rosenthal RJ, Friedman RL, Phillips EH, editors. The pathophysiology of pneumoperitoneum; 1998. Berlin Heidelberg New York: Springer Verlag. p. 115–130.
5. Diamant M, Benumof JL, Saidman LJ. Hemodynamics of increased intraabdominal pressure interaction with hypovolemia and and halotane anesthesia. Anesthesiology 1978;48:23–7.

Laparoscopy in the Acute Abdomen

Dennis L. Fowler

▶ **Key Controversy**

A. Diagnostic laparoscopy in the acute abdomen
  - Free air and generalized peritonitis
  - Acidosis/sepsis in the critically ill ICU patient
B. Therapeutic laparoscopy in the acute abdomen
  - Perforated viscus
  - Small bowel obstruction

4.1
Introduction

Laparoscopy offers the potential for accurate diagnosis and minimally invasive treatment. In patients with an acute abdominal condition, it is sometimes difficult to make an accurate diagnosis clinically, and, at times, it is even difficult to make an accurate diagnosis radiographically. At first glance it appears that laparoscopy would be an ideal method to evaluate these patients with an acute abdominal condition of unknown cause, and should provide an accurate diagnosis. Further, some of these patients are quite sick from their acute abdominal condition, and therapeutic laparoscopy might confer the benefits of a less invasive procedure.

Despite the potential benefit of diagnosing or treating acute abdominal conditions laparoscopically, there are several potential issues with using laparoscopy in patients with an acute abdomen. The disease process may create an environment in the abdomen that makes laparoscopy difficult or impossible, i.e., massively distended intestine or diffuse fibrinopurulent exudates. Additionally, the tension pneumoperitoneum might increase the translocation of bacteria into the circulation, or the CO_2 might reduce the ability of the peritoneum to effectively deal with an infectious process. Because of these issues, there is controversy about whether acute abdominal conditions should or should not be approached laparoscopically.

Controversies regarding the laparoscopic treatment of acute cholecystitis and appendicitis will be discussed in detail later in this book in the chapters on cholecystectomy (Chap. 20) and appendectomy (Chap. 29). This chapter will focus on the controversies around diagnostic laparoscopy in the acute abdomen, the effect of laparoscopy on peritonitis, laparoscopy for perforated viscus, and laparoscopic treatment of small bowel obstruction.

4.2
Discussion

4.2.1
Diagnostic Laparoscopy in the Acute Abdomen

4.2.1.1
Free Air and Generalized Peritonitis

In some patients with an acute abdomen, the diagnosis may be relatively straightforward, either on the basis of clinical findings or an imaging study such as computed tomography (CT) scan or ultrasound. For example, if the history is typical for appendicitis and the patient has peritonitis only in the right lower quadrant, the diagnosis of appendicitis is likely and may be further confirmed with a CT scan. In these patients, laparoscopy may not be needed to make a diagnosis, but could simply be used to confirm the diagnosis and treat the patient. However, in patients who have a less typical history but have evidence of an acute abdominal condition (findings of generalized peritonitis or "free air" on plain X-rays/CT scan), a diagnostic laparoscopy may yield an accurate diagnosis in a high percentage of patients.

Laparoscopy via a trocar at the umbilicus will allow visualization of both the upper and lower quadrants of the abdominal cavity. After inserting the laparoscope into the abdomen, the surgeon can identify the area of the abdomen with the most inflammation. This can be identified by the erythematous changes in the peritoneum and the presence of fluid and purulent exudates. Although a thorough examination is important, the area with the most inflammation should lead the surgeon to the underlying problem (perforated ulcer, appendicitis, ovarian torsion, diverticulitis, infarcted intestine, etc.). Numerous studies have documented that laparoscopy yields an accurate diagnosis in 85–100% of patients with an acute abdomen [1–3]. However, there is a small percentage of cases in which the inflammatory process is so severe that it might preclude identification of the source. Additionally, there are a small number of cases in which the etiology of the condition is not apparent, even in the absence of severe inflammation. Nonetheless, if performed with appropriate care and technique, it is unlikely that this failed attempt at diagnosis will result in harm to the patient.

Several investigators have raised questions about the effect of CO_2 laparoscopy on the physiologic response to peritonitis [4–8]. In these animal studies, there was evidence that CO_2 pneumoperitoneum adversely affected the ability of the peritoneum to prevent bacteremia and endotoxemia if the peritonitis had its onset more than 12 h prior to intervention. Additionally, the morphology of the mesothelium was altered by the CO_2 pneumoperitoneum. Further, in one of these studies the CO_2 depressed lipopolysaccharide-stimulated cytokine release by macrophages, possibly reducing the efficiency of the response to the insult [7]. Other animal studies have concluded that there is no deleterious effect from the CO_2 pneumoperitoneum [9–10]. The latter study actually raises the possibility that the CO_2 pneumoperitoneum might provide a beneficial effect in the response to the peritonitis by attenuating the acute phase inflammatory response. Several clinical studies have concluded that there is not a significant adverse effect caused by CO_2 pneumoperitoneum [11–13]. These studies looked at the outcome after using laparoscopy for diagnosis and treatment of perforated ulcers. Hence, there is little, if any, evidence that laparoscopy should not be performed in the presence of peritonitis.

4.2.1.2
Acidosis/Sepsis in the Critically Ill Intensive Care Unit Patient

The critically ill patient in the intensive care unit (ICU) who has acidosis without an identifiable cause is a diagnostic challenge. Often the patient is too sick to move to the radiology department for X-rays, angiography, or a CT scan, but intestinal ischemia is often a possibility and should be ruled in or out. Bedside diagnostic laparoscopy is a safe and accurate technique in selected patients [14–17]. Although it should not be used in patients with a tensely distended abdomen (because of the lack of space in the peritoneal cavity in which to work laparoscopically), it has been used safely in otherwise critically ill patients who require ventilatory and pressor support. These series all documented a reduction in negative exploratory laparotomy rates as well as facilitating timely surgical intervention when indicated.

As stated, the use of diagnostic laparoscopy yields significant benefits in terms of making an accurate diagnosis. But the benefits of using laparoscopy in the acute abdomen extend well beyond the high diagnostic accuracy. If the treatment of the underlying cause of the acute abdominal condition can be performed laparoscopically, there may be outcome benefits. But even if the surgeon cannot complete the surgical treatment laparoscopically, the use of diagnostic laparoscopy as the first part of the procedure allows the surgeon to localize the disease process and then place a laparotomy incision close to the site of the disease. This will usually allow the use of a smaller incision than would have been necessary if the initial exploration had been done with a laparotomy. Additionally, all quadrants of the abdomen can be well seen and irrigated during the laparoscopic portion of the procedure.

4.2.2
Therapeutic Laparoscopy in the Acute Abdomen

4.2.2.1
Perforated Viscus

The use of laparoscopy to treat the underlying cause of peritonitis has been challenged on the same bases as diagnostic laparoscopy. However, the three referenced articles regarding the use of laparoscopy for the treatment of perforated ulcers all suggest that in most patients, the outcome is not adversely affected by using laparoscopy [11–13]. The one exception is in the hemodynamically unstable patient. In this situation, the patient may not tolerate the hemodynamic effects of the pneumoperitoneum, and laparotomy should be used if the patient cannot be stabilized prior to surgery.

It is particularly in the patients with free intraperitoneal air that the diagnosis of the underlying pathology may not be made prior to surgery. Laparoscopy allows the surgeon to identify the site of the perforation before deciding whether a laparotomy will be needed. If the disease process can be treated by laparoscopy, then an unnecessary laparotomy can be avoided. If a laparotomy is required, the laparotomy can be minimized and place over the site of perforation. This is particularly helpful in the situation where the perforation is expected in the upper gastrointestinal tract, but is found in the sigmoid colon. However, depending on the experience of the surgeon, most cases of surgical peritonitis can be successfully treated with a laparoscopic approach. The site of the perforation should be treated with a technique similar to open surgery. For a perforated ulcer in the foregut, a Graham patch remains the usual treatment. For a perforated colon with peritonitis, a resection with or without a stoma would be the indicated procedure.

4.2.2.2
Small Bowel Obstruction

The use of laparoscopy to treat small bowel obstruction is desirable for several reasons. Not only might there be less ileus postoperatively, there might be fewer adhesions developing after adhesiolysis if done laparoscopically. However, the presence of the distended intestine proximal to the site of obstruction may make visualization of the site of obstruction more difficult or impossible as well as increase the chance of injury of the intestine. Suter et al. found that if the bowel was dilated to more than 4 cm in diameter, the chance of conversion to open surgery was increased [18]. When successful, however, they found that laparoscopic adhesiolysis resulted in a quicker resumption of diet, fewer complications, and a shorter hospital stay than in the converted patients. Other investigators have had variable success in resolving small bowel obstruction laparoscopically (46–84%) [19–20]. Levard et al. reported 308 patients from a multisite study, and they were successful in treating the bowel obstruction laparoscopically in 54% of cases [21]. This may be representative of the real world success rate because of the multisite nature of the study and because of the larger number of patients. Fischer and Doherty reviewed all the reported series of laparoscopic adhesiolysis for bowel obstruction [22]. They found in their review that surgeons were successful in relieving the small bowel obstruction with laparoscopy in 67.8% of cases (range 35–87%). Reasons for conversion in the remaining 32.2% included: (1) inability to find the site of obstruction (41.3%), (2) strangulation (22.6%), (3) laparoscopically created intestinal injury (18%), (4) suspected tumor (6.5%), and (5) other reasons (18.5%). Overall, 5.8% of laparoscopically attempted cases resulted in an intestinal perforation. Based on these findings, it seems reasonable to initiate the surgical treatment of small bowel obstruction with laparoscopy in all patients without a tensely distended abdomen.

4.3
Summary

— Laparoscopy in patients with an acute abdominal condition yields an accurate diagnosis in a high percentage of patients (87–100%).
— Diagnostic laparoscopy in patients with an acute abdominal condition helps the surgeon plan the surgical approach in one of two ways.
  – The surgeon may proceed with laparoscopic treatment if indicated and technically possible.
  – If laparoscopic treatment is not technically possible, the surgeon may minimize the length of an abdominal incision by positioning the incision directly over the site of the disease process.
— Bedside laparoscopy in the ICU is safe and accurate for evaluating patients with suspected intestinal ischemia or intra-abdominal sepsis.
— Laparoscopy is safe for diagnosis and treatment of patients with a perforated viscus as long as the patient is hemodynamically stable.

— Laparoscopy is safe and effective for the treatment of small bowel obstruction if the abdomen is not tensely distended and the adhesions are not extensive.

References

1. Navez B, Tassetti V, Scohy JJ, et al. Laparoscopic management of acute peritonitis. Br J Surg 1998;85:32–6.
2. Chung RS, Diaz JJ, Chari V. Efficacy of routine laparoscopy for the acute abdomen. Surg Endosc 1998;12:219–22.
3. Sanna A, Adani GL, Anania G, et al. The role of laparoscopy in patients with suspected peritonitis: experience of a single institution. J Laparoendosc Adv Surg Tech 2003;13:17–9.
4. Bloechle C, Emmermann A, Achilles E, et al. Effect of a pneumoperitoneum on the extent and severity of peritonitis induced by gastric ulcer perforation in the rat. Surg Endosc 1995;9:898–900.
5. Bloechle C, Emmermann A, Strate T, et al. Laparoscopic vs open repair of gastric perforation and abdominal lavage of associated peritonitis in pigs. Surg Endosc 1998;12:212–8.
6. Bloechle C, Kluth D, Holstein AF, et al. A pneumoperitoneum perpetuates severe damage to the ultrastructural integrity of parietal peritoneum in gastric perforation-induced peritonitis in rats. Surg Endosc 1999;13:683–8.
7. West MA, Baker J, Bellingham J. Kinetics of decreased LPS-stimulated cytokine release by macrophages exposed to CO_2. J Surg Res 1996;63:269–74.
8. West MA, Hackam DJ, Baker J, et al. Mechanism of decreased in vitro murine macrophage cytokine release after exposure to carbon dioxide: relevance to laparoscopic surgery. Ann Surg 1997;226:179–82.
9. Clary EM, Bruch SM, Lau CL, et al. Effects of pneumoperitoneum on hemodynamic and systemic immunologic responses to peritonitis in pigs. J Surg Res 2002;108:32–8.
10. Hanly EJ, Mendoza-Sagaon M, Murata K, et al. CO_2 pneumoperitoneum modifies the inflammatory response to sepsis. Ann Surg 2003;237:343–50.
11. Robertson GS, Wemyss-Holden SA, Maddern GJ. Laparoscopic repair of perforated peptic ulcers. The role of laparoscopy in generalized peritonitis. Ann R Coll Surg Engl 2000;82:6–10.
12. Lau JY, Lo SY, Ng EK, et al. A randomized comparison of acute phase response and endotoxemia in patients with perforated peptic ulcers receiving laparoscopic or open patch repair. Am J Surg 1998;186:325–7.
13. Katkhouda N, Mavor E, Mason RJ, et al. Laparoscopic repair of perforated duodenal ulcers: outcome and efficacy in 30 consecutive patients. Arch Surg 1999;134:845–50.
14. Gagne DJ, Malay MB, Hogle NJ, et al. Bedside diagnostic minilaparoscopy in the intensive care patient. Surgery 2002;131:491–6.
15. Brandt CP, Priebe PP, Echhauser ML. Diagnostic laparoscopy in the intensive care patient: avoiding the nontherapeutic laparotomy. Surg Endosc 7:168–71.
16. Orlando R, Crowell KI. Laparoscopy in the critically ill. Surg Endosc 1997;11:1072–4.

17. Forde K, Treat M. The role of peritoneoscopy (laparoscopy) in the evaluation of the acute abdomen in critically ill patients. Surg Endosc 1992;6:219–21.

18. Suter M, Zermatten P, Halkie N, et al. Laparoscopic management of mechanical small bowel obstruction: are there predictors of success or failure? Surg Endosc 2000;14:478–83.

19. Navez B, Arimont JM, Guiot P. Laparoscopioc approach in acute small bowel obstruction. A review of 68 patients. Hepatogastroenterology 1998;45:132–40.

20. Chosidow D, Johanet H, Montariol T, et al. Laparoscopy for acute small-bowel obstruction secondary to adhesions. J Laparoendosc Adv Surg Tech 2000;10:155–9.

21. Levard H, Boudet MJ, Msika S, et al. Laparoscopic treatment of acute small bowel obstruction: a multicentre retrospective study. Aust N Z J Surg 2001;71:641–6.

22. Fischer CP, Doherty D. Laparoscopic approach to small bowel obstruction. Semin Laparosc Surg 2002;9:40–5.

Commentary

PHILIP S. BARIE

Fowler has outlined the potential utility of laparoscopy for the diagnosis and treatment of the acute abdomen for "selected patients." Therein lies the problem. It has been a decade since laparoscopic cholecystectomy became commonplace, yet in that period we have yet to develop definitive evidence of efficacy for the diagnosis and management of the acute abdomen, even for perforated appendicitis [1]. Anecdotes and selected case series abound [2, 3], but even historical controls are usually not reported. Appendicitis notwithstanding, randomized, controlled clinical trials of relevant endpoints are still lacking [4]. With respect to laparoscopy, that it can be done does not necessarily mean that it should be done. Moreover, caution must be taken in extrapolating the results obtained for "garden-variety" emergencies of stable patients to those of critically ill, hemodynamically unstable patients in the ICU.

The argument is sometimes made that laparoscopy can avoid the perils of intrahospital transport for the unstable patient, implying that visualization can be excellent during laparoscopy at the bedside, while avoiding the putative substantial risks of transport. This argument is specious. Intrahospital transport is safely possible even when patients are receiving vasoactive medications or being ventilated with high levels of positive end-expiratory pressure [5]. A formal diagnostic laparoscopy for intra-abdominal infection requires several changes in position during the procedure (Trendelenberg position, reverse Trendelenberg, bilateral decubitus positions) to enable meticulous inspection of the bowel [6], which is difficult-to-impossible at the bedside.

Visibility can be impeded by several other factors. The 2-mm laparoscope, which can facilitate peritoneoscopy under local anesthesia, transmits less light than larger instruments, and visibility can be suboptimal. Intracavitary pressures of 12–15 mmHg from CO_2 insufflation can compress the inferior vena cava, reducing cardiac output if the patient is hypovolemic. It may be necessary to reduce distending pressures to 5–7 mmHg to support hemodynamics while at the same time impeding visibility. It is also reported that absorption of CO_2 from the peritoneum may worsen acidosis or precipitate myocardial ischemia [7]. Moreover, recent abdominal incisions or penetrating wounds may not be gas-tight, making it difficult to maintain gas insufflation for optimum visibility. Furthermore, as pointed out by Fowler, intestinal ischemia can be difficult to diagnose by laparoscopy. Life-threatening ischemia can be non-transmural, lending a deceptively benign appearance to an exceedingly dangerous situation.

There is evidence that laparoscopy, or specifically CO_2 pneumoperitoneum may promote the persistence of infection. There is some evidence that laparoscopic management of perforated appendicitis may increase the risk of persistent or recurrent intra-abdominal infection [1]. Pneumoperitoneum with either CO_2 or N_2O has been reported to increase bacterial counts of *Escherichia coli* [8] and *Bacteroides fragilis* [9] in experimental peritonitis, although it is unproven whether the phenomena are due to a growth-promoting effect, or inhibition of peritoneal host defenses and clearance of bacteria.

Owing to the paucity of Class I data, published evidence-based guidelines are necessarily weak, but published guidelines do exist [10]. Preoperatively, all patients should be assessed for the coexistence of cardiac, pulmonary, hepatic, renal, or vascular disease. If appropriate perioperative measures and surgical techniques are employed, laparoscopy with pneumoperitoneum may be undertaken in patients with peritonitis. Monitoring of end-tidal CO_2 concentration is mandatory. The lowest intra-abdominal pressure that allows adequate exposure of the operative field should be used. In patients with cardiopulmonary disease or hemodynamic instability, intraoperative and postoperative arterial blood gas monitoring is recommended. Intraoperative sequential intermittent pneumatic compression of the lower extremities is recommended for all prolonged laparoscopic procedures.

Common sense, and objective evidence of how sick the patient is, should guide the decision to attempt laparoscopy for management of the acute abdomen. For example, failure rates are higher when perforated peptic ulcers greater than 1 cm diameter are sutured laparoscopically [11]. Paradoxically, the sicker the patient is, the less favorable a candidate he or she may be for a minimally-invasive surgical approach. Failure rates for laparoscopic repair of perforated peptic ulcer are higher with increased severity of illness, as assessed by the APACHE II score [12]. Unfortunately, comparable studies of outcomes of other acute abdominal pathologies have not been reported.

References

1. Sauerland S, Lefering R, Neugebauer EA. Laparoscopic versus open surgery for suspected appendicitis. Cochrane Database Syst Rev 2002;1:CD001546.
2. Gagne DJ, Malay MB, Hogle NJ, Fowler DL. Bedside diagnostic minilaparoscopy in the intensive care unit. Surgery 2002;131:491–6.
3. Hackert T, Kienle P, Weitz J, et al. Accuracy of diagnostic laparoscopy for early diagnosis of abdominal complications after cardiac surgery. Surg Endosc 2003;17:1671–4.
4. Branicki FJ. Abdominal emergencies: diagnostic and therapeutic laparoscopy. Surg Infect 2002;3:269–82.
5. Szem JW, Hydo LJ, Fischer E, et al. High risk intrahospital transport of critically ill patients: safety and outcome of the necessary „road trip". Crit Care Med 1995;23:1660–6.
6. Geis WP, Kim HC. Use of laparoscopy in the diagnosis and treatment of patients with surgical abdominal sepsis. Surg Endosc 1995;9:178–82.
7. Clary EM, Bruch AM, Lau CL, et al. Effects of pneumoperitoneum on hemodynamic and systemic immunologic responses to peritonitis in pigs. J Surg Res 2002;108:32–8.
8. Sare M, Demirkiran AE, Alibey E, Durmaz B. Effect of abdominal insufflation on bacterial growth in experimental peritonitis. J Laparoendosc Adv Surg Tech A 2001;11: 285–9.
9. Sare M, Demirkiran AE, Tastekin N, Durmaz B. Effects of laparoscopic models on anaerobic bacterial growth with *Bacteroides fragilis* in experimentally induced peritonitis. J Laparoendosc Adv Surg Tech A 2003;13:175–9.
10. Neudecker J, Sauerland S, Neugebauer E, et al. The European Association for Endoscopic Surgery clinical practice guideline on the pneumoperitoneum for laparoscopic surgery. Surg Endosc 2002;16:1121–43.
11. Lau WY, Leung KL, Kwong KH, et al. A randomized study comparing laparoscopic versus open repair of perforated peptic ulcer using suture or sutureless technique. Ann Surg 1996;224:131–8.
12. Lee FY, Leung KL, Lai PB, et al. Selection of patients for laparoscopic repair of perforated peptic ulcer. Br J Surg 2001;88:133–6.

Laparoscopy in Special Conditions: Previous Abdominal Surgery, Pregnancy and Liver Disease

Payam Massaband, Myriam J. Curet

▶ **Key Controversy**

A. Location of initial access
B. Choice of access technique
C. Performance of laparoscopic adhesiolysis

5.1
Previous Abdominal Surgery

5.1.1
Introduction

Initially, patients with previous abdominal surgery were discouraged from laparoscopic surgery because of the increased risk of bowel injury caused by needle or trocar insertion. In addition, laparoscopic adhesiolysis was feared to be more dangerous and time consuming than open adhesiolysis. However, 30–50% of patients presenting for laparoscopic surgery have had previous abdominal operations [1–3], which would eliminate many patients from experiencing the benefits of a minimally invasive surgery. With increased experience and new instrumentation, laparoscopic surgery can be offered to patients with previous abdominal surgery with excellent results. Controversies exist in the best choice for initial access, the location of initial access and in how to perform laparoscopic adhesiolysis safely.

5.1.2
Discussion

5.1.2.1
Location of Initial Access

Previous abdominal surgery is not an absolute predictor of peritoneal adhesions. In autopsy studies, 75–90% of patients with previous abdominal surgery had adhesions. Not all adhesions were located at the previous abdominal surgery site. Furthermore, as many as 25% of patients without a history of abdominal surgery had adhesions [4]. Clinical studies have shown that as high as one-third of patients with previous abdominal surgery had no adhesions [5–9].

Patients with previous abdominal surgery pose two specific problems: (1) obtaining safe access in order to initiate pneumoperitoneum, and (2) performing safe adhesiolysis to gain adequate exposure to operative field. As we have mentioned, presence and location of adhesions are not predictable. Some authors recommend preoperative ultrasound for localization of adhesions and determination of safe entry points [10–12]. It is more likely, however, for adhesions to be located near sites of prior surgery. For this reason, some advocate placement of the initial trocar in a site far from previous scars. Although it is advantageous for the first trocar to be placed in a position from which surgery may be performed, this is not necessary. In the upper quadrants, placement is safest in the midclavicular line [7]. In the lower quadrants, the trocars are best placed lateral to the epigastric vessels but sufficiently medial to avoid the colon [13]. Palmer's point is along the left midclavicular line, 3 cm caudal to the costal margin or the right upper quadrant and has been advocated by Corson et al. [14]. Halpern has recommended the right upper quadrant in patients with pelvic surgery [9, 13].

5.1.2.2
Choice of Access Technique

The blind access approach with Veress needle has been associated with a high rate of complications, regardless of patients past surgical history. Blind insertion is associated with most vascular injuries and a majority of bowel injuries related to access [10, 15–21]. These risks are higher if the patient has had prior laparotomy even when a small gauge syringe was used to determine the presence of adhesions [22].

The historical alternative to the blind approach is the "open" laparoscopy approach first described by Hasson [23]. This allows identification of adherent bowel and dissection of the bowel away from the abdominal wall. Some surgeons use an open technique routinely because of the decreased risk of vascular or visceral injury. The prevalence of almost all vascular and most visceral injuries are decreased with the open technique [9, 10, 20, 21, 24, 25]. The open technique may be technically difficult when performed through a previous umbilical scar – careful dissection is necessary. Reports of insertion of a Hasson trocar in the right iliac fossa, right upper quadrant, or subxiphoid area have suggested fewer complications and easier insertion [2, 7, 17, 26]. Though associated with longer operative times [2], the time decreases with the experience of the surgeon [9] and avoiding morbidity is time well spent.

Newer approaches of gaining access to the abdominal cavity involve the use of special optical trocars that allow the user to view the tissue layers of the abdominal wall as they are being traversed. Pioneered by Melzer and colleagues [27, 28], there have been several modifications to date and the data regarding the safety, efficacy, and advantages over other techniques have been inconclusive. Several studies have supported the use of optical access trocars, even in patients with prior abdominal surgery [14, 29–32]. There have been few reported major complications with optical access trocars but a review of FDA and manufacturer databases revealed a significant number of visceral and vascular injuries [33]. Though the total number of patients is unknown, this study makes it clear that optical access trocars may not be as safe as is implied by the lack of reports in the literature to the contrary.

There is clearly no perfect method for gaining access to the abdominal cavity. The overall incidence of major complications is low, even for patients with prior abdominal surgery. We prefer open laparoscopy in cases of prior surgery. If there is any suggestion of adherent bowel or unclear abdominal wall anatomy, a different site should be chosen for entry.

5.1.2.3
Performance of Laparoscopic Adhesiolysis

Once safe access is obtained, adequate visualization of the abdomen to insert the remaining ports and to perform the planned surgery must be obtained. If adhesions are present, they may be circumvented by angling the laparoscope around the edge or through fenestrations in the adhered omentum [9, 13]. Adequate visualization of the operative field often requires adhesiolysis, though. Numerous techniques are available. Blunt finger dissection through the initial trocar site when open laparoscopy is used may be adequate. The trocar and camera may be used for blunt dissection. When the adhesions are too dense to separate with gentle traction, sharp or cautery dissection may be used. It is best to follow the line of tissue adherence to avoid blood loss and adjacent tissue damage. As in open surgery, traction-counter-traction may be used to help develop the desired plane. If cautery is used for adhesiolysis, care must be taken to avoid injury to adjacent organs, which can result from inadequate visualization or transmission of heat beyond target tissue. Ports should be placed as necessary for adequate visualization and retraction, regardless of the necessity of these ports for the desired surgery. The surgical ports may be placed later.

Lysis of all visible adhesions is unnecessary. Only adhesions that interfere with trocar placement and with performance of the intended operation should be dissected [9]. Additional adhesiolysis adds to surgical time and risks without benefit. Once adequate adhesiolysis is complete, the area should be inspected carefully for hemostasis and evidence of bowel injury. If found, these complications should be treated immediately. If laparoscopic repair is not feasible, conversion to the open procedure should be performed without hesitation. Missed bowel injury is a significant and preventable cause of added morbidity and mortality associated with laparoscopic surgery [14, 34, 35].

The effect of adhesions depends on the planned laparoscopic procedure and the site of the previous surgery. Many studies have attempted to identify risk factors for conversion to open surgery [18, 36–42]. Previous abdominal surgery has not been uniformly implicated. In some studies, however, previous abdominal surgery and specifically upper abdominal surgery has been associated with conversion when laparoscopic cholecystectomies were studied [3, 40, 43, 44]. Many reports of patients with prior abdominal surgery who have undergone laparoscopic surgery successfully have been published, however. Specifically, laparoscopic cholecystectomies [3, 5, 12, 45] and laparoscopic antireflux procedures [46–49] have been studied. All studies report minimal conversion rates and only one study [3] found significantly increased complications after subgroup analysis of patients with prior upper abdominal surgery. All other studies reported no significant differences in morbidity. Furthermore, these patients experience the advantages of minimally invasive surgery, including decreased hospital stay and less postoperative pain.

5.1.3
Summary

— Previous abdominal surgery is not a contraindication to attempting a procedure laparoscopically. Patients should be warned of the increased risk for bowel injury, the possible need for additional trocars, and the increased risk for conversion.
— Preoperative planning is important and includes assessing the geographic relationship between the proposed surgery and the abdominal scar, initial entry at a distance from previous scars, and the use of the open technique for access and careful adhesiolysis.
— Surgeons should be sufficiently experienced in less complicated cases before attempting laparoscopy in patients who may have extensive adhesions.

5.2
Laparoscopic Surgery in Liver Disease

▶ **Key Controversies**

A. Laparoscopic surgery in patients with compensated cirrhosis
B. Laparoscopic surgery in patients with uncompensated cirrhosis

5.2.1
Introduction

For years the conventional wisdom was that liver disease, and cirrhosis in particular, were contraindications to performing laparoscopic surgery. In 1992 a consensus conference discouraged laparoscopic cholecystectomy in cirrhotic patients [50]. As surgeons became technically more adept, many of the conditions that were once considered contraindications to laparoscopic surgery are being reconsidered. Liver disease is no exception.

5.2.2
Discussion

5.2.2.1
Laparoscopic surgery in patients with compensated cirrhosis

Cirrhotic patients are at increased risk of morbidity and mortality, regardless of type of surgery [51, 52]. Patients with cirrhosis have multiple systemic problems including malnutrition, coagulopathies, ascites, and renal dysfunction. Often, metabolism of drugs administered during surgery is diminished. In addition, hepatic blood flow is altered in these patients. Patients with cirrhosis typically are unable to compensate for the decrease in portal blood flow seen with anesthesia, which can be further exacerbated by perioperative complications. Historically high morbidity and mortality rates in these patients have improved as better anesthetics, improved surgical technique, more thorough preoperative assessment, and better postoperative intensive care unit management have become available [51].

Reasons for the initial concerns regarding laparoscopic surgery in particular involved the bleeding risks during dissection and trauma to umbilical varices during port placement. More recent concerns have involved CO_2 pneumoperitoneum and its effects on liver physiology. Basic research regarding the effects of CO_2 pneumoperitoneum and its effects on liver physiology has been performed on cirrhotic rats. Pneumoperitoneum in rats decreases portal venous return, additive to that seen with anesthesia [53]. Normal rats are able to increase hepatic arterial blood flow to compensate for the decrease. Cirrhotic rats are unable to make up for this loss and therefore have decreased blood flow during laparoscopy [53].

There is a higher incidence of biliary disease in cirrhotic patients [54]. The increased incidence and the desire to offer the benefits of laparoscopic surgery to this population led to the eventual use of laparoscopy on patients in whom the diagnosis of cirrhosis had not yet been established or those with well-compensated liver disease. Starting with retrospective reviews of patients who were found to have cirrhosis during or after laparoscopic surgery, there has been an accumulating body of evidence supporting the safety and advantages of laparoscopy in liver disease, especially with regard to cholecystectomy in patients with Child's class A or B cirrhosis [55, 60]. Evaluation of cirrhotic patients undergoing cholecystectomy demonstrated decreased blood transfusion rates, morbidity, wound infections, and hospital stay in the group of patients treated laparoscopically [61–63]. In fact, comparison of laparoscopic cholecystectomy in cirrhotics with matched non-cirrhotic controls reveals minimally increased bleeding risk with little to no increase in conversion rate or perioperative mortality [55, 64–67]. Yeh et al. have reported the largest series of these retrospective studies. Though they report similar 30-day mortality rates, the perioperative mortality rate was increased in the cirrhotic group [57]. In any event, the mortality rate is lower than the historical mortality rates of cirrhotic patients undergoing cholecystectomy [52, 68]. Yeh et al. report improvement of conversion rates and decreased blood loss as the experience of the surgeon increased. A retrospective study of laparoscopic and open appendectomies in patients with cirrhosis demonstrated similar results as seen in cirrhotic patients undergoing laparoscopic cholecystectomy, with decreased wound bleeding and fewer wound infections after laparoscopic surgery, compared with those undergoing open appendectomy. In addition, postoperative pain levels and hospital stay were also less in the laparoscopic group [69].

Laparoscopy has also been shown to preserve immune response, when compared with open surgery [70–74]. This finding has also been replicated in a randomized, prospective study of patients with chronic liver disease [75]. Proponents cite preserved immune response as the reason for the decreased wound infection rate in cirrhotics undergoing laparoscopic surgery.

Several authors have recommended meticulous operative technique to improve outcome. The umbilical trocar should be placed in such a way as to avoid umbilical varices, if they exist. The subxiphoid port should be placed more laterally to avoid the falciform ligament [55].

Given the concerns of altered hepatic blood flow and inadequate compensation for decreased portal blood flow in cirrhotic patients undergoing a pneumoperitoneum, attention has focused on the use of gasless laparoscopy in these patients. Giraudo et al. have compared pneumoperitoneum at different pressures and gasless laparoscopy. They found that gasless laparoscopy and low pressure pneumoperitoneum caused a lower increase in the liver function tests than conventional pressure laparoscopy [76]. Some have used gasless laparoscopic surgery to perform liver resections in patients with cirrhosis. Itamoto et al. advocate the use of gasless laparoscopy in addition to a 5 cm "mini" laparotomy for liver resection in these patients who would otherwise not be candidates for major hepatectomy [77].

5.2.2.2
Laparoscopic Surgery in Patients with Uncompensated Cirrhosis

Although the results for improved outcomes with laparoscopic surgery are valid, the bulk of the data thus far have been accumulated with Child's A or B cirrhotics. It is not clear whether these outcomes may be applied to Child's C patients. Clearly the decision to proceed to surgery is difficult when dealing with decompensated cirrhosis, as morbidity and mortality rates in these patients are prohibitive. There are four cases of laparoscopic cholecystectomy performed on Child's C patients reported in the literature, with one mortality [61, 64, 78]. The mortality was in a patient awaiting cardiac transplantation [64]. Many authors have recommended maximizing medical management of cirrhotics and attempting to improve Child's class prior to surgery. Important future studies will assess the risks of surgery involving Child's C patients and the potential improvement in outcome without pneumoperitoneum. It is possible that the decrease in hepatic blood flow seen with gasless laparoscopy may be more clinically relevant in patients with borderline hepatic function. Advantages of laparoscopy that are specific to this group of patients may emerge. For example, decreased adhesion formation may lead to less blood loss during transplantation, as these patients frequently go on to require liver transplants.

5.2.3
Summary

- Cirrhotic patients are at increased risk for significant morbidity and mortality following any surgery. Laparoscopic surgery may pose unique risks associated with the increased intra-abdominal pressure and decreased hepatic blood flow.
- There is increasing evidence to suggest that laparoscopic procedures, especially in patients with Child's class A or B cirrhosis, may decrease morbidity and mortality compared with those of open surgery.

— Gasless laparoscopy may be a preferable method of operative approach in patients with compromised hepatic function.
— As yet the role of laparoscopy in patients with uncompensated cirrhosis is unknown and a minimally invasive approach in these patients should be addressed cautiously.

5.3
Pregnancy

▶ **Key Controversies**

A. Clinical significance of intraoperative physiologic changes
B. Guidelines during laparoscopic surgery in pregnant patients
C. Arterial line
D. Intraoperative maternal–fetal monitoring
E. Laparoscopic surgery during the third trimester
F. Tocolytics

5.3.1
Introduction

As with previous abdominal surgery and liver disease, pregnancy was initially considered an absolute contraindication to laparoscopic surgery. Persistent questions regarding the effects of CO_2 pneumoperitoneum, such as decreased venous return, uterine blood flow, and maternal–fetal acidosis, prevented the application of laparoscopy to pregnant patients. As high as 0.75% of pregnant patients require non-obstetric surgery [79, 80]. The low total number of pregnant patients who undergo surgery makes it impossible for statistically significant studies to be performed. Despite this, or perhaps because of it, guidelines regarding the use of laparoscopy in pregnancy have been published [81]. Even as the questions regarding the physiology of laparoscopy during pregnancy are answered, some areas of controversy persist, including (1) the clinical significance of intraoperative physiologic changes, (2) the efficacy of the recommended guidelines, and (3) the feasibility of laparoscopic surgery during the third trimester of pregnancy.

Studies in the gynecologic literature regarding laparoscopy for potential ectopic pregnancy reveal many subsequent normal intrauterine pregnancies and deliveries. Regardless of the trimester in which laparoscopy was performed, there was no evidence for increased fetal loss or adverse long-term outcomes [82–86]. As a result, surgeons began performing laparoscopic appendectomies and cholecystectomies on pregnant patients in 1991 [87–89].

5.3.2
Discussion

5.3.2.1
Clinical Significance of Intraoperative Physiologic Changes

Concerns regarding the deleterious effects of laparoscopic surgery on the mother and fetus include possible maternal hemodynamic changes and instability secondary to decreased venous return and cardiac output [90–93]. Increased abdominal pressure may lead to decreased uterine blood flow, increased intrauterine pressure, fetal hypoxia and acidosis [90–92, 94–96]. The use of carbon dioxide can potentiate this fetal acidosis and may result in maternal acidosis. Several animal studies have been performed to address the severity of these changes and the effects on mother and fetus. Despite documentation of severe fetal acidosis, one long-term study found that all ewes delivered full-term, healthy lambs [96]. Several studies have found that nitrous oxide and helium pneumoperitoneum cause less fetal and maternal acidosis and less fetal tachycardia. These findings suggest that alternate insufflating gasses may be safer but corroborating studies on pregnant patients are lacking [90, 95, 97–106].

Clinical studies have supported the concept that the intraoperative detrimental physiologic changes seen with carbon dioxide pneumoperitoneum do not result in poor fetal or maternal outcomes. When laparoscopic surgery is compared with the open counterpart, the safety is comparable and the benefits of laparoscopic surgery are realized by both mother and fetus. In addition to the usual decreased pain and hospital stay, laparoscopic patients ambulate earlier, which decreases the already significant risk of deep venous thrombosis. Another advantage is the decreased fetal depression with decreased narcotic use [81, 91, 107–111]. Some studies [80] report decreased birth weight with any surgery, due to intrauterine growth retardation or prematurity. Rojansky et al. [111] found that premature delivery or need for tocolysis, intrauterine growth retardation, and miscarriage rate only occurred with the open group. A long-term study [84] found that one child who was prenatally determined to be small for gestational age conformed to the growth chart at birth. Amos et al [112] have been the only authors to present significant adverse outcomes, with fetal loss in four of seven patients. Possibly due to the morbidity of the presenting conditions (three patients with pancreatitis and one with ruptured appendix), these results have not been replicated in the literature. The cautious approach to surgery is necessary, however, because surgeons may not be reporting adverse outcomes and controlled trials are not practical.

5.3.2.2
Guidelines During Laparoscopic Surgery in Pregnant Patients

To date, over 300 laparoscopic cholecystectomies during pregnancy have been reported. Because of this increase, guidelines regarding the use of laparoscopy in pregnancy have been published [81]. These include recommendations on positioning, degree of intraabdominal pressure, thromboembolic prophylaxis, use of arterial lines and intraoperative fetal monitoring.

Left lateral positioning is recommended during open surgery to decrease the uterine pressure on the inferior vena cava. This position is even more important during laparoscopic surgery where the pneumoperitoneum can also contribute to decreased venous return. Minimizing the degree of reverse Trendelenburg and lowering insufflation pressure are also recommended [91, 92, 113–116]. Although the evidence is nonexistent, most authors recommend pressures less than 12 mmHg [81, 84, 108, 117]. No controversy exists over the recommendation that prophylaxis against deep venous thrombosis be used. In addition to the decreased venous return and stasis, pregnant patients have increased hematologic risk for clot formation [115, 118].

Unanswered questions exist regarding the potential harmful effects of fetal exposure to smoke and carbon monoxide emission from cautery. The possibility of harmful effects and the difficulty with finding scientific evidence to the contrary has led to recommendations to evacuate smoke immediately and to limit the duration of surgery as much as possible [84, 108].

5.3.2.3
Arterial Line

There is controversy regarding whether end-tidal CO_2 ($ETCO_2$) monitoring is sufficient for measuring intraoperative acidosis. Early studies suggested routine arterial blood gases for all pregnant patients undergoing laparoscopic surgery. These recommendations were based on animal studies and an early human study with bad outcomes [101, 112, 119]. Since then, there have been many studies supporting the use of capnography for monitoring acidosis, finding that $ETCO_2$ correlates well with arterial blood gases. Based on these studies, the recommendations are to keep $ETCO_2$ between 32 and 36 mmHg by varying minute ventilation [91, 92, 94, 96, 120].

5.3.2.4
Intraoperative Maternal–Fetal Monitoring

Most authors currently recommend preoperative and postoperative fetal monitoring only [91, 92, 121]. Some authors recommend intraoperative monitoring even in the case of a nonviable fetus, reasoning that fetal distress can be treated by immediate desufflation [84, 115, 117]. If intraoperative monitoring is desired, the transvaginal route is preferred because it does not interfere with the operative field and the signal is not lost when pneumoperitoneum is established [118, 122]. The decision to monitor intraoperatively should be made on a case-by-case basis taking fetal age, maternal health, and underlying surgical disease into account.

5.3.2.5
Laparoscopic Surgery During the Third Trimester

Although any type of surgery at any time during pregnancy poses risks to both fetus and mother, initial recommendations regarding the timing of surgery during pregnancy involved the balance between teratogenesis and miscarriage early in pregnancy with preterm labor, premature delivery and large, obstructive uterus in later pregnancy. For these reasons, the second trimester is recommended as the safest time for surgery [108]. Current evidence suggests that if surgery becomes necessary, it can be performed laparoscopically with minimal risks, regardless of gestational age [79, 84, 91, 92, 97, 108, 123–132].

During the third trimester, the size of the gravid uterus may pose difficulty with access and visualization. We recommend use of open laparoscopy for gaining access to the abdominal cavity, although reports of a Veress needle inserted in the right upper quadrant safely have been published. Generally, trocar placement has to be modified with progressing uterine size, by moving them cephalad. The camera port should be placed no lower than the fundus of the uterus for laparoscopic cholecystectomy. Some authors recommend placement of the camera port in the subxiphoid region for laparoscopic appendectomy. These modifications can help improve intraoperative visualization.

5.3.2.6
Tocolytics

The major risk in the third trimester involves preterm labor and premature delivery. The fear of premature contractions and delivery has led some authors to use prophylactic tocolysis. The results of these investigations are inconclusive [122, 133–135]. Tocolytic use is not benign and the rate of premature contraction varies widely depending on the disease process and surgery. In one study, 40% of patients with appendicitis had contractions preoperatively while none of the patients with biliary disease had contractions. Postoperatively, 8% of patients undergoing cholecystectomy had contractions, as opposed to 52% of patients undergoing adnexal surgery. In general, the data support the use of tocolytics for patients who are having preterm labor. Prophylactic use of tocolytics only for high-risk patients avoids treating patients unnecessarily, but is yet unsupported by the literature [79, 114, 136, 137].

5.3.3
Summary

— There are not many studies addressing the long-term effects of laparoscopic surgery on the fetus.
— Although there is no evidence for long-term consequences, surgery should be avoided during pregnancy, if possible. If surgery is necessary, the evidence supports the safe use of laparoscopic surgery, regardless of fetal age. Published guidelines should be followed until more data are available.

5.4
General Conclusions

Previous surgery, liver disease, and pregnancy should no longer be considered contraindications to laparoscopic surgery. Surgeons should exercise good judgment in patient selection, use meticulous surgical techniques, and prepare thoroughly for the planned procedure. Patients should be advised of the increased risks involved. With these caveats in mind, these patients can still experience the advantages of minimally invasive surgery without increased risks.

References

1. Parsons JK, Jarrett TJ, Chow GK, et al. The effect of previous abdominal surgery on urological laparoscopy. J Urol 2002;168:2387–90.
2. Patel M, Smart D. Laparoscopic cholecystectomy and previous abdominal surgery: a safe technique. Aust N Z J Surg 1996;66:309–11.
3. Schirmer BD, Dix J, Schmieg RE Jr., et al. The impact of previous abdominal surgery on outcome following laparoscopic cholecystectomy. Surg Endosc 1995;9:1085–9.
4. Weibel MA, Majno G. Peritoneal adhesions and their relation to abdominal surgery. A postmortem study. Am J Surg 1973;126:345–53.

5. Wongworawat MD, Aitken DR, Robles AE, et al. The impact of prior intra-abdominal surgery on laparoscopic cholecystectomy. Am Surg 1994;60:763–6.
6. Levrant SG, Bieber EJ, Barnes RB. Anterior abdominal wall adhesions after laparotomy or laparoscopy. J Am Assoc Gynecol Laparosc 1997;4:353–6.
7. Kumar SS. Laparoscopic cholecystectomy in the densely scarred abdomen. Am Surg 1998;64:1094–6.
8. Halpern NB. Laparoscopic cholecystectomy in pregnancy: a review of published experiences and clinical considerations. Semin Laparosc Surg 1998;5:129–34.
9. Halpern NB. Access problems in laparoscopic cholecystectomy: postoperative adhesions, obesity, and liver disorders. Semin Laparosc Surg 1998;5:92–106.
10. Borzellino G, De Manzoni G, Ricci F. Detection of abdominal adhesions in laparoscopic surgery. A controlled study of 130 cases. Surg Laparosc Endosc 1998;8:273–6.
11. Caprini JA, Arcelus JA, Swanson J. et al. The ultrasonic localization of abdominal wall adhesions. Surg Endosc 1995;9:283–5.
12. Miller K, Holbling N, Hutter J, et al. Laparoscopic cholecystectomy for patients who have had previous abdominal surgery. Surg Endosc 1993;7:400–3.
13. Halpern NB. The difficult laparoscopy. Surg Clin North Am 1996;76:603–13.
14. Corson SL, Chandler JG, Way LW. Survey of laparoscopic entry injuries provoking litigation. J Am Assoc Gynecol Laparosc 2001;8:341–7.
15. Munro MG. Laparoscopic access: complications, technologies, and techniques. Curr Opin Obstet Gynecol 2002;14:365–74.
16. Champault G, Cazacu F, Taffinder N. Serious trocar accidents in laparoscopic surgery: a French survey of 103,852 operations. Surg Laparosc Endosc 1996;6:367–70.
17. Gersin KS, Heniford BT, Arca MJ, et al. Alternative site entry for laparoscopy in patients with previous abdominal surgery. J Laparoendosc Adv Surg Tech A 1998;8:125–30.
18. Mayol J, Garcia-Aguilar J, Ortiz-Oshiro E, et al. Risks of the minimal access approach for laparoscopic surgery: multivariate analysis of morbidity related to umbilical trocar insertion. World J Surg 1997;21:529–33.
19. McKernan JB, Champion JK. Access techniques: Veress needle –initial blind trocar insertion versus open laparoscopy with the Hasson trocar. Endosc Surg Allied Technol 1995;3:35–8.
20. Nuzzo G, Giuliante F, Tebala GD, et al. Routine use of open technique in laparoscopic operations. J Am Coll Surg 1997;184:58–62.
21. Sigman HH, Fried GM, Garzon J, et al. Risks of blind versus open approach to celiotomy for laparoscopic surgery. Surg Laparosc Endosc 1993;3:296–9.
22. Lecuru F, Leonard F, Philippe Jais J, et al. Laparoscopy in patients with prior surgery: results of the blind approach. JSLS 2001;5:13–6.
23. Hasson HM. A modified instrument and method for laparoscopy. Am J Obstet Gynecol 1971;110:886–7.
24. Hasson HM, Rotman C, Rana N, et al. Open laparoscopy: 29-year experience. Obstet Gynecol 2000;96:763–6.
25. Hanney RM, Carmalt HL, Merrett N, et al. Use of the Hasson cannula producing major vascular injury at laparoscopy. Surg Endosc 1999;13:1238–40.
26. Diez J, Delbene R, Ferreres A. The feasibility of laparoscopic cholecystectomy in patients with previous abdominal surgery. HPB Surg 1998;10:353–6.
27. Melzer A, Weiss U, Roth K, et al. Visually controlled trocar insertion by means of the „optical scalpel". Endosc Surg Allied Technol 1993;1:239–42.

28. Melzer A, Riek S, Roth K, et al. Endoscopically controlled trocar and cannula insertion. Endosc Surg Allied Technol 1995;3:63–8.

29. String A, Berber E, Foroutani A, et al. Use of the optical access trocar for safe and rapid entry in various laparoscopic procedures. Surg Endosc 2001;15:570–3.

30. Catarci M, Carlini M, Gentileschi P, et al. Major and minor injuries during the creation of pneumoperitoneum. A multicenter study on 12,919 cases. Surg Endosc 2001;15:566–9.

31. Marcovich R, Del Terzo MA, Wolf JS Jr. Comparison of transperitoneal laparoscopic access techniques: Optiview visualizing trocar and Veress needle. J Endourol 2000;14:175–9.

32. Wolf JS Jr. Laparoscopic access with a visualizing trocar. Tech Urol 1997;3:34–7.

33. Sharp HT, Dodson MK, Draper ML, et al. Complications associated with optical-access laparoscopic trocars. Obstet Gynecol 2002;99:553–5.

34. El-Banna M, Abdel-Atty M, El-Meteini M, et al. Management of laparoscopic-related bowel injuries. Surg Endosc 2000;14:779–82.

35. Schrenk P, Woisetschlager R, Rieger R, et al. Mechanism, management, and prevention of laparoscopic bowel injuries. Gastrointest Endosc 1996;43:572–4.

36. Alponat A, Kum CK, Koh BC, et al. Predictive factors for conversion of laparoscopic cholecystectomy. World J Surg 1997;21:629–33.

37. Fried GM, Barkun JS, Sigman HH, et al. Factors determining conversion to laparotomy in patients undergoing laparoscopic cholecystectomy. Am J Surg 1994;167:35–41.

38. Liu CL, Fan ST, Lai EC, et al. Factors affecting conversion of laparoscopic cholecystectomy to open surgery. Arch Surg 1996;131:98–101.

39. Liu SI, Siewert B, Raptopoulos V, et al. Factors associated with conversion to laparotomy in patients undergoing laparoscopic appendectomy. J Am Coll Surg 2002;194:298–305.

40. Schrenk P, Woisetschlager R, Rieger R, et al. A diagnostic score to predict the difficulty of a laparoscopic cholecystectomy from preoperative variables. Surg Endosc 1998;12:148–50.

41. Sikora SS, Kumar A, Saxena R, et al. Laparoscopic cholecystectomy–can conversion be predicted? World J Surg 1995;19:858–60.

42. Yu SC, Chen SC, Wang SM, et al. Is previous abdominal surgery a contraindication to laparoscopic cholecystectomy? J Laparoendosc Surg 1994;4:31–5.

43. Hutchinson CH, Traverso LW, Lee FT. Laparoscopic cholecystectomy. Do preoperative factors predict the need to convert to open? Surg Endosc 1994;8:875–80.

44. Jorgensen JO, Hunt DR. Laparoscopic cholecystectomy. A prospective analysis of the potential causes of failure. Surg Laparosc Endosc 1993;3:49–53.

45. Frazee RC, Roberts JW, Symmonds R, et al. What are the contraindications for laparoscopic cholecystectomy? Am J Surg 1992;164:491–5.

46. Awad ZT, Anderson PI, Sato K, et al. Laparoscopic reoperative antireflux surgery. Surg Endosc 2001;15:1401–7.

47. Curet MJ, Josloff RK, Schoeb O, et al. Laparoscopic reoperation for failed antireflux procedures. Arch Surg 1999;134:559–63.

48. DePaula AL, Hashiba K, Bafutto M, et al. Laparoscopic reoperations after failed and complicated antireflux operations. Surg Endosc 1995;9:681–6.

49. Szwerc MF, Wiechmann RJ, Maley RH et al. Reoperative laparoscopic antireflux surgery. Surgery 1999;126:723–9.

50. National Institutes of Health. Gallstones and laparoscopic cholecystectomy. NIH Consens State Sci Statements 1992;10:1–28.
51. Rizvon MK, Chou CL. Surgery in the patient with liver disease. Med Clin North Am 2003;87:211–27.
52. Mansour A, Watson W, Shayani V, et al. Abdominal operations in patients with cirrhosis: still a major surgical challenge. Surgery 1997;122:730–6.
53. Tsuboi S, Kitano S, Yoshida T, et al. Effects of carbon dioxide pneumoperitoneum on hemodynamics in cirrhotic rats. Surg Endosc 2002;16:1220–5.
54. Maggi A, Solenghi D, Panzeri A, et al. Prevalence and incidence of cholelithiasis in patients with liver cirrhosis. Ital J Gastroenterol Hepatol 1997;29:330–5.
55. Leone N, Garino M, De Paolis P, et al. Laparoscopic cholecystectomy in cirrhotic patients. Dig Surg 2001;18:449–52.
56. Tuech JJ, Pessaux P, Regenet N, et al. Laparoscopic cholecystectomy in cirrhotic patients. Surg Laparosc Endosc Percutan Tech 2002;12:227–31.
57. Yeh CN, Chen MF, Jan YY. Laparoscopic cholecystectomy in 226 cirrhotic patients. Experience of a single center in Taiwan. Surg Endosc 2002;16:1583–7.
58. D'Albuquerque LA, de Miranda MP, Genzini T, et al. Laparoscopic cholecystectomy in cirrhotic patients. Surg Laparosc Endosc 1995;5:272–6.
59. Gugenheim J, Casaccia M Jr., Mazza D, et al. Laparoscopic cholecystectomy in cirrhotic patient. HPB Surg 1996;10:79–82.
60. Sleeman D, Namias N, Levi D, et al. Laparoscopic cholecystectomy in cirrhotic patients. J Am Coll Surg 1998;187:400–3.
61. Yerdel MA, Koksoy C, Aras N, et al. Laparoscopic versus open cholecystectomy in cirrhotic patients: a prospective study. Surg Laparosc Endosc 1997;7:483–6.
62. Saeki H, Korenaga D, Yamaga H, et al. A comparison of open and laparoscopic cholecystectomy for patients with cirrhosis. Surg Today 1997;27:411–3.
63. Poggio JL, Rowland CM, Gores GJ, et al. A comparison of laparoscopic and open cholecystectomy in patients with compensated cirrhosis and symptomatic gallstone disease. Surgery 2000;127:405–11.
64. Clark JR, Wills VL, Hunt DR. Cirrhosis and laparoscopic cholecystectomy. Surg Laparosc Endosc Percutan Tech 2001;11:165–9.
65. Jan YY, Chen MF. Laparoscopic cholecystectomy in cirrhotic patients. Hepatogastroenterology 1997;44:1584–7.
66. Morino M, Cavuoti G, Miglietta C, et al. Laparoscopic cholecystectomy in cirrhosis: Contraindication or privileged indication? Surg Laparosc Endosc Percutan Tech 2000;10:360–3.
67. Angrisani L, Lorenzo M, Corcione F, et al. Gallstones in cirrhotics revisited by a laparoscopic view. J Laparoendosc Adv Surg Tech A 1997;7:213–20.
68. Thulstrup AM, Sorensen HT, Vilstrup H. Mortality after open cholecystectomy in patients with cirrhosis of the liver: A population-based study in denmark. Eur J Surg 2001;167:679–83.
69. Tsugawa K, Koyanagi N, Hashizume M, et al. A comparison of an open and laparoscopic appendectomy for patients with liver cirrhosis. Surg Laparosc Endosc Percutan Tech 2001;11:189–94.
70. Trokel MJ, Bessler M, Treat MR, et al. Preservation of immune response after laparoscopy. Surg Endosc 1994;8:1385–8.

71. Gleason NR, Blanco I, Allendorf JD, et al. Delayed-type hypersensitivity response is better preserved in mice following insufflation than after laparotomy. Surg Endosc 1999;13:1032–4.

72. Gitzelmann CA, Mendoza-Sagaon M, Talamini MA, et al. Cell-mediated immune response is better preserved by laparoscopy than laparotomy. Surgery 2000;127:65–71.

73. Allendorf JD, Bessler M, Whelan RL, et al. Postoperative immune function varies inversely with the degree of surgical trauma in a murine model. Surg Endosc 1997;11:427–30.

74. Allendorf JD, Bessler M, Whelan RL, et al. Better preservation of immune function after laparoscopic-assisted vs. open bowel resection in a murine model. Dis Colon Rectum 1996;39 (10 Suppl):S67–S72.

75. Lausten SB, Ibrahim TM, El-Sefi T, et al. Systemic and cell-mediated immune response after laparoscopic and open cholecystectomy in patients with chronic liver disease. a randomized, prospective study. Dig Surg 1999;16:471–7.

76. Giraudo G, Brachet Contul R, Caccetta M, et al. Gasless laparoscopy could avoid alterations in hepatic function. Surg Endosc 2001;15:741–6.

77. Itamoto T, Katayama K, Miura Y, et al. Gasless laparoscopic hepatic resection for cirrhotic patients with solid liver tumors. Surg Laparosc Endosc Percutan Tech 2002;12:325–30.

78. Lacy AM, Balaguer C, Andrade E, et al. Laparoscopic cholecystectomy in cirrhotic patients. Indication or contradiction? Surg Endosc 1995;9:407–8.

79. Visser BC, Glasgow RE, Mulvihill KK, et al. Safety and timing of nonobstetric abdominal surgery in pregnancy. Dig Surg 2001;18:409–17.

80. Mazze RI, Kallen B. Reproductive outcome after anesthesia and operation during pregnancy: a registry study of 5405 cases. Am J Obstet Gynecol 1989;161:1178–85.

81. Society of American Gastrointestinal Endoscopic Surgeons (SAGES). Guidelines for laparoscopic surgery during pregnancy. Surg Endosc 1998;12:189–90.

82. Lemaire BM, van Erp WF. Laparoscopic surgery during pregnancy. Surg Endosc 1997;11:15–8.

83. Mazze RI, Kallen B. Appendectomy during pregnancy: A Swedish registry study of 778 cases. Obstet Gynecol 1991;77:835–40.

84. Rizzo AG. Laparoscopic surgery in pregnancy: long-term follow-up. J Laparoendosc Adv Surg Tech A 2003;13:11–5.

85. Samuelsson S, Sjovall A. Laparoscopy in suspected ectopic pregnancy. Acta Obstet Gynecol Scand 1972;51:31–5.

86. Thomas SJ, Brisson P. Laparoscopic appendectomy and cholecystectomy during pregnancy: six case reports. JSLS 1998;2:41–6.

87. Arvidsson D, Gerdin E. Laparoscopic cholecystectomy during pregnancy. Surg Laparosc Endosc 1991;1:193–4.

88. Pucci RO, Seed RW. Case report of laparoscopic cholecystectomy in the third trimester of pregnancy. Am J Obstet Gynecol 1991;165:401–2.

89. Weber AM, Bloom GP, Allan TR et al. Laparoscopic cholecystectomy during pregnancy. Obstet Gynecol 1991;78 (5 Pt 2):958–9.

90. El-Minawi MF, Wahbi O, El-Bagouri IS, et al. Physiologic changes during CO_2 and N_2O pneumoperitoneum in diagnostic laparoscopy. A comparative study. J Reprod Med 1981;26:338–46.

91. Shay DC, Bhavani-Shankar K, Datta S. Laparoscopic surgery during pregnancy. Anesthesiol Clin North Am 2001;19:57–67.
92. Steinbrook RA. Anaesthesia, minimally invasive surgery and pregnancy. Best Pract Res Clin Anaesthesiol 2002;16:131–43.
93. Motew M, Ivankovich AD, Bieniarz J, et al. Cardiovascular effects and acid-base and blood gas changes during laparoscopy. Am J Obstet Gynecol 1973;115:1002–12.
94. Barnard JM, Chaffin D, Droste S, et al. Fetal response to carbon dioxide pneumoperitoneum in the pregnant ewe. Obstet Gynecol 1995;85:669–74.
95. Fitzgerald SD, Andrus CH, Baudendistel LJ, et al. Hypercarbia during carbon dioxide pneumoperitoneum. Am J Surg 1992;163:186–90.
96. Curet MJ, Vogt DA, Schob O, et al. Effects of CO_2 pneumoperitoneum in pregnant ewes. J Surg Res 1996;63:339–44.
97. Al-Fozan H, Tulandi T. Safety and risks of laparoscopy in pregnancy. Curr Opin Obstet Gynecol 2002;14:375–9.
98. Curet MJ, Weber DM, Sae A, et al. Effects of helium pneumoperitoneum in pregnant ewes. Surg Endosc 2001;15:710–4.
99. Gardner JG, Trus TL, Laycock WS, et al. Converting from carbon dioxide to nitrous oxide pneumoperitoneum. Surg Endosc 1995;9:1034–5.
100. Hunter JG, Staheli J, Oddsdottir M, et al. Nitrous oxide pneumoperitoneum revisited. Is there a risk of combustion? Surg Endosc 1995;9:501–4.
101. Hunter JG, Swanstrom L, Thornburg K. Carbon dioxide pneumoperitoneum induces fetal acidosis in a pregnant ewe model. Surg Endosc 1995;9:272–9.
102. Ivankovich AD, Miletich DJ, Albrecht RF, et al. Cardiovascular effects of intraperitoneal insufflation with carbon dioxide and nitrous oxide in the dog. Anesthesiology 1975;42:281–7.
103. Mazze RI. Nitrous oxide during pregnancy. Anaesthesia 1986;41:897–9.
104. Neuberger TJ, Andrus CH, Wittgen CM, et al. Prospective comparison of helium versus carbon dioxide pneumoperitoneum. Gastrointest Endosc 1996;43:38–41.
105. Schob OM, Allen DC, Benzel E, et al. A comparison of the pathophysiologic effects of carbon dioxide, nitrous oxide, and helium pneumoperitoneum on intracranial pressure. Am J Surg 1996;172:248–53.
106. Tsereteli Z, Terry ML, Bowers SP, et al. Prospective randomized clinical trial comparing nitrous oxide and carbon dioxide pneumoperitoneum for laparoscopic surgery. J Am Coll Surg 2002;195:173–80.
107. Affleck DG, Handrahan DL, Egger MJ, et al. The laparoscopic management of appendicitis and cholelithiasis during pregnancy. Am J Surg 1999;178:523–9.
108. Bisharah M, Tulandi T. Laparoscopic surgery in pregnancy. Clin Obstet Gynecol 2003;46:92–7.
109. Oelsner G, Stockheim D, Soriano D, et al. Pregnancy outcome after laparoscopy or laparotomy in pregnancy. J Am Assoc Gynecol Laparosc 2003;10:200–4.
110. Reedy MB, Kallen B, Kuehl TJ. Laparoscopy during pregnancy: A study of five fetal outcome parameters with use of the swedish health registry. Am J Obstet Gynecol 1997;177:673–9.
111. Rojansky N, Shushan A, Fatum M. Laparoscopy versus laparotomy in pregnancy: a comparative study. J Am Assoc Gynecol Laparosc 2002;9:108–10.
112. Amos JD, Schorr SJ, Norman PF, et al. Laparoscopic surgery during pregnancy. Am J Surg 1996;171:435–7.

113. Costantino GN, Vincent GJ, Mukalian GG, et al. Laparoscopic cholecystectomy in pregnancy. J Laparoendosc Surg 1994;4:161–4.

114. Lanzafame RJ. Laparoscopic cholecystectomy during pregnancy. Surgery 1995;118:627–33.

115. Morrell DG, Mullins JR, Harrison PB. Laparoscopic cholecystectomy during pregnancy in symptomatic patients. Surgery 1992;112:856–9.

116. Steinbrook RA, Brooks DC, Datta S. Laparoscopic cholecystectomy during pregnancy. Review of anesthetic management, surgical considerations. Surg Endosc 1996;10:511–5.

117. Glasgow RE, Visser BC, Harris HW, et al. Changing management of gallstone disease during pregnancy. Surg Endosc 1998;12:241–6.

118. Curet MJ, Allen D, Josloff RK, et al. Laparoscopy during pregnancy. Arch Surg 1996;131:546–51.

119. Cruz AM, Southerland LC, Duke T, et al. Intraabdominal carbon dioxide insufflation in the pregnant ewe. Uterine blood flow, intraamniotic pressure, and cardiopulmonary effects. Anesthesiology 1996;85:1395–402.

120. Bhavani-Shankar K, Steinbrook RA, Brooks DC, et al. Arterial to end-tidal carbon dioxide pressure difference during laparoscopic surgery in pregnancy. Anesthesiology 2000;93:370–3.

121. Wishner JD, Zolfaghari D, Wohlgemuth SD, et al. Laparoscopic cholecystectomy in pregnancy. A report of 6 cases and review of the literature. Surg Endosc 1996;10:314–8.

122. Graham G, Baxi L, Tharakan T. Laparoscopic cholecystectomy during pregnancy: a case series and review of the literature. Obstet Gynecol Surv 1998;53:566–74.

123. Stepp KJ, Tulikangas PK, Goldberg JM, et al. Laparoscopy for adnexal masses in the second trimester of pregnancy. J Am Assoc Gynecol Laparosc 2003;10:55–9.

124. Sen G, Nagabhushan JS, Joypaul V. Laparoscopic cholecystectomy in third trimester of pregnancy. J Obstet Gynaecol 2002;22:556–7.

125. Mohamed H, Maiti S, Phillips G. Laparoscopic management of ectopic pregnancy: a 5-year experience. J Obstet Gynaecol 2002;22:411–4.

126. Fatum M, Rojansky N. Laparoscopic surgery during pregnancy. Obstet Gynecol Surv 2001;56:50–9.

127. de Perrot M, Jenny A, Morales M, et al. Laparoscopic appendectomy during pregnancy. Surg Laparosc Endosc Percutan Tech 2000;10:368–71.

128. Lachman E, Schienfeld A, Voss E, et al. Pregnancy and laparoscopic surgery. J Am Assoc Gynecol Laparosc 1999;6:347–51.

129. Conron RW Jr., Abbruzzi K, Cochrane SO, et al. Laparoscopic procedures in pregnancy. Am Surg 1999;65:259–63.

130. Barone JE, Bears S, Chen S, et al. Outcome study of cholecystectomy during pregnancy. Am J Surg 1999;177:232–6.

131. Andreoli M, Servakov M, Meyers P, et al. Laparoscopic surgery during pregnancy. J Am Assoc Gynecol Laparosc 1999;6:229–33.

132. Curet MJ. Special problems in laparoscopic surgery. Previous abdominal surgery, obesity, and pregnancy. Surg Clin North Am 2000;80:1093–110.

133. Allen JR, Helling TS, Langenfeld M. Intraabdominal surgery during pregnancy. Am J Surg 1989;158:567–9.

134. Hunt MG, Martin JN, Jr., Martin RW, et al. Perinatal aspects of abdominal surgery for nonobstetric disease. Am J Perinatol 1989;6:412–7.
135. Kort B, Katz VL, Watson WJ. The effect of nonobstetric operation during pregnancy. Surg Gynecol Obstet 1993;177:371–6.
136. Geisler JP, Rose SL, Mernitz CS, et al. Non-gynecologic laparoscopy in second and third trimester pregnancy: Obstetric implications. Jsls 1998;2:235–8.
137. McKellar DP, Anderson CT, Boynton CJ, et al. Cholecystectomy during pregnancy without fetal loss. Surg Gynecol Obstet 1992;174:465–8.

Commentary

Markus Schäfer, Pierre-Alain Clavien

The successful advent of laparoscopy has challenged many traditional surgical dogmas and restrictions during the last 15 years. Increasing surgical experience, better anesthesiological management, preoperative and postoperative care, as well as improved technical equipment, have greatly broadened operative indications while simultaneously limiting former contraindications. Growing evidence from clinical and basic research has improved our knowledge concerning the effects of the CO_2 pneumoperitoneum and its clinical impact. Nevertheless, patients with previous abdominal surgery, liver disease, and special conditions such as pregnancy need careful attention in order to prevent poor outcome.

Previous Abdominal Surgery

Adhesion formation represents a nearly unavoidable consequence after (open) abdominal surgery. Not only are chronic pain, ileus formation and female infertility the main clinical issues, but adhesions may considerably impede surgical abdominal re-interventions [1].

Safe access to the abdominal cavity remains one of the most crucial steps in laparoscopic surgery that may be impaired by previous abdominal surgery and obesity. Although the reported incidence of trocar and Veress needle injuries is very low and ranges from 0.03% to 0.2%, vascular and hollow viscus organ perforations are associated with an increased morbidity [2, 3]. There is still some ongoing controversy concerning the best access technique; however, we clearly favor the open access as proposed by Hasson [4]. The *open access* does not fully obviate any injury of intra-abdominal structures, but lesions are more frequently identified immediately and thereby properly treated. The use of blunt trocars further minimizes the risk of perforation injuries. The surgeon's belief that the open technique is more time consuming and associated with an increased gas leakage could not have been verified. In order to avoid additional skin incisions, many surgeons tend to use previous incision sites and scars. This widespread custom may be fatal, since parietal adhesion formation predominantly occurs exactly at those localizations! Therefore, the first trocar should always be placed far away from a previous incision using the open technique [2].

Intra-abdominal adhesiolysis is an important prerequisite to perform the planned operation at the target organ. Adhesiolysis needs to be performed carefully, but the precise extent remains to be elucidated. Whereas in open surgery complete release of all adhesions has been preferred for many years, some authors in the laparoscopic era have stressed that only adhesions that interfere with the trocar placement and hiding the target organ must be freed. Blunt dissection using the surgeon's finger or the camera should be abandoned. From our point of view, the use of bipolar cautery and/or ultrasonic dissection devices is most appropriate for a meticulous dissection that prevents bleeding and unintentional transmission of heat.

Liver Disease

Patients with liver disease are at increased risk to develop postoperative complications [5]. A careful *preoperative* evaluation is therefore mandatory to assess the patient's individual risk. The severity of liver pathology (e.g., degree of steatosis, extent of cirrhosis) and functional capacity (e.g., synthesis of coagulation factors or serum bilirubin level) are major factors influencing postoperative risks. Child's classification has been validated by numerous studies to predict the risk of mortality with excellent accuracy (Child A 10%, Child B 30%, Child C 80%) [6]. As a consequence, Child C liver cirrhosis has been widely accepted as a contraindication for elective surgery. Patients with Child A or B cirrhosis can safely be operated by a laparoscopic approach. Preexisting ascites must be treated aggressively preoperatively since it is associated with an increased postoperative morbidity and also makes the operation more difficult. Newly occurring ascites during the postoperative course must immediately analyzed to rule out inadvertent intestinal perforation and bacterial peritonitis.

Laparoscopic surgery is particularly characterized by its decreased tissue trauma of the abdominal wall and the use of a CO_2 pneumoperitoneum, whereas the surgical intervention at the target organ remains unchanged. Careful trocar insertion and dissection are mandatory to avoid bleeding complications from intra-abdominal organs and the abdominal wall with its possible varices. The successful surgical control of bleeding complications related to portal hypertension may be difficult to achieve with laparoscopic devices. The advantages of the decreased tissue trauma have been demonstrated in several series with patients undergoing laparoscopic cholecystectomy and appendectomy. Those patients revealing a Child A or B cirrhosis had a decreased blood loss and wound infection rate compared with patients with open surgery. There is also some evidence that decreasing the tissue trauma has a beneficial impact preserving the immune response. The current experience with Child C patients is very limited and the results are not convincing.

The CO_2 pneumoperitoneum induces numerous *transitory* pathophysiological changes, both in humans and animals [7]. In particular, impaired visceral blood flow that is caused by increased intra-abdominal pressure, hypercarbia-induced vasoconstriction and decreased cardiac output, has been documented in healthy and cirrhotic patients and animals. Since liver cirrhosis decreases compensatory arterial hepatic blood flow, some serious concerns have been raised that the limited hepatic blood flow significantly impairs liver function. However, there is a large discrepancy between measurable pathophysiological changes and its clinical impact on morbidity and mortality rates in daily clinical practice. The patient's functional reserves and compensatory mechanisms as well as a careful anesthesiological management can protect most organ systems against clinically relevant damages. Gasless laparoscopy that has been proposed instead of CO_2 pneumoperitoneum, never gained widespread use due to the limited view and the need for an abdominal wall lifting system.

Pregnancy

It is estimated that 0.2–0.5% of pregnant women need surgery for acute abdominal disorder, whereby appendectomy, cholecystectomy and adnexal procedures are the commonest operations [8]. Elective operations are generally postponed until postterm taking into account the risks for both, mother and fetus. The *rate of fetal loss* has decreased during recent years, actually ranging from 0–10% [8].

Laparoscopy adversely influences pregnancy by the use of CO_2 pneumoperitoneum and difficulties to safely access the abdominal cavity. Maternal and fetal hemodynamics, acid-base balance and organ blood flow may be further impaired by adverse effects of anesthetic agents and postoperative medication. The risk of thromboembolism is increased due venous stasis and altered coagulation. The growing uterus displaces particularly small and large bowel, and is itself at risk for perforation injuries gaining access to the peritoneal cavity.

Since the early 1990s, laparoscopy has been increasingly used during pregnancy, whereby there is good evidence that laparoscopy can safely be performed at any trimester [9]. The first trocar must always inserted using the open (Hasson) technique in order to prevent any lesion of the intestine and uterus. Trocar placement must be adapted to the gestational age with its growing uterus and organ displacement. In order to less impair venous back flow and stasis of the lower extremities, patients need to be placed in a left lateral position and the intra-abdominal pressure should not exceed 10 mmHg. The surgeon must be well trained and experienced in advanced laparoscopic techniques. Although no intraoperative fetal monitoring is necessary, preoperative and postoperative management and monitoring by an experienced obstetrician remains a crucial prerequisite.

References

1. Swank DJ, Swank-Bordewijk SC, Hop WC, et al. Laparoscopic adhesiolysis in patients with chronic abdominal pain: a blinded randomized controlled multi-centre trial. Lancet 2003;361:1247–51.
2. Schäfer M, Lauper M, Krähenbühl L. Trocar and Veress needle injuries during laparoscopic surgery. Surg Endosc 2001;15:275–80.
3. Schäfer M, Lauper M, Krähenbühl L. A nation's experience of bleeding complications during laparoscopy. Am J Surg 2000;180:73–7.
4. Bonjer HJ, Hazebroek EJ, Kazemier G, et al. Open versus closed establishment of pneumoperitoneum in laparoscopic surgery. Br J Surg 1997;84:599–602.
5. Rizvon MK, Chou CL. Surgery in the patient with liver disease. Med Clin North Am 2003;87:211–27.
6. Mansour A, Watson W, Shayani V, et al. Abdominal operations in patients with cirrhosis: still a major surgical challenge. Surgery 1997;122:730–5.
7. Schäfer M, Krähenbühl L. Effect of laparoscopy on intraabdominal blood flow. Surgery 2001;129:385–9.
8. Visser BC, Glasgow RE, Mulvihill KK, Mulvihill SJ. Safety and timing of nonobstetric abdominal surgery during pregnancy. Dig Surg 2001;18:409–17.
9. Society of the American Gastrointestinal Endoscopic Surgeons (SAGES). Guidelines for laparoscopic surgery during pregnancy. Surg Endosc 1998;12:189–90.

Laparoscopy in Abdominal Trauma

MICHEL B. ABOUTANOS, RAO IVATURY

> ▶ **Key Controversies**
>
> A. Indications
> – Diagnostic laparoscopy
> – Therapeutic Laparoscopy
> B. Cost-effectiveness of laparoscopy in abdominal trauma

6.1
Introduction

The role of laparoscopy in the evaluation and management of abdominal trauma has been the subject of numerous studies and debates [1–8]. Little argument exists in the role (utility) of laparoscopy in the unstable patient. Similarly, the utility of laparoscopy in blunt trauma is very limited [5, 9, 10]. The accuracy of diagnostic peritoneal lavage (DPL), the emergence of ultrasonography (US) as a screening tool in the emergency department, and the accurate definition of organ injuries on spiral computed tomography (CT) scan have limited the use of laparoscopy as a primary diagnostic tool in blunt abdominal trauma. Laparoscopy can be used as an adjunct to CT scan, especially in the presence of peritoneal fluid and the absence of solid organ injuries [5, 10].

The greatest challenge in abdominal trauma is the optimal management of penetrating abdominal injuries in a stable patient with doubtful intraperitoneal trajectory (tangential abdominal and lower thoracic wounds). A policy of mandatory exploration results in a 30–40% negative laparotomy rate. This is unacceptable in today's vast diagnostic armamentarium [local wound exploration (LWE), DPL, US, CT, and laparoscopy]. In both retrospective and prospective studies, significant postoperative complication rates (21–43%) resulted from these negative laparotomies [11–16]. Over the last decade laparoscopy established its role in the evaluation and management of penetrating abdominal trauma, and challenged various dicta including (1) mandatory laparotomy for all penetrating injuries, (2) mandatory laparotomy upon documentation of peritoneal violation, (3) mandatory laparotomy upon documentation of diaphragmatic and solid organ injuries, and recently (4) mandatory laparotomy upon suspicion or diagnosis of hollow organ and retroperitoneal injuries. The controversies remain regarding whether laparoscopy can minimize unnecessary laparotomies while avoiding missed injuries, and whether it can safely manage these injuries in a cost-effective manner without significant complications.

6.2
Discussion

6.2.1
Indications

6.2.1.1
Diagnostic Laparoscopy (DL)

In the non-operative management of penetrating abdominal injuries, various modalities have been used, including observation, LWE, DPL, US, and even CT scan. However, the reported rates of nontherapeutic laparotomies associated with these standard modalities remain high (5%–39%) [12, 17–24].

The role of laparoscopy in the diagnosis of penetrating abdominal injuries was clearly established in the last decade. However, its potential value has been advocated in the English literature since 1976 [25]. The advantages of laparoscopy over other modalities include its ability to determine violation of the peritoneum, to directly visualize injured organs, to assess ongoing hemorrhage, and to carry out therapeutic measures. It has been shown through numerous studies to be a safe, sensitive (94%) and specific (98%) procedure for the evaluation and treatment of the stable patient with abdominal trauma [26, 27]. In a multicenter retrospective analysis of 510 stable patients with penetrating injuries (316 stab wounds with penetration of anterior fascia, 194 gunshot wounds with doubtful intraperitoneal trajectory), laparotomy was avoided in 303 (59.4%) patients. The overall incidence of non-therapeutic laparotomy was 10.2% [28]. Several studies have also shown that 40–60% of laparotomies can be safely avoided with the use of laparoscopy in selected stable patients with penetrating injuries [1, 4, 24, 29]. Despite the growing evidence that laparoscopy is a safe and feasible modality which can play a major role in the evaluation and management of the stable patient with penetrating abdominal trauma, considerable skepticism over its use still exist [1–6, 14, 30–34]

The main controversy is in the ability of laparoscopy to diagnose *all* significant injuries, including intestinal injuries and retroperitoneal injuries. Studies have shown laparoscopy to be highly accurate in the diagnosis of peritoneal penetration. Moreover, together with thorocoscopy, laparoscopy has become the diagnostic tool of choice for diaphragmatic injuries when compared with other non-operative modalities [2, 3, 4]. The shortcomings of diagnostic laparoscopy are in retroperitoneal and hollow viscus injuries [1, 3, 25]. Reports of missed splenic lacerations, mesenteric hematomas and small bowel injuries were noted in earlier studies [2, 3, 17] with up to 41% missed injury rate per patient [2, 3, 17, 33, 35]. A decade ago, one of us (RI) reported bowel injury identification at the time of laparoscopic examination to be only 20 % [1]. These early findings lead many to limit the diagnostic utility of laparoscopy to lower thoracic and upper quadrant abdominal stab wounds.

We believe the shortcomings of laparoscopy will be overcome with the exponential advancement of laparoscopic technology and dedicated training. The prior reports of laparoscopy's inability to visualize organs such as the spleen or pancreas or to adequately run the bowel and elicit the presence of hollow viscus injuries are being challenged [1–3, 17, 36]. The ability to run the bowel, mobilize the colon, enter the lesser sac and evaluate the pancreas and the posterior gastric surface have been described [37]. Most recently, Choi and Lim reported zero missed injuries in their diagnostic and therapeutic evaluation of 78 trauma patients where 40 small bowel injuries were accurately identified, along with three splenic, seven colonic, and three pancreatic injuries. Their success was attributed to advanced skills in laparoscopy and their ability to carry out extensive abdominal laparoscopic exploration [36].

We strongly emphasize that in the absence of proficiently running the small bowel and mobilizing the retroperitoneal colon, bowel perforation cannot be ruled out with 100% accuracy. Therefore, a celiotomy (or miniceliotomy with segmental evisceration and inspection) is mandated to avoid the potential fatal complication of missed bowel injury [28, 32, 36, 38].

Another controversy is whether DL offers an advantage over the standard diagnostic modalities (LWE, DPL) in terms of its predictive value regarding the need for therapeutic laparotomy. This does not appear to be the case in blunt trauma. However, it seems that laparoscopy carries a selective advantage in the evaluation of penetrating abdominal injuries, where all other diagnostic modalities fall short. Fabian et al. reported that 49% of patients with penetrating anterior and lateral abdominal injuries who underwent LWE with noted violation of the anterior fascia did not have peritoneal penetration upon laparoscopic evaluation [2]. Furthermore, when fascial penetration is present, LWE still carries a negative laparotomy rate of nearly 50%. When intraabdomial injuries are clearly demonstrated, greater than 25% are insignificant, resulting in a high rate of nontherapeutic laparotomies [2, 18]. LWE is not advocated for lower chest wounds.

DPL in blunt trauma has proved excellent in large series achieving positive predictive value (PPV), negative predictive value (NPV) and non-therapeutic laparotomy (NTL) percentages of 99, 98–99, and 6%, respectively [39, 40]. The use of DPL in penetrating trauma is less satisfactory. Reliance upon DPL using standard criteria for positivity (RBC count of 100,000/ml3) results in unacceptably high rates of missed injuries with an NPV of only 75–88% [41, 42]. When the RBC count is lowered to 1,000–50,000/ml3, a 50% or higher NTL rate is noted for lower chest wounds [21]. Diagnostic laparoscopy appears to offer a clear advantage with respect to predictive value in the evaluation of penetrating injuries [9]. DLs high rate of success (sensitivity 96.2%, NPV 95.5%) in predicting non-therapeutic laparotomy when it is negative validates the policy of observation following a normal DL. With a specificity and a PPV of 100%, a positive diagnostic laparoscopy will lead to a therapeutic laparotomy [9].

6.2.1.2
Therapeutic Laparoscopy

Many authors deem it inadvisable to perform therapeutic laparoscopy based on injuries seen at diagnostic laparoscopy [9]. This was based on the concept that injuries to the small intestine, colon, and retroperitoneum are frequently missed [2], and those missed are frequently associated with other significant injuries [1, 4, 5, 9, 29]. Therefore, a positive DL can lead to a therapeutic laparotomy, but not necessarily to a therapeutic laparoscopy. Therapeutic laparoscopy was initially limited to repair diaphragmatic injuries (sutures, staples or mesh), hemostasis of low grade splenic and liver lacerations, and autotransfusion of collected blood from the hemoperitoneum [3, 28, 43, 44].

With rapid advancement in video technology and technical expertise, we believe there will be an inevitable progression towards the use of laparoscopy as a therapeutic tool in the selective management of stable patients with abdominal trauma. The largest initial experience with therapeutic laparoscopy was reported in 1997 by Zantut et al., where 26 of 28 patients had successful therapeutic procedures (16 diaphragmatic repair, 6 hepatic repair, 3 gastrostomy repair and 1 cholecystectomy) [28]. Other reports have included repair and resection of full thickness gastric, small bowel and colonic injuries (via either sutures or staplers), splenectomies, and distal pancratectomies [3, 28, 32, 45–49]. Intraparenchymal injection of fibrin glue have been used successfully for deep solid visceral injuries [50]. Recently, Choi and Lim reported the largest experience of therapeutic laparoscopy (43 total laparoscopic, 20 laparoscopically assisted, and 2 hand-assisted laparoscopic procedures) [36]. In addition to a splenectomy, a distal pancreatectomy and 4 Hartmann's procedures, primary closure of 15 small bowel, 8 gastric, and 4 colonic injuries were all successfully performed with total unassisted laparoscopic surgery. Hand-assisted laparoscopic splenectomy and distal pancreatectomy were used in two patients with severe adhesions [36].

It must be emphasized that competency in basic laparoscopy is the minimum requirement before attempting therapeutic laparoscopy. Both trauma management and advanced laparoscopic skills are essential

6.2.2
Cost Effectiveness

The economic benefit of laparoscopy versus celiotomy or other diagnostic modalities has also been a topic of debate. The key issue is whether laparoscopy, in the evaluation of the stable trauma patient, is justified from an economic standpoint especially when other options for diagnosis and treatment are available. A strict comparison between laparoscopy and laparotomy becomes more important as the therapeutic advantage of laparoscopy over other modalities becomes more and more accepted.

In a recent study performed at our institution, 23 patients who underwent mandatory celiotomy were compared with 31 patients who underwent laparoscopic evaluation. The surgical costs were found to be the same. However, the hospital costs and length of stay were significantly reduced [34]. Taner et al. found a 1.78-fold increase in hospital costs in patients undergoing non-therapeutic laparotomy compared with those of diagnostic laparoscopy alone [24]. In their cost analysis of diagnostic laparoscopy verses laparotomy in evaluation of penetrating abdominal injuries, Marks et al. found laparoscopy resulted in an overall savings of US$1,059 per laparoscopy performed when compared with laparotomy [51].

Similar results showing decreases in morbidity, negative or non-therapeutic laparotomy rates (30–60% reduction) and hospital stays (from 5 to 2 days on average) have been reported by several authors [1, 2, 14, 34, 51–56]. These studies and outcomes point to the cost effectiveness of diagnostic laparoscopy in the evaluation of the hemodynamically stable patient.

On the other hand, Fabian et al. found routine laparoscopic evaluation would have increased their institution's charges for care of penetrating trauma victims by more than US$50,000 on an annual basis [2]. This study, however, was criticized on the basis that hospital charges have no relation to actual costs. The heavy use of disposable instrumentation was also noted as unnecessary and costly [32, 34, 51].Technological advances have now allowed most institutions to utilize less costly standard laparoscopic equipment.

6.3
Summary

— The accumulated evidence indicates that diagnostic laparoscopy has a major role to play in the evaluation and treatment of selected patient with penetrating abdominal injuries.
— Diagnostic laparoscopy can greatly minimize unnecessary laparotomies while avoiding missed injuries. However, mandatory celiotomy is still the treatment of choice where advanced skills in laparoscopy are lacking.
— Therapeutic laparoscopy is feasible. However a proficiency in both trauma management and advanced laparoscopic skills is necessary.
— The accumulated evidence indicates that diagnostic laparoscopy can be cost effective in the diagnoses of penetrating injuries.

References

1. Ivatury R, Simon R, Stahl W. A critical evaluation of laparoscopy in penetrating abdominal trauma. J Trauma 1993;34:822–8.
2. Fabian T, Croce M, Stewart B, et al. A prospective analysis of diagnostic laparoscopy in trauma. Ann Surg 1993;217:557–65.
3. Livingston D, Tortella B, Blackwood J, et al. The role laparoscopy in abdominal trauma. J Trauma 1992;33:471–5.
4. Ivatury R, Simon R, Weksler J, et al. Laparoscopy in the evaluation of the intrathoracic abdomen after penetrating injury. J Trauma 1992;33:101–9.
5. Townsend M, Flauncbaum L, Choban P, et al. Diagnostic laparoscopy as an adjunct to selective conservative management of solid organ injuries after blunt abdominal trauma. J Trauma 1993;35:647–51.
6. Sosa J, Arrillaga A, Puente I, et al. laparoscopy in 121 consecutive patients with abdominal gunshot wounds. J Trauma 1995;39:501–4.
7. Salvino C, Esposito T, Marshall W, et al. The role of diagnostic laparoscopy in the management of trauma patients: a preliminary assessment. J Trauma 1993;34:506–13.
8. Correa-Zantut L, Rodriguez A, Birolini D. Laparoscopy as a diagnostic tool in the evaluation of trauma. Panam J Trauma 1990;2:6–12.
9. Elliott D, Rodriguez A, Moncure M, et al. The accuracy of diagnostic laparoscopy in trauma patients: a prospective, controlled study. Int Surg 1998;83:294–8.
10. Ivatury R, Zantut L, Yelon J. Trauma care in the new millennium. Laparoscopy in the new century. Surg Clin North Am 1999;79:1291–5.
11. Weiglt J, Kingman R. Complications of negative laparotomy for trauma. Am J Surg 1988;156:544.
12. Renz B, Feliciano D. Unnecessary laparotomy for trauma: a prospective study of morbidity. J Trauma 1995;38:350–6.
13. Leppaniemi A, Salo J, Haapiainen R. Complications of negative laparotomy for truncal stab wounds. J Trauma 1995;38:54–8.

14. Sosa J, Baker M, Puente F, et al. Negative laparotomy in abdominal gunshot wounds: potential impact of laparoscopy. J Trauma 1995;38:194–7.

15. Lowe R, Boyd D, Folk F, et al. The negative laparotomy for abdominal trauma. J Trauma 1972;12:853–61.

16. Poole G, Thomae K, Hauser C. Laparoscopy in trauma. Surg Clin North Am 1996;76:547–56.

17. Brandt C, Priebe P, Jacobs D. Potential of laparoscopy to reduce non-therapeutic trauma laparotomies. Am Surg 1994;60:416–20.

18. Demetriades D, Rabinowitz B. Indication for operation in abdominal stab wounds. Ann Surg 1987;205:129–32.

19. Drost T, Rosemurgy A, Kearney R, et al. Diagnostic peritoneal lavage: limited indications due to evolving concepts in trauma care. Am Surg 1991;57:126–8.

20. Henneman P, Marx J, Moore E, et al. Diagnostic peritoneal lavage: accuracy in predicting necessary laparotomy following blunt and penetrating trauma. J Trauma 1990;30:1345–55.

21. Oreskovich M, Carrico C. Stab wounds of the anterior abdomen: analysis of a management plan using local wound exploration and quantitative peritoneal lavage. Ann Surg 1983;198:411–9

22. Miller F, Cryer H, Chilikuri S, et al. Negative findings on laparotomy for trauma. South Med J 1989;82:1231–4.

23. Sozuer E, Akyurak N, Kafali M, et al. Diagnostic peritoneal lavage in blunt abdominal trauma victims. Eur J Emerg Med 1998;5:231–4.

24. Taner A, Topgul K, Kucukel F, et al. Diagnostic laparoscopy decreases the rate of unnecessary laparotomies and reduces costs in trauma patients. J Laparoendosc Adv Surg Tech A 2001;11:207–11.

25. Gazzaniga A, Stanton W, Bartlett R. Laparoscopy in the diagnosis of blunt and penetrating injuries to the abdomen. Am J Surg 1976;131:315–8.

26. Renz B, Feleciano D. the length of hospital stay after an unnecessary laparotomy for trauma: a prospective study. J Trauma 1996;40:187–90.

27. Ross S, Dragon G, O'Malley K, et al. Morbidity of negative celiotomy in trauma. Injury 1995;26:393–4.

28. Zantut L, Ivatury R, Smith S, Kawahara N, et al. Diagnostic and therapeutic laparoscopy for penetrating abdominal trauma: a multicenter experience. J Trauma 1997;42:825–31.

29. Guth A, Pachter H. Laparoscopy for penetrating thoracoabdominal trauma: pitfalls and promises. JSLS 1998;2:123–7.

30. Zantut L, Rodriguez A, Birolini D. Laparoscopy as a diagnostic tool in the evaluation of trauma. Panam J Trauma. 1990;2:6.

31. Ivatury R, Simon R, Stahl W. Selective celiotomy for missile wounds of the abdomen based on laparoscopy. Surg Endosc 1994;8:366.

32. Smith R, Fry W, Morabito D, et al. Therapeutic laparoscopy in trauma. Am J Surg 1995;170:632–7.

33. Rossi P, Mullins D, Thal E. Role of laparoscopy in the evaluation of abdominal trauma. Am J Surg 1993;166:707–11.

34. DeMaria E, Dalton J, Gore D, et al. Complementary roles of laparoscopic abdominal exploration and diagnostic peritoneal lavage for evaluating abdominal stab wounds: a prospective study. J Laparoendosc Adv Surg Tech A 2000;10:131–6.

35. Mazuski J, Shaoiro M, Kaminski D. Diagnostic laparoscopy for evaluation of penetrating abdominal trauma. J Trauma 1997;42:163.

36. Choi Y, Lim K. Therapeutic laparoscopy for abdominal trauma. Surg Endosc 2003;17:421–7.

37. Gorecki P, Cottam D, Angus G, et al. Diagnostic and therapeutic laparoscopy for trauma: a technique of safe and systemic exploration. Surg Laparosc Endosc Percutan Tech 2002;12:195–8.

38. Muckart DJ, Thomson SR. Undetected injuries a preventable cause of increased morbidity and mortality. Am J Surg 1991;162:457–60.

39. Fisher R, Beverlin B, Engrav L, et al. Diagnostic peritoneal lavage: fourteen years and 2586 patients later. Am J Surg 1978;136:701–4.

40. Alyono D, Morrow C, Perry J. Reappraisal of diagnostic peritoneal lavage criteria for operation in penetrating and blunt trauma. Surgery 1982;92:751–7.

41. Moore E, Moore J, Van Duzer-Moore S, et al. Mandatory laparotomy for gunshot wounds penetrating the abdomen. Am J Surg 1980;140:847–51.

42. Thal E, May R, Beesinger D. Peritoneal lavage: its unreliability in gunshot wounds of the lower chest and abdomen. Arch Surg 1980;115:430–3.

43. Koehler R, Smith R. Thoracoscopic repair of missed diaphragmatic injury in penetrating trauma: case report. J Trauma 1994;37:424–7. [Comment in J Trauma 1994;37:515].

44. Smith R, Meister P, Tsoi E, et al. Laparoscopically guided blood salvage and autotransfusion in splenic trauma: a case report. J Trauma 1993;34:313–4.

45. Gandhi R, Stringel G. Laparoscopy in pediatric abdominal trauma. JSLS 1997;1:349–51.

46. Gunning K, Moont M, Surgue M. Laparoscopic repair of penetrating intraabdominal injuries. Br J Surg 1995;82:920.

47. Hauser C, Poole G, Thomae K. Laparoscopic surgery and the management of traumatic hemoperitoneum in stable patients. Surg Endosc 1996;10:694–5.

48. Frantzides C, Ludwig K, Aprahmanian C, et al. Laparoscopic closure of gastric stab wounds: a case report. Surg Laparosc Endosc 1993;3:63–6.

49. Mathonnet M, Peyrou P, Gainant A, et al. Role of laparoscopy in blunt perforations of the small bowel. Surg Endosc 2003;17:641–5.

50. Salvino C, Esposito T, Smith D, et al. Laparoscopic injection of fibrin glue to arrest intraparenchymal abdominal hemorrhage: an experimental study. J Trauma 1993;35:762–6.

51. Marks J, Youngleman D, Berk T. Cost analysis of diagnostic laparoscopy vs. laparotomy in the evaluation of penetrating abdominal trauma. Surg Endosc 1997;11:272–6.

52. Carey J, Koo R, Miller R, et al. Laparoscopy and thorocoscopy in evaluation of abdominal trauma. Am Surg 1995;61:92–5.

53. Henderson V, Organ C, smith R. Negative trauma celiotomy. Am Surg 1993;59:365–70.

54. Peterson S, Sheldon G. Morbidity of a negative finding at laparotomy in abdominal trauma. Surg Gynecol Obstet 1979;148:23–6.

55. Ryan M, Leighton T, Pianim N, et al. Medical economic consequences of gang-related shootings. Am Surg 1993;59:831–3.

56. Smith R, Tsoi E, Fry W, et al. Laparoscopy is cost effective in the evaluation of abdominal trauma. Surg Endosc 1993;7:137.

Commentary

DEMETRIOS DEMETRIADES

Laparoscopy and minimally invasive surgery in general have revolutionized the practice of surgery. This enthusiasm could not leave trauma surgery untouched. Starting in the late 1980s and early 1990s numerous studies evaluated laparoscopy in both, blunt and penetrating abdominal trauma. The commentator himself was caught in the excitement and got actively involved in the new technology. Unfortunately, it proved a classic case of technology desperately looking for application.

Advanced CT scan technology has practically eliminated any role of laparoscopy in blunt trauma, except in the rare Intensive Care Unit cases with suspected bowel ischemia or acalculous cholecystitis. Its role in penetrating trauma is more controversial. The major limitations of diagnostic laparoscopy are related to the inability to diagnose reliably hollow viscus perforations or retroperitoneal injuries. More recent studies suggested that experienced laparoscopists can "run" the bowel reliably and identify all injuries. However, the majority of trauma surgeons do not possess this advanced level skills and should not practice it lightly. Some authors use diagnostic laparoscopy to assess peritoneal violation in patients with stab wounds or gunshot wounds to the anterior abdomen. However, peritoneal violation does not necessarily mean a significant intra-abdominal injury. In the case of stab wounds up to 30% of patients with proven peritoneal penetration do not have any significant injury requiring surgical repair.

At this point, the only proven indication for diagnostic laparoscopy is in the evaluation of suspected diaphragmatic injuries. In our center, this is the only indication for diagnostic laparoscopy in trauma. It is our protocol to evaluate routinely all patients with left thoracoabdomianl penetrating injuries who have no peritoneal signs. In our experience 24% of these asymptomatic injuries had an occult diaphragmatic injury. The incidence was similar in anterior, lateral and posterior injuries. Most of the patients with diaphragmatic injuries had a normal chest radiography or a non-specific hemothorax. Injuries to the right thoracoabdominal area require a less vigorous evaluation because of the "buttressing" effect of the liver, which protects against a diaphragmatic hernia. However, we have seen patients with visceral herniation after right anterior right thoracoabdominal wounds. We currently recommend the laparoscopic evaluation of these patients.

Laparoscopy evaluation of the diaphragm should be done semi-electively, ideally at least 6 to 8 h postinjury. Clinical observation during this period rules out any associated hollow viscus perforation and any diaphragmatic injury can safely be repaired laparoscopically, without the need for open laparotomy.

Bedside diagnostic laparoscopy with or without gas insufflation has been suggested as an attractive alternative to a formal laparoscopy under general anesthesia. Our experience with this approach and with 2-mm or 3-mm scopes has been unsatisfactory because of significant patient discomfort and poor visual field. Future technological advances may make this option practical and avoid the risks and expenses of general anesthesia.

Therapeutic laparoscopy in trauma is currently limited to the repair of diaphragmatic injuries. There is experimental evidence that suture-repair or staple-repair is equally effective. Although therapeutic laparoscopy has been reported for hepatic, splenic and hollow viscus repairs, this approach is still not an acceptable standard or practice and it should be limited in centers with special experience and as part of study evaluations. As correctly pointed out by Drs. Ivatury and Aboutanos, proficiency in both trauma management and advanced laparoscopic skills is critical for these therapeutic applications.

Laparoscopy in Abdominal Malignancy

John Wayman, Glyn G. Jamieson

> ## Key Controversy
>
> A. Risks of laparoscopy in abdominal malignancy
> B. Role of laparoscopy in abdominal malignancy
>   – Planning
>   – Therapeutic

7.1
Introduction

The laparoscopic approach is an important development in the investigation and treatment of abdominal malignancy. However, as a diagnostic tool it is invasive and its value over and above existing non-invasive imaging techniques must be clear to outweigh its potentially detrimental effects.

As a therapeutic tool laparoscopy offers the benefits of minimalization of surgical trauma but this needs to be balanced against any compromise of oncological principles and it needs also to be compared critically with the results of conventional surgery. The role of laparoscopy in malignant disease can be interpreted differently by enthusiasts and non-enthusiasts. Its role should be driven by clinical need and determined by actual rather than potential benefit and certainly not by enthusiasm for new technology. Conversely, progress should not be inhibited by leaders of opinion in surgery who remain more comfortable with conventional operative approaches and are reluctant to embrace new technology.

7.2
Discussion

7.2.1
Risks of Laparoscopy in Abdominal Malignancy

Even though a procedure is seen as minimally invasive, liberal use of such a procedure in cancer patients should raise some concern. Little is known about the long-term effects of laparoscopy on the course of malignant disease in humans. There is evidence of an attenuation of the immune response to surgery following laparoscopic procedures [1]. Animal studies provide ample evidence that pneumoperitoneum impairs cellular [2] and humoral [3] immune responses. The effect of laparoscopy on the human immune system has been compared with that of open surgery in several randomized trials. All trials documented profound effects of laparoscopy on both the systemic cellular [4] and the humoral [5] immune response with suppression of intraperitoneal cell-mediated immunity [6] compared with the pre-operative immune status. Systemic immunity appears to be better preserved after laparoscopic surgery than after open surgery but some studies found the effects of laparoscopy were no different from those of laparotomy [5, 7, 8]. Thus there is good evidence that laparoscopy influences patients' immune responses but, on the other hand, there is no evidence to support the notion that this has any clinical importance in terms of patient outcome [9].

There are many reports of tumor seeding during laparoscopy as demonstrated by incisional (port-site) metastases and development of peritoneal dissemination [10]. There is anecdotal evidence of rapid peritoneal tumor spread following laparoscopy [11]. The insufflation associated with laparoscopy may have a significant effect on the invasive capacity of tumor cells and promote tumor growth. It has been suggested as a factor in the incidence of port-site metastases seen in patients following laparoscopic resection for malignancy [12–16]. There is experimental evidence, which appears to support this. Exposure of a colonic adenocarcinoma cell line to either a CO_2 or helium pneumoperitoneum causes an increase in tumor cell invasiveness, which is abolished by the presence of an inhibitor of matrix metalloproteases [17]. The invasive capacity of a pancreatic cell line is augmented by helium and CO_2 pneumoperitoneum associated with increased gelatinase activity [18]. In the rat model, port-site wound metastases were significantly increased using air, CO_2 and N_2O insufflation compared with use of helium [19]. Tumor implantation also appears to be promoted by the presence of intraperitoneal blood during rodent laparoscopy [20].

There is conflicting evidence as to whether escape of aerosolized tumor cells around the trocar or through the port site (the so-called "chimney effect") results in implantation. Experimental evidence suggests that port site metastases are more common where gas could escape around the trocar [21, 22]. Other in vitro and in vivo studies including studies in patients with pancreatic cancer have failed to confirm such findings [23, 24].

Although one international survey suggests that incisional metastases occur more commonly than would have been expected following open surgery [25], large controlled single center studies suggest that the incidence is no different [26, 27]. Peritoneal implantation undoubtedly can occur if there is disruption of tumor and this may be especially likely with inexpert laparoscopic manipulation and extraction [28]. When compared with conventional surgery, expert laparoscopic colorectal surgery for colonic cancer has not been associated with an increase in the incidence of intraperitoneal cancer cell spillage [29]. Ultimately wound recurrence seems to be more related to tumor biology, stage and the degree of manipulation [30, 31]. Criticism that laparoscopy itself leads to an unacceptable incidence of port-site metastases is, on the balance of evidence, unfounded.

7.2.2
Role of Laparoscopy in Abdominal Malignancy

7.2.2.1
Planning Laparoscopy

The advantages of planning laparoscopy should be balanced carefully against the potential risks. Widely accepted standards of treatment for many malignancies have not been established. If the therapeutic strategy is always surgical exploration then preoperative staging is unnecessary. However, where there are considerable non-operative treatment strategies available, staging procedures must be sufficiently accurate to allow correct assignment of cases to specific treatment protocols.

Historically it has not been uncommon for "open and close" laparotomies to be performed when diseases have been under-staged by conventional imaging. With refinements of technique and technology of computed tomography (CT), magnetic resonance imaging and ultrasound, this has become a rarity. Nevertheless, cases with undetected small hepatic metastases or peritoneal deposits are still sometimes encountered at preliminary laparotomy [32]. Planning or "staging" laparoscopy has proved useful in planning treatment and has been a proven benefit in identifying radiologically undetected hepatic and peritoneal metastases.

Used in this way, laparoscopy replaces the preliminary assessment at the commencement of a laparotomy for resection of an organ. If a laparoscopy causes a significant change in management to a non-operative treatment, then such an approach allows better allocation of resources and better preparation of patients and spares patients the morbidity of a more major surgical insult. In some situations such accuracy of preoperative staging may not be necessary. While there may be a significant discrepancy between laparoscopic and CT findings, this does not necessarily lead to alterations in management plans [33]. In such conditions as gastric and pancreatic cancer, the decision whether surgery is to be curative or palliative is often an intraoperative decision, and whether surgery was curative or palliative may only become known with pathological findings postoperatively. Furthermore, resection may remain a management plan despite the presence of small hepatic, peritoneal or nodal deposits.

Even in centers that practice staging laparoscopy, open and close laparotomies can still occur [34]. Laparoscopy may miss deep liver lesions, which are detected by palpation. The addition of laparoscopic ultrasound may substitute for the lack of tactile sensitivity in laparoscopy, enabling detection of deeply placed lesions [35]. In certain centers, the use of laparoscopic ultrasound sound has improved the assessment of nodal involvement and local invasion and has proved useful in planning treatment particularly for patients with pancreatic and peri-ampullary tumors [36, 37]. In some centers, the routine use of laparoscopic ultrasound has enhanced the role of staging laparoscopy leading to a reduction yet further in non-therapeutic laparotomies, improved resectability rates and optimization of palliation [38, 39]. Yet, in other centers, 96% accuracy of staging is achieved by CT and ultrasound scan alone, perhaps obviating the need for more invasive procedures [40, 41].

With advances in conventional imaging the pursuit of occult intra-abdominal dissemination may become less of a priority of staging protocols. With modern conventional imaging, the presence of local invasion by pancreatic cancer is the most influential in deciding operability and often the most difficult parameter to determine preoperatively by laparoscopy [36, 41]. Other, less invasive diagnostic modalities such as color Doppler are more effective than laparoscopy in the assessment of local invasion by pancreatic and biliary malignancy and may be a more useful and relevant tool for planning treatment [42].

The use of peritoneal cytology at the time of staging laparoscopy has been advocated to add to the technique and provide a further marker of prognosis [43]. Even molecular diagnosis can be made of laparoscopic peritoneal washings [44, 45], which may reveal more information on prognosis. Some practice "extended diagnostic laparoscopy" [46]. This involves not merely inspection but dissection, laparoscopic ultrasound, peritoneal lavage and biopsy. This has been reported to result in a modification of therapeutic strategy in up to 40% of patients [46–48]. However, as yet there does not appear to be strong evidence to support such individualized treatment strategies. In gastric cancer, for example, peritoneal washings may be performed but the technology risks exceeding our ability to correctly interpret the information provided. Positive peritoneal cytology may identify a poor prognosis group but it is not established whether these patients should be excluded from surgery. In certain situations, this information may aid the decision making process but its overall impact has not been established.

Competition between adjuncts to laparoscopy and improvements in conventional imaging means we need to constantly re-balance the roles of these diagnostic tools. More so than any other investigation, because of its invasive nature, laparoscopy should be planned to answer specific questions in a particular case. While laparoscopy can detect subtle macroscopic malignant disease missed on other investigations, as the precision of other investigations improve along with the expertise of their interpretation, individual centers will need to decide for themselves how much additional value is gained from laparoscopy. A selective approach to planning laparoscopy is practiced successfully in many centers [34, 49, 50]. Use of the technique may sensibly be restricted to patients in whom there is a specific suspicion of intra-abdominal dissemination in situations where a palliative open procedure would be inappropriate. The evolution of the role laparoscopy as a therapeutic tool in abdominal malignancy may lead to yet further adjustment of its preoperative role.

7.2.2.2
Therapeutic Laparoscopy

The potential benefits of a laparoscopic approach are well known from surgery for benign disease. Minimizing surgical trauma has the potential of less pain, less respiratory compromise, early restoration of bowel function, earlier mobilization and earlier discharge for patients. In addition laparoscopic techniques often allow excellent visualization and may, in skilled hands, minimize tumor manipulation [51].

In a palliative setting, laparoscopic gastrojejunostomy for obstructing distal gastric cancer or pancreatic head cancer reportedly can be performed with less immune suppression, lower morbidity and earlier recovery of gastrointestinal function compared with open surgery [52]. Laparoscopic biliary bypass may be performed with similar success [53, 54]. This may be particularly appropriate in the setting of a pre-operative staging laparoscopy, which demonstrates unresectable disease [55]. There seems little argument against a laparoscopic approach for palliative procedures other than the availability of the necessary laparoscopic expertise.

Case series suggest that the results of laparoscopically assisted distal gastrectomy are broadly similar to open surgery although complications have been high with a reported anastomotic leak rate of up to14% [56, 57]. There is significantly less postoperative pain, less respiratory compromise, more rapid recovery of gastrointestinal function, earlier mobilization and shorter postoperative stay [58–60]. This improves the cost-effectiveness of surgery with the additional costs of the laparoscopic procedure easily offset by reduced hospital costs [61]. Quality-of-life assessments suggested that patients had significantly better results when compared with conventional surgery [62]. However, there is some evidence that these benefits are at the expense of longer operating times and smaller lymph node yield [63]. Proof of the oncological effectiveness of the laparoscopic approach will only come with longer-term follow-up. Currently this data is sparse but equivalent long-term survival is reported anecdotally with relatively advanced gastric cancers [64].

The laparoscopic approach has encouraged a new wave of surgical inventiveness. Further developments and modifications of technique have expanded the role of laparoscopic surgery in abdominal malignancy. The "hand assist" techniques make extended lymph node dissection and intracorporeal anastomosis more feasible and easier than with laparoscopy alone [65, 66]. Laparoscopic local resection, intragastric local resection and combined laparoscopic endoscopic resection are part of an ever-increasing range of options for the surgical treatment of gastric tumors [67, 68].

There seems to be no conventional surgery that is not feasible laparoscopically. Therefore there seems little reason for this approach not to be considered in all cases. Thus it has been reported in esophageal cancer [69], gastric cancer [66, 70, 71], liver tumors [72], pancreatic cancer [73] and small bowel tumors [74]. In almost all circumstances series reported have varied from the anecdotal to small. The limiting factor is technical expertise and to a certain extent appropriate equipment. As well as the duration and early complications of surgery, for surgery performed with curative intent technical expertise will be reflected in the oncological adequacy of surgery. While even the role of radical lymphadenectomy is disputed in conventional surgery, long-term follow-up studies are necessary to prove the adequacy of laparoscopic resection for malignancy.

7.3
Summary

— There is no reason, in principle to consider a laparoscopic approach inappropriate for the diagnosis and treatment of abdominal malignancy.
— There is no convincing evidence of an increased incidence of port-site metastatses or acceleration of disease, specific to the laparoscopic approach.
— The value of planning laparoscopy should be carefully considered in individual cases and not regarded as a necessity.
— There is no reason to think that oncological standards, however they may be defined, cannot be maintained by the laparoscopic approach to surgery.
— Long-term comparative follow-up survival data are required before the case for laparoscopic surgery for abdominal malignancy can be considered proven.

— Ultimately the results achievable for laparoscopic resection of abdominal malignancy, like conventional surgery, is likely to be related to expertise rather than the approach itself.

References

1. Hartley JE, Mehigan BJ, Monson JR. Alterations in the immune system and tumor growth in laparoscopy. Surg Endosc 2001;15:305–13.
2. Gitzelmann CA, Mendoza-Sagaon M, Talamini MA, et al. Cell-mediated immune response is better preserved by laparoscopy than laparotomy. Surgery 2000;127:65–71.
3. Iwanaka T MS Arkovitz MS, Arya G, Ziegler MM. Evaluation of operative stress and peritoneal macrophage function in minimally invasive operations. J Am Coll Surg 1997;184:357–63.
4. Leung KL, Lai PB, Ho RL, et al. Systemic cytokine response after laparoscopic-assisted resection of rectosigmoid carcinoma: a prospective randomized trial. Ann Surg 2000;231:506–11.
5. Perttila J, Salo M, Ovaska J, et al. Immune response after laparoscopic and conventional Nissen fundoplication. Eur J Surg 1999;165:21–8.
6. Gupta A, Watson DI. Effect of laparoscopy on immune function. Br J Surg 2001;88:1296–306.
7. Hewitt PM, Ip SM, Kwok SP, et al. Laparoscopic-assisted vs. open surgery for colorectal cancer: comparative study of immune effects. Dis Colon Rectum 1998;41:901–9.
8. Squirrell DM, Majeed AW, Troy G, et al. A randomized, prospective, blinded comparison of postoperative pain, metabolic response, and perceived health after laparoscopic and small incision cholecystectomy. Surgery 1998;123:485–95.
9. Urbach DR, Swanstrom LL, Hansen PD. The effect of laparoscopy on survival in pancreatic cancer. Arch Surg 2002;137:191–9.
10. Bouvy ND, Marquet RL, Jeekel H, Bonjer HJ. Impact of gas(less) laparoscopy and laparotomy on peritoneal tumor growth and abdominal wall metastases. [Comment]. Ann Surg 1996;224:694–700.
11. Gave AA, Hopkins MA. Laparoscopy and unsuspected intra-abdominal malignancy with rapid peritoneal spread. Surg Endosc 2001;15:518.
12. Bouvy ND, Marquet RL, Jeekel J, Bonjer HJ. Laparoscopic surgery is associated with less tumour growth stimulation than conventional surgery: an experimental study. [Comment]. Br J Surg 1997;84:358–61.
13. Ishida H, Murata N, Yamada H, et al. Influence of trocar placement and CO_2 pneumoperitoneum on port site metastasis following laparoscopic tumor surgery. Surg Endosc 2000;14:193–7.
14. Wu JS, Jones DB, Guo LW, et al. Effects of pneumoperitoneum on tumor implantation with decreasing tumor inoculum. Dis Colon Rectum 1998;41:141–6.
15. Le Moine MC, Navarro F, Burgel JS, et al. Experimental assessment of the risk of tumor recurrence after laparoscopic surgery. Surgery 1998;123:427–31.
16. Volz J, Volz-Koster S, Kanis S, et al. Modulation of tumor-induced lethality after pneumoperitoneum in a mouse model. Cancer 2000;89:262–6.

17. Ridgway PF, Smith A, Ziprin P, et al. Pneumoperitoneum augmented tumor invasiveness is abolished by matrix metalloproteinase blockade. Surg Endosc 2002;16:533–6.

18. Ridgway PF, Ziprin P, Jones TL, et al. Laparoscopic staging of pancreatic tumors induces increased invasive capacity in vitro. Surg Endosc 2003;17:306–10.

19. Neuhaus SJ, Watson DI, Ellis T, et al. Wound metastasis after laparoscopy with different insufflation gases. Surgery 1998;123:579–83.

20. Neuhaus SJ, Ellis, G.G. Jamieson GG and Watson DI. Experimental study of the effect of intraperitoneal heparin on tumour implantation following laparoscopy. [Comment]. Br J Surg 1999;86:400–4.

21. Reilly WT, Nelson H, Schroeder G, et al. Wound recurrence following conventional treatment of colorectal cancer. A rare but perhaps underestimated problem. Dis Colon Rectum 1996;39:200–7.

22. Tseng LN, Berends FJ, Wittich P, et al. Port-site metastases. Impact of local tissue trauma and gas leakage. Surg Endosc 1998;12:1377–80.

23. Whelan RL, Sellers GJ, Allendorf JD, et al. Trocar site recurrence is unlikely to result from aerosolization of tumor cells. Dis Colon Rectum 1996;39 (10 Suppl):S7–13.

24. Reymond MA, Wittekind C, Jung A, et al. The incidence of port-site metastases might be reduced. Surg Endosc 1997;11:902–6.

25. Paolucci V, Schaeff B, Schneider M, Gutt C. Tumor seeding following laparoscopy: international survey. [Comment]. World J Surg 1999;23:989–95.

26. Shoup M, Brennan MF, Karpeh MS, et al. Port site metastasis after diagnostic laparoscopy for upper gastrointestinal tract malignancies: an uncommon entity. Ann Surg Oncol 2002;9:632–6.

27. Pearlstone DB,. Feig BW and Mansfield PF. Port site recurrences after laparoscopy for malignant disease. Semin Surg Oncol 1999;16:307–12.

28. Mayer C, Miller DM and. Ehlen TG. Peritoneal implantation of squamous cell carcinoma following rupture of a dermoid cyst during laparoscopic removal. Gynecol Oncol 2002;84:180–3.

29. Kim SH, Milsom JW, Gramlich TL, et al. Does laparoscopic vs. conventional surgery increase exfoliated cancer cells in the peritoneal cavity during resection of colorectal cancer? Dis Colon Rectum 1998;41:971–8.

30. Pearlstone DB, Mansfield PF, Curley SA, et al. Laparoscopy in 533 patients with abdominal malignancy. Surgery 1999;125:67–72.

31. Wang PH, Yuan CC, Lin G, Ng HT, Chao HT. Risk factors contributing to early occurrence of port site metastases of laparoscopic surgery for malignancy. Gynecol Oncol 1999;72:38–44.

32. von Bubnoff AC, Schneider AR, Breer H, Arnold JC and Riemann, JF. Significance of staging laparoscopy in pancreatic carcinoma: a case report. [In German]. Z Gastroenterol 2001;39 Suppl:35–40.

33. Yano M, Tsujinaka T, Shiozaki H, et al. Appraisal of treatment strategy by staging laparoscopy for locally advanced gastric cancer. World J Surg 2000;24:1130–5.

34. Bhalla R, Formella L, Kerrigan DD. Need for staging laparoscopy in patients with gastric cancer. Br J Surg 2000;87:362–73.

35. Hunerbein M, Rau B, Schlag PM. Laparoscopy and laparoscopic ultrasound for staging of upper gastrointestinal tumours. Eur J Surg Oncol 1995;21:50–5.

36. John TG, Wright A, Allan PL, et al. Laparoscopy with laparoscopic ultrasonography in the TNM staging of pancreatic carcinoma. World J Surg 1999;23:870–81.

37. Murugiah M, Paterson-Brown S, Windsor JA, Miles WF, Garden OJ. Early experience of laparoscopic ultrasonography in the management of pancreatic carcinoma. Surg Endosc 1993;7:177–81.
38. Goudas LA, Brams DM, Birkett DH. The use of laparoscopic ultrasonography in staging abdominal malignancy. Semin Laparosc Surg 2000;7:78–86.
39. Goletti O, Buccianti P, Chiarugi M, et al. Laparoscopic sonography in screening metastases from gastrointestinal cancer: comparative accuracy with traditional procedures. Surg Laparosc Endosc Percutan Tech 1995;5:176–82.
40. Bottger T, Engelman R, Seifert JK, Low R, Junginger T. Preoperative diagnostics in pancreatic carcinoma: would less be better? Langenbecks Arch Surg 1998;383:243–8.
41. Bottger TC, Boddin J, Duber C, et al. Diagnosing and staging of pancreatic carcinoma-what is necessary? Oncology 1998;55:122–9.
42. Smits NJ, Reeders JW. Imaging and staging of biliopancreatic malignancy: role of ultrasound. Ann Oncol 1999;10 Suppl 4:20–4.
43. Hayes N, Wayman J, Wadehra V, et al. Peritoneal cytology in the surgical evaluation of gastric carcinoma. Br J Cancer 1999;79:520–4.
44. Fujiwara Y, Takiguchi S, Mori T, et al. The introduction of preoperative staging laparoscopy and molecular diagnosis of peritoneal lavages for the treatment of advanced gastric cancer. Gan to Kagaku Ryoho 2002;29:2279–81.
45. Iwasaki Y, Arai K, Kimura Y, et al. Preoperative diagnostic laparoscopy with local anesthesia and lavage telomerase activity for advanced gastric cancer. Gan to Kagaku Ryoho 2002;29:2275–8.
46. Feussner H, Omote K, Fink U, Walker SJ, Siewert JR. Pretherapeutic laparoscopic staging in advanced gastric carcinoma. [Comment]. Endoscopy 1999;31:342–7.
47. Hunerbein M, Rau B, Hohenberger P, Schlag PM. The role of staging laparoscopy for multimodal therapy of gastrointestinal cancer. Surg Endosc 1998;12:921–5.
48. Asencio F, Aguilo J, Salvador JL, et al. Video-laparoscopic staging of gastric cancer. A prospective multicenter comparison with noninvasive techniques. Surg Endosc 1997;11:1153–8.
49. Rumstadt B, Schwab M, Schuster K, Hagmuller E, Trede M. The role of laparoscopy in the preoperative staging of pancreatic carcinoma. J Gastrointest Surg 1997;1:245–50.
50. Lavonius MI, Laine S, Salo S, Sonninen P, Ovaska J. Role of laparoscopy and laparoscopic ultrasound in staging of pancreatic tumours. Ann Chir Gynaecol 2001;90:252–5.
51. Yahchouchy-Chouillard E, Etienne JC, Fagniez PL, Adam R, Fingerhut A. A new «no-touch» technique for the laparoscopic treatment of gastric stromal tumors. Surg Endosc 2002;16:962–4.
52. Choi YB. Laparoscopic gatrojejunostomy for palliation of gastric outlet obstruction in unresectable gastric cancer. Surg Endosc 2002;16:1620–6.
53. Scott-Conner CE. Laparoscopic biliary bypass for inoperable pancreatic cancer. Semin Laparosc Surg 1998;5:185–8.
54. Charukhchyan SA, Lucas GW. Lesser sac endoscopy and laparoscopy in pancreatic carcinoma definitive diagnosis, staging and palliation. Am Surg 1998;64:809–14.
55. Croce E, Olmi S, Azzola M, Russo R, Golia M. Surgical palliation in pancreatic head carcinoma and gastric cancer: the role of laparoscopy. Hepatogastroenterology 1999;46:2606–11.

56. Fujiwara M, Kodera Y, Kasai Y, et al. Laparoscopy-assisted distal gastrectomy with systemic lymph node dissection for early gastric carcinoma: a review of 43 cases. J Am Coll Surg 2003;196:75–81.
57. Ballesta Lopez C, Ruggiero R, Poves I, Bettonica C, Procaccini E. The contribution of laparoscopy to the treatment of gastric cancer. Surg Endosc 2002;16:616–9.
58. Shimizu S, Uchiyama A, Mizumoto K, et al. Laparoscopically assisted distal gastrectomy for early gastric cancer: is it superior to open surgery? Surg Endosc 2000;14:27–31.
59. Kitano S, Shiraishi N, Fujii K, et al. A randomized controlled trial comparing open vs laparoscopy-assisted distal gastrectomy for the treatment of early gastric cancer: an interim report. Surgery 2002;131 Suppl:S306–11.
60. Adachi Y, Shiraishi N, Shiromizu A, et al. Laparoscopy-assisted Billroth I gastrectomy compared with conventional open gastrectomy. Arch Surg 2000;135:806–10.
61. Adachi Y, Shiraishi N, Ikebe K, et al. Evaluation of the cost for laparoscopic-assisted Billroth I gastrectomy. Surg Endosc 2001;15:932–6.
62. Adachi,Y, Suematsu T, Shiraishi N, et al. Quality of life after laparoscopy-assisted Billroth I gastrectomy. Ann Surg 1999;229:49–54.
63. Mochiki,E, Nakabayashi T, Kamimura H, et al. Gastrointestinal recovery and outcome after laparoscopy-assisted versus conventional open distal gastrectomy for early gastric cancer. World J Surg 2002;26:1145–9.
64. Goh PM, Khan AZ, So JB, et al. Early experience with laparoscopic radical gastrectomy for advanced gastric cancer. Surg Laparosc Endosc Percutan Tech 2001;11:83–7.
65. Tanimura S, Higashino M, Fukunaga Y, Osugi H. Hand-assisted laparoscopic distal gastrectomy with regional lymph node dissection for gastric cancer. Surg Laparosc Endosc Percutan Tech 2001;11:155–60.
66. Chau CH, Siu WT, Li MK. Hand-assisted D2 subtotal gastrectomy for carcinoma of stomach. Surg Laparosc Endosc Percutan Tech 2002;12:268–72.
67. Ludwig K, Wilhelm L, Scharlau U, Amtsberg G and Bernhardt J. Laparoscopic-endoscopic rendezvous resection of gastric tumors. Surg Endosc 2002;16:1561–5.
68. Ohgami M, Otani Y, Furukawa T, et al. Curative laparoscopic surgery for early gastric cancer: eight years experience. Nippon Geka Gakkai Zasshi 2000;101:539–45.
69. Okushiba S, Ohno K, Itoh K, et al. Hand-assisted endoscopic esophagectomy for esophageal cancer. Surg Today 2003;33:158–61.
70. Reyes CD, Weber KJ, Gagner M, Divino CM. Laparoscopic vs open gastrectomy. A retrospective review. Surg Endosc 2001;15:928–31.
71. Tanimura S, Higashino M, Fukunaga Y, Osugi H. Laparoscopic gastrectomy with regional lymph node dissection for upper gastric cancer. Gastric Cancer 2003;6:64–8.
72. Descottes B, Lachachi F, Sodji M, et al. Early experience with laparoscopic approach for solid liver tumors: initial 16 cases. Ann Surg 2000;232:641–5.
73. Gagner M, Pomp A. Laparoscopic pylorus-preserving pancreatoduodenectomy. Surg Endosc 1994;8:408–10.
74. Ehrmantraut W, Sardi A, Laparoscopy-assisted small bowel resection. Am Surg 1997;63:996–1001.

Commentary

ABDALLA ZARROUG and MICHAEL G. SARR

Wayman and Jamieson present a concise, unbiased overview of laparoscopy in the staging and therapy of intra-abdominal malignancies. Although this topic remains "steeped" in controversy, the real question is "What is the Controversy?" Does the controversy center around the philosophy of *THE BEST* treatment or does it relate to the (patho)physiology of laparoscopy itself. These are not unimportant questions and get at the heart of the matter – some based on science, some based on philosophy, some based on financial considerations, and some still based on ignorant closed-mindedness. We will address these "controversies" in two categories: diagnostic/staging "planning" laparoscopy, and therapeutic laparoscopy.

Diagnostic/Staging Laparoscopy

The authors nicely outline the overriding concept that staging laparoscopy should be reserved for those situations in which the results of the laparoscopy would potentially change the ultimate *surgical* therapy, i.e., celiotomy versus non-operative palliation or resection versus palliation. I will use pancreatic cancer as an example of a *philosophical approach*. Few would argue that multiple small peritoneal metastases in patients with pancreatic cancer portend a dismal prognosis (mean survival 6 months), and in this situation, palliation of jaundice without a celiotomy (endoscopic stent) seems best [1]. In contrast, patients with colorectal cancer benefit little (if at all) from staging laparoscopy because of the development of local complications (obstruction, bleeding) within the large intestine that require operative intervention; these local complications are not readily amenable to non-operative palliative measures.

However, consider the patient with locally unresectable pancreatic cancer (vascular involvement, distant nodes) but without peritoneal or liver metastases. Some surgeons would argue that because locally unresectable disease means incurable disease, non-operative palliation is the *BEST* treatment. In contrast, other groups have a *different philosophy*, i.e., locally unresectable disease often has a definable response to palliative chemo-radiation therapy, survival approaches 12–14 months, and these patients are *better* palliated with an operative palliation (hepaticojejunostomy, prophylactic gastrojejunostomy), which provides a much more durable biliary decompression as well as preventing gastric outlet obstruction (prophylactic gastrojejunostomy) [2]. There are reasonable arguments for each approach. The former group would support the extended staging laparoscopy [3], while the latter group would support a limited staging laparoscopy [4].

Finally, how about the concept of peritoneal cytology? If Warshaw's theory [5] that a positive staging peritoneal cytology can be shown to signify incurable disease (not "unresectable" but rather "incurable" disease) then a positive cytology at the time of staging laparoscopy (or rather staging peritoneal cytology) would prevent an incurable resection and stimulate use of the *BEST* palliative therapy (operative versus non-operative as described above). These arguments can be applied to gastric and hepatobiliary neoplasms as well.

What about an institutional approach to laparoscopy based on *financial considerations*? Consider a large hospital with a very tightly scheduled operating room with a patient scheduled for a staging laparoscopy/pancreatoduodenectomy. What happens to operating room efficiency and cost if the planned 6–7 h operation turns into a 30-min positive laparoscopy. Who uses the room next? Also, is a 10% chance of finding unresectable, incurable disease and avoiding celiotomy an acceptable rate to justify the cost of laparoscopy in the other 90% of patients? What if the staging laparoscopy needs to be done as a separate operation several days before potential operation (operating room cost, anesthesia, etc.)? In these times when our budgets are limited and the global cost to society *is* an important variable in the availability of healthcare, these considerations are "controversial" in some environments and less so in others.

However, within this arena, we all need to *maintain an open mind*. Introduction of new chemotherapeutic options or other adjuvant treatments (immunotherapy, hyperthermia, etc.) may change the paradigm. For instance, considerable interest recently has been focused on treatment options for patients with gastric cancer with minimal (but present) peritoneal disease. Intraperitoneal chemotherapy with hyperthermia may offer a reasonable response justifying gastrectomy in the absence of obstruction or bleeding. Other new (as yet unproven) advances are on the horizon and may change the current philosophy.

Therapeutic Laparoscopy

Concerning the (patho)physiology of laparoscopy, it is now clear that the original worry of an inordinate incidence of port-site metastases after laparoscopic resection of colon cancer has proven to be an old "spouses" tale – except possibly for gallbladder cancer, which is predisposed to implantation in port sites (but also in open incisions).

But what about long-term outcome of laparoscopic resection for cancer? Multiple confirmatory studies of a lack of any objective detrimental effect of a laparoscopic approach in long-term survival are still in progress, but all the preliminary work by technically proficient surgeons certainly suggests an equal outcome. With these studies in mind, the consideration put forth by Wayman and Jamieson that outcome will probably depend of operator expertise, and not by the *biology* of a laparoscopic approach, seems justified. Currently, advanced laparoscopic resections are limited to certain centers with technically advanced laparoscopic surgeons. However, the increasing interest in teaching of advanced laparoscopic techniques to surgical residents and fellows will populate the general surgical community over the next decade such that technically advanced laparoscopists (maybe better termed laparologists) will be the rule rather than the exception, obviating an argument against laparoscopic resection for fear of "technical incompetence". In addition, introduction of new technology will undoubtedly allow us to carry out "bigger" minimally invasive procedures – witness the ease of resection with the Harmonic Scalpel (Ethicon Corp., Cincinnati, OH, USA) versus the hook cautery, the ease of extracorporeal suturing and knot tying with the Endostitch (US Surgical Corp., Norwalk, CT, USA) and Suture Assistant (Ethicon Corp.), even the possibility of robotic technology to increase the degrees of freedom of the laparoscopic instruments, abolition of tremor, and three-dimensional, bifocal imaging

Thus, is the controversy really a controversy? Probably not, but despite our often preconceived beliefs (some unfortunately set in stone), the future will continue to evolve; and we, as well, need to give up our ignorance and embrace the new science – and probably modify also our philosophy based on therapeutic advances that benefit the patient.

References

1.   Shepherd HA, Royle G, Ross HPR, Arthur M, Colin-Jones D. Endoscopic biliary endoprosthesis in the palliation of malignant obstruction of the distal common bile duct: a randomized trial. Br J Surg 1988;75:1166–8.
2.   Luque de Leon E, Tsiotos GG, Balsiger B, Barnwell J, Burgart LJ, Sarr MG. Staging laparoscopy for pancreatic cancer should be used to select the best means of palliation and not only to maximize resectability rate. J Gastrointest Surg 1999;3:111–8.
3.   Conlon KC, Dougherty E, Klimstra DS, Coit DG, Turnbull ADM, Brennan MF. The value of minimal access surgery in the staging of patients with potentially resectable peripancreatic malignancy. Ann Surg 1996;223:134–40.
4.   Fernandez-del Castillo C, Rattner DW, Warshaw AL. Further experience with laparoscopy and peritoneal cytology in the staging of pancreatic cancer. Br J Surg 1995;82, 1127–9.

5. Makary MA, Warshaw AL, Centeno BA, Willet CG, Sigala H, Fernandez-del Castillo C. Implications of peritoneal cytology for pancreatic cancer management. Arch Surg 1998;133:361–5.

8

Hand-Assisted Laparoscopic Surgery

GORDIE K. KABAN, DONALD R. CZERNIACH, DEMETRIUS E.M. LITWIN

► **Key Controversies**

    A. Are postoperative outcomes of HALS equivalent to a laparoscopic approach?
    B. Does HALS reduce the conversion rate to open surgery?
    C. Is HALS a "bridge" for surgeons performing advanced laparoscopic procedures?
    D. Does HALS reduce operative time compared to laparoscopic surgery?
    E. Does HALS share the immunologic advantage seen in laparoscopic surgery?

8.1
Introduction

Hand-assisted laparoscopic surgery (HALS) is a product of the evolution of peritoneal access techniques that has taken place over the last 15 years. Prior to the introduction of HALS in the mid 1990s, the laparoscopic surgeon's armamentarium was limited to the use of instruments placed through small access ports. HALS, however, has challenged and expanded our fundamental definition of minimal access surgery by using incisions larger than those traditionally used in laparoscopic procedures. In HALS, the surgeon's hand replaces an inanimate laparoscopic instrument, returning the direct tactile feedback and manual dexterity that is noticeably absent in conventional laparoscopic surgery. Often considered a hybrid approach or a middle ground along the spectrum between open and laparoscopic surgery, HALS is emerging as a distinct access technique in many surgical specialties.

8.1.1
Hand-Assist Devices and Principles for Use

Innovation in the area of hand-assist devices has generated a number of unique products based on the original concept of maintaining pneumoperitoneum with the surgeon's hand inside the peritoneal cavity. Early attempts at HALS involved inserting the hand through a small fascial incision with pneumoperitoneum sequestered around the hand with towel clips and moist sponges [1]. The first device used for HALS was the extracorporeal pneumo-peritoneum access bubble [2], which was followed by several devices that, through unique innovations, allowed reliable maintenance of intra-abdominal pressure while providing excellent operative versatility.

There are currently six devices available for HALS:

1. HandPort (Smith and Nephew Endoscopy, Andover, MA, USA)
2. Gelport (Applied Medical, Rancho Santa Margarita, CA, USA)
3. LapDisc (Ethicon Endosurgery, Cincinnati, OH, USA)
4. Omniport (Advanced Surgical Concepts, Dublin, Ireland)
5. Intromit (Applied Medical, Rancho Santa Margarita, CA, USA)
6. Pneumosleeve (Dexterity Inc., Roswell, GA, USA)

Although there are many potential benefits of HALS, each device has specific properties that can be advantageous or restrictive, depending on the procedure. As a consequence, a surgeon contemplating HALS should be familiar with several of these devices.

The principles for the application of a HALS device are simple. First, the surgeon should adhere to the concept of port-site triangulation and avoid placing the device directly over the target organ. The fascial incision should be measured and made to approximate the surgeon's glove size. Ideally, the incision should be placed in a location that would be conveniently enlarged for open conversion if necessary. The surgeon is most comfortable when using the non-dominant hand through the device for retraction and finger dissection, leaving the dominant hand free for laparoscopic dissection. In general, HALS devices are used most effectively when the operating surgeon uses the device as a simple laparoscopic port, while recognizing the design nuances that are unique to each device.

8.2
Discussion

8.2.1
Are Postoperative Benefits of HALS Equivalent to a Purely Laparoscopic Approach?

There is growing evidence from prospective trials that for certain procedures, laparoscopic surgery can shorten hospital stay, reduce analgesic use and shorten time to resumption of activity [3–6]. The most controversial area regarding HALS is whether the postoperative benefits of a purely laparoscopic procedure are preserved when a hand-assisted approach is used. The most apparent differences between HALS and the conventional laparoscopic technique are the larger incision size required for the hand, the potential for more vigorous visceral retraction and manipulation, and the tension and stretch placed on the abdominal wall by the HALS device [7]. The cumulative effect of these differences on operative and postoperative outcomes is the subject of controversy. Although not established through clinical studies, most surgeons would agree that HALS is of little benefit and may even be detrimental in any procedure that can be routinely performed using only 5-mm and 10-mm incisions, such as laparoscopic cholecystectomy, appendectomy or splenectomy. Currently fueling the use of a hand-assisted approach is the fact that the fascial incision necessary for HALS is similar in length to the so-called utility incision that is crucial to many advanced laparoscopic procedures. This utility incision is made during or at the conclusion of the laparoscopic procedure, in order to perform an anastomosis or remove a large or intact specimen. This incision has been shown to be of similar size (7–8 cm) as that needed for placement of a HALS device [8], making the procedures equivalent with regard to the morbidity of the incision. Laparoscopic procedures that require a utility incision, such as colectomy, splenectomy and nephrectomy are therefore considered to be best suited for the HALS technique.

The best evidence regarding the equivalence of HALS and laparoscopic procedures is derived from three prospective trials [7–9] and other comparative retrospective studies [10, 11] primarily in the area of colorectal surgery. The HALS Study Group multicenter trial randomized and prospectively compared HALS ($n=22$) and standard laparoscopic ($n=18$) surgery for benign and incurable colorectal disease [8]. They were able to demonstrate equivalence with regard to length of hospital stay, return of bowel function, and postoperative pain and functional recovery. In the only other study of this caliber, Targarona et al. [7] prospectively randomized patients to HALS ($n=27$) or conventional laparoscopic colon resection ($n=27$). Return of bowel sounds, time to refeeding, major and minor morbidity, and length of hospital stay were equivalent in both groups. In further support of HALS, they were able to prove oncologic equivalence with intraoperative cytology, lymph node harvesting, and specimen length. The HALS approach in total colectomy in the setting of benign disease has also been shown to be similar to laparoscopic surgery in early postoperative outcomes by Nakajiima et al. [10]. In a retrospective analysis of a small number of consecutive patients (HALS $n=12$, laparoscopic $n=11$), they were able to show similar postoperative recovery (duration of epidural analgesia, bowel sounds, diet, hospital stay) with similar morbidity rates between both groups. These studies suggest that when HALS is used for colectomy, the postoperative benefits of a minimally invasive approach are not compromised.

In live donor nephrectomy, a hand-assisted approach has been adopted for the purpose of reducing warm ischemia times by expeditious extraction of the kidney through the hand-assist device. When performed completely laparoscopically, a utility incision must be made at the conclusion of the case to remove the donor kidney. Several retrospective studies have promoted the advantages of HALS for live donor nephrectomy, with claims of equivalent postoperative outcomes [12–14]. In the only trial of its kind, a prospective, randomized study of hand-assisted donor nephrectomy versus open donor nephrectomy was able to demonstrate a 47% reduction in analgesic use, a 35% reduction in hospital stay, and a 73% reduction in pain at 6 weeks follow-up [15]. Although a laparoscopic nephrectomy arm was not included in this trial, the results are good evidence that HALS, as a minimally invasive technique, provides real benefits compared with open surgery.

Laparoscopic splenectomy has become routine for removal of the normal-sized spleen at many centers. In the setting of splenomegaly, especially massive splenomegaly, however, the physical constraints of the enlarged spleen commonly require the creation of a utility incision for splenic removal. The three largest retrospective series to date evaluating the use of the hand-assist technique in the setting of splenomegaly suggest similar postoperative outcomes to laparoscopic splenectomy [11, 16, 17]. Targarona et al., comparing hand-assisted splenectomy (n=20) with conventional laparoscopic splenectomy (n=36), found that the HALS technique was associated with statistically less morbidity (36% vs 10%) and a shorter hospital stay (6.3±3.3 days vs 4±1.2 days). The two groups were comparable in terms of age, diagnosis and average spleen weight (1425±884 g vs 1753±1124 g) [16]. Rosen et al. [18], compared 14 hand-assisted splenectomies (average spleen weight 1516 g) to a consecutive group of 31 laparoscopic splenectomies (average weight 1031 g). Length of hospital stay 5.4 days vs 4.2 days and complication rates of 36% vs 16% were higher in the HALS group, but not statistically different. This preliminary retrospective data is encouraging, and lends further weight to the equivalence of the HALS technique.

Despite case series demonstrating the feasibility of HALS in other areas such as hepatic resection [19, 20], aorto-bifemoral bypass [21, 22], and pancreatic surgery [23] there are no current studies comparing open and laparoscopic cohorts.

8.2.2
Does HALS Reduce the Conversion Rate to Open Surgery?

One of the advantages of a hand-assisted technique is the ability of the surgeon to regain the tactile sense and versatility of their own hand, a concept that is taken for granted in open surgery. Some have suggested that the presence of the surgeon's hand intraperitoneally improves visual–spatial orientation [24], and therefore performance of laparoscopic tasks, although this opinion is not unanimous [25]. These theoretical benefits may have translated into a reduction in the conversion rate in some studies when compared with those of purely laparoscopic procedures. When used for colonic resection, Targarona et al. were able to achieve a conversion rate of 7% with HALS, compared with 23% in the laparoscopic group [7]. The HALS Study Group trial did find a lower conversion rate with HALS (14% vs 22%) but without statistical significance [8]. Kercher et al. reviewed 49 consecutive patients undergoing laparoscopic splenectomy for massive splenomegaly (length >17 cm, weight >600 g). They were able to eliminate open conversion in 5 patients with the use of a hand-assist device, and used HALS exclusively for seven patients with spleen lengths greater than 22 cm. A reduction in conversion rates is further supported in other retrospective splenectomy series [11, 17].

8.2.3
Is HALS a "Bridge" for Surgeons Performing Advanced Laparoscopic Procedures?

It has been suggested that HALS represents a hybrid between open and laparoscopic surgery, and therefore may be a logical facilitator for the less experienced surgeon making the transition to more advanced laparoscopic cases. Even for the seasoned laparoscopist, HALS may allow the completion of the challenging case without conversion to laparotomy. Although there is no direct evidence to support this, several authors have concluded that the hand-assist technique can in fact shorten the learning curve for difficult laparoscopic procedures [17, 26]. Describing their first 10 cases of laparoscopic (hand-assisted) live donor nephrectomies, Bemelman et al. concluded that even at the beginning of the learning curve, operative times (median 140 min) were reduced as compared to published, conventional laparoscopic donor nephrectomy [27]. HALS as a "bridge" or learning tool for new laparoscopic surgeons is an appealing notion that has yet to be substantiated.

8.2.4
Does HALS Reduce Operative Time Compared to Laparoscopic Surgery?

There are conflicting reports regarding the ability of HALS to significantly reduce operative times when the hand-assist approach is used, and this appears to be procedure-dependent. Data from the two prospective randomized trials comparing HALS with laparoscopic colon resection, where the HALS device was used from the onset of the case, did reveal shorter operative times; however the difference was not statistically significant [7, 8]. A reduction in operative time in splenectomy is inconsistent with some studies showing a benefit and others no difference [11, 16].

In contrast, hand-assisted nephrectomy data is more congruous. In a recent retrospective study, a 27% reduction in operative time (270 min vs 197 min) was demonstrated in a comparison of laparoscopic and HALS live donor nephrectomy [28]. Other small retrospective comparisons have further supported this advantage over laparoscopic surgery [12, 13, 29, 30]. No prospective randomized trials comparing HALS and laparoscopic nephrectomy have been performed to answer this question more definitively.

8.2.5
Does HALS Share the Immunologic Advantage Seen in Laparoscopic Surgery?

An attenuated inflammatory and immune response following laparoscopic versus open surgical procedures is well documented in both animal and human studies [31–34]. The surgical insult, thought to be less severe in laparoscopic procedures, results in a blunted immunologic response as measured by serum levels of several cytokines including C-reactive protein (CRP) and interleukin-6 (IL-6). Despite current data suggesting similarity of clinical outcomes between HALS and laparoscopic surgery, little is known about how HALS fits into the spectrum of surgical trauma. In the only published human clinical study addressing this issue, HALS colectomy in comparison with laparoscopic colectomy was found to result in a significant increase in CRP and IL-6 levels at several early postoperative time points [7]. Whether HALS more closely resembles open surgery or laparoscopic surgery in degree of immune response is still a matter of debate. Preliminary data from the University of Massachusetts has demonstrated a significant difference between the immunologic response in both hand-assisted and laparoscopic nephrectomy versus open nephrectomy in a porcine model (unpublished data). These data suggests that HALS more closely mimics laparoscopic surgery as measured by immunologic markers. The controversy surrounding this issue promises to further define our concept of minimally invasive surgery.

8.3
Summary

— Evidence from prospective and retrospective clinical studies of colectomy, splenectomy and live donor nephrectomy suggest that HALS is similar to laparoscopic surgery with respect to return of bowel function, length of hospital stay, and postoperative pain.

— Although HALS can result in shorter operative times and can reduce conversions to open surgery, its role as a bridge to advanced procedures for the less experienced laparoscopic surgeon remains to be established.

— More investigation is required into the inflammatory and immune response following HALS to determine whether it resembles laparoscopic surgery in the degree of surgical insult.

— Prospective, randomized clinical trials comparing hand-assisted, laparoscopic and open procedures are necessary to determine where HALS will fit in the spectrum of minimally invasive techniques.

References

1. Kusminsky R, Boland J, Tiley E, et al. Hand-assisted laparoscopic splenectomy. Surg Laparosc Endosc 1995;5:463–7.
2. Cuschieri A, Shapiro S. Extracorporeal pneumoperitoneum access bubble for endoscopic surgery. Am J Surg 1995;170:391–4.
3. Milsom J, Bohm B, Hammerhofer K, et al. A prospective, randomized trial comparing laparoscopic versus conventional techniques in colorectal cancer surgery: a preliminary report. J Am Coll Surg 1998;187:55–7.
4. Bringman S, Ramel S, Heikkinen TJ, et al. Tension-free inguinal hernia repair: TEP versus mesh-plug versus Lichtenstein: a prospective randomized controlled trial. Ann Surg 2003;237:142–7.
5. Lacy AM, Garcia-Valdecasas JC, Delgado S, et al. Laparoscopy-assisted colectomy versus open colectomy for treatment of non-metastatic colon cancer: a randomised trial. Lancet 2002;359:2224–9.
6. Kitano S, Shiraishi N, Fujii K, et al. A randomized controlled trial comparing open vs laparoscopy-assisted distal gastrectomy for the treatment of early gastric cancer: an interim report. Surgery 2002;131 (1 Suppl):S306–11.
7. Targarona E, Gracia E, Garriga J, et al. Prospective randomized trial comparing conventional laparoscopic colectomy with hand-assisted laparoscopic colectomy. Surg Endosc 2002;16:234–9.
8. HALS Study Group. Hand-assisted laparoscopic surgery for colorectal disease. A prospective randomized trial. Surg Endosc 2000;14:896–901.
9. Southern Surgeon's Club Study Group. Handoscopic surgery. A prospective multicenter trial of a minimally invasive technique for complex abdominal surgery. Arch Surg 1999;134:477–86.
10. Nakajiima K, Lee S, Cocilovo C, et al. Laparoscopic total colectomy: hand-assisted versus standard technique. Surg Endosc 2004;18:582–6.
11. Rosen M, Brody F, Walsh M, et al. Hand-assisted laparoscopic splenectomy vs conventional laparoscopic splenectomy in cases of splenomegaly. Arch Surg 2002;137:1348–52.
12. Ruiz-Deya G, Cheng S, Palmer E, et al. Open donor, laparoscopic donor, and hand-assisted donor nephrectomy: a comparison of outcomes. J Urol 2001;166:1270–4.

13. Wolf J, Moon T, Nakada S. Hand-assisted laparoscopic nephrectomy: comparison to standard laparoscopic nephrectomy. J Urol 1998;160:22–7.

14. Stifelman M, Hull D, Sosa R, et al. Hand-assisted laparoscopic donor nephrectomy: a comparison with the open approach. J Urol 2001;166:444–8.

15. Wolf J, Merion R, Leichtman A. Randomized controlled trial of hand-assisted laparoscopic versus open surgical live donor nephrectomy. Transplantation 2001;72:284–90.

16. Targarona E, Balague C, Cerdan G, et al. Hand-assisted laparoscopic splenectomy (HALS) in cases of splenomegaly. Surg Endosc 2002;16:426–30.

17. Borrazzo EC, Daly JM, Morrisey KP, et al. Hand-assisted laparoscopic splenectomy for giant spleens. Surg Endosc 2003;17:918–20.

18. Rosen M, Brody F, Walsh M, et al. Hand-assisted laparoscopic splenectomy vs conventional laparoscopic splenectomy in cases of splenomegaly. Arch Surg 2002;137:1348–52.

19. Antonetti M, Killelea B, Orlando R IIIrd. Hand-assisted laparoscopic liver surgery. Arch Surg 2002;37:407–12.

20. Fong Y, Jarnagin W, Conlon K, et al. Hand-assisted laparoscopic liver resection. Lessons learned from an initial experience. Arch Surg 2000;135:854–9.

21. Arous E, Nelson P, Yood S, et al. Hand-assisted laparoscopic aortobifemoral bypass grafting. J Vasc Surg 2000;31: 1142–8.

22. Da Silva L, Kolvenbach R, Pinter L. The feasibility of hand-assisted laparoscopic aortic bypass using a low transverse incision. Surg Endosc 2001;16:173–6.

23. Cuschieri A. Laparoscopic hand-assisted surgery for hepatic and pancreatic disease. Surg Endosc 2000;14:991–6.

24. Targarona E, Gracia E, Rodriquez M, et al. Hand-assisted laparoscopic surgery. Arch Surg 2002;138:133–40.

25. Rosser J. Hand-assisted laparoscopic surgery – invited critique. Arch Surg 2003;138:141.

26. Meijer DW, Bannenberg JJ, Jakimowicz JJ. Hand-assisted laparoscopic surgery, an overview. Surg Endosc 2000;14:891–5.

27. Bemelman W, van Doorn R, Th. De Wit L, et al. Hand-assisted laparoscopic donor nephrectomy. Surg Endosc 2001;15:442–4.

28. Lindstrom P, Haggman M, Wadstrom J. Hand-assisted laparoscopic surgery (HALS) for live donor nephrectomy is more time- and cost-effective than standard laparoscopic nephrectomy. Surg Endosc 2002;16:422–5.

29. Gershbein AB, Fuchs GJ. Hand-assisted and conventional laparoscopic live donor nephrectomy: a comparison of two contemporary techniques. J Endourol 2002;16:509–13.

30. Slakey DP, Hahn JC, Rogers E, et al. Single-center analysis of living donor nephrectomy: hand-assisted laparoscopic, pure laparoscopic, and traditional open. Prog Transplant 2002;12:206–11.

31. Schwenk W, Jacobi C, Mansmann U, et al. Inflammatory response after laparoscopic and conventional colorectal resections-results of a prospective randomized trial. Langenbecks Arch Surg 2000;385:2–9.

32. Maruszynski M, Pojda Z. Interleukin 6 (IL-6) levels in monitoring of surgical trauma. Surg Endosc 1995;9:882–5.

33. Allendorf J, Bessler M, Whelan R, et al. Better preservation of immune function after laparoscopic-assisted vs. open bowel resection in a murine model. Dis Colon Rectum 1996;39:S67–72.
34. Jacobi C, Ordeman J, Zieren U, et al. Increased systemic inflammation after laparaotomy vs laparoscopy in an animal model of peritonitis. Arch Surg 1998;133:258–262.

Commentary 1

WILLEM A. BEMELMAN, DIRK J. GOUMA

This chapter on *Controversies in Hand-Assisted Laparoscopic Surgery* is an excellent reflection of the current status of "handoscopic" surgery. The five Key Controversies mentioned are indeed the most important issues of controversy and the authors successfully summarized the current literature and data on these issues, ending up with a few open questions. The future and in particular randomized trials will provide the final answer. However, there are some aspects that need some more clarification.

The success of hand-assisted surgery depends largely on the quality of the hand port. Currently at least six devices are available and so far none of these has been proven superior. In our institute, several devices have been used for CE registration in splenectomy, live kidney donor nephrectomy, sigmoidectomy and total (procto) colectomy [1, 2]. Essentially, there are two types of ports. Those that work with an adhesive flange and those that work with other means to ensure an effective seal. All devices proved to work well in animals or slim patients without any troublesome skin fold, particularly if the procedure is short. In daily practice, however, long procedures and obese patients challenge the efficacy of these devices.

The devices with adhesives flanges (Intromit and Dexterity device) have the disadvantages that the seal often loosens due to movement of the hand, due to skin folds and as result of perspiration of the skin, particularly in advanced time consuming laparoscopic surgery. The Handport and Omniport are excellent devices ensuring a reliable seal, however the former is rather bulky. The Lapdisc looks rather neat and efficient, but the valve is very difficult to rotate when the hand is inside, particularly when the glove is fatty, which is more common in adipose patients. The Gelport works well, but is bulky, which is a disadvantage placing the device in a Pfannenstiel position in a fat patient. Studies that compare the potential advantages of these different devices are not yet available.

The authors state that most comparative studies indicate that results of pure laparoscopy and those of hand-assisted laparoscopy are equivalent. Likewise, other studies indicate that open surgery and hand-assisted surgery have similar results, e.g., immunologic response, pain and hospital stay, in hand-assisted and open restorative proctocolectomy [3, 4]. Possibly, it is true that conversion rates are lower in hand-assisted surgery for colonic cancer. However, both the randomized trial of Targarona et al. and the HALS study group report conversion rates >20% in the laparoscopic group indicating either poor patient selection or a learning curve effect. Experienced laparoscopic colorectal surgeons report much lower conversion rates. So, the available randomized comparisons of hand-assisted versus pure laparoscopy are probably biased by a learning-curve effect, which has been the reason to apply handports in the first place. However, conversion rates in hand-assisted live donor nephrectomy are very low, and, even in case of major bleeding, conversion was averted [5].

Although both procedures can be done very efficient purely laparoscopically, live donor nephrectomy and total (procto) colectomy are good indications for hand-assisted surgery because of speed and safety [4, 6]. As mentioned already by Kaban and co-authors these patients do need the limited abdominal incision at the end of the procedure anyhow. The most important time-gain is established during the dissection phase. On the other hand, for the experienced laparoscopic surgeon, the time-gain is more limited. Other well-established indications for hand-assisted surgery are limited other than to avert conversion occasionally.

We should also realize that if the difference between open and laparoscopic surgery is already limited for a particular surgical procedure, the difference between hand-assisted and the total laparoscopic approach will also be limited at least in terms of the benefits of a shorter hospital stay and earlier return to bowel function. It might be that the extent of the procedure also reflects the potential gain of any minimal invasive approach. The definitive role of hand-assisted laparosopic surgery needs to be defined in more detail in the near future.

References

1. Meijer DW, Bannenberg JJ, Jakimowicz JJ. Hand-assisted laparoscopic surgery: an overview. Surg Endosc 2000;14:891–5.
2. Maartense S, Bemelman WA, Meijer DW, Gouma DJ. Hand-assisted laparoscopic surgery (HALS): a report of 150 procedures. Surg Endosc 2004;18:397–401.
3. Dunker MS, ten Hove T, Bemelman WA, Slors JFM, Gouma DJ, va Deventer SJH. Interleukin-6. C-reactive protein and expression of human leukocyte antigen-DR on peripheral blood mononuclear cells in patients after laparoscopic versus conventional bowel resection: a randomized study. Dis Colon Rectum 2003;46:1238–44.

4. Maartense S, Dunker MS, Slors JF, Cuesta MA, Gouma DJ, van Deventer SJ, et al. Laparoscopic-assisted versus open restorative proctocolectomy with ileal pouch anal anastomosis a randomized trial. Ann Surg 2004; 240(6):984–992.
5. Maartense S, Bemelman WA. Renal clip dislodgement during hand-assisted laparoscopic live donor nephrectomy. Surg Endosc 2003;11:1851.
6. Maartense S, Idu M, Bemelman FJ, Balm R, Surachno S, Bemelman WA. Hand-assisted laparoscopic living (unrelated) donor nephrectomy: a safe and fast procedure to perform left as well as right-sided nephrectomies. Br J Surg 2004;91:344–8.

Commentary 2

ARA DARZI

I read this chapter from Dr. Kaban and his colleagues with great interest regarding the application of hand-assist technology in laparoscopic surgery. The chapter starts by highlighting the advantages of hand-assist laparoscopic surgery and also the different technologies that are available to us, including some of the new generation devices. It also refers to the number of studies that have been carried out by the group, including a randomized controlled trial demonstrating that hand-assist surgery does not take away the advantages of laparoscopic surgery. It also highlights that the conversion rate from hand-assist surgery to open surgery is less than that from laparoscopic to open surgery, which in itself suggests that certainly in the hands of a beginner, hand-assist surgery might provide, with the bridging technology, the skills of laparoscopic surgery. Another statement to support this is included in the form that hand-assist surgery does reduce the operative time for minimally invasive colorectal surgery.

Overall, it is a very thorough look at the technology of hand-assist surgery highlighting some of its advantages and also dealing with the myth of some of its disadvantages.

Hand-assisted laparoscopic surgery is one novel technology, which will transform major re-sectional surgery towards minimally invasive approaches. It has been used for colorectal surgery, nephrectomies, and more recently in vascular surgery. A number of randomized controlled trials have demonstrated the advantages of hand-assist surgery over and above open surgery without the loss of the main advantages of laparoscopic surgery. It will also provide the bridging tool for those who are starting with advanced laparoscopic surgery because of the tactile feedback.

Needlescopic Surgery

Eric C. Poulin, Christopher M. Schlachta, Joe Mamazza

▶ **Key Controversies**

A. Definition of needlescopic surgery
B. Equipment limitations
C. Limited applications
D. Objective outcomes not better

9.1
Introduction

"The Ultimate Craftsman is the one who leaves no trace"
Sun Tzu and the Art of War

During the 1990s, surgeons became convinced that the superior patient benefits of laparoscopic surgery could be attributed in large part to the reduction of operative trauma. The reduction of operative trauma was mediated by access to body cavities through small (5–12 mm) trocar sites and the use of long slender instruments that kept the surgeons' hands outside of the chest or abdomen. This reduced the handling of tissues and organs, and almost eliminated traction on the muscles of the abdominal wall and the various intracavitary organs and mesenteries. Many basic science studies have chronicled the advantages of this technology on most trauma markers and the immune system. Minimally invasive surgery is considered by most accounts to be relatively immune friendly [1].

It was therefore predictable that the next step in the evolution of minimally invasive surgery would be to further reduce trauma by using smaller instruments in the quest for even better outcomes. These efforts are referred to as needlescopic, minilaparoscopic or microlaparoscopic surgery. However, there are currently fewer than 100 articles in the peer-reviewed literature on the topics of needlescopic minilaparoscopic or microlaparoscopic surgery, including case reports and excluding gynecological indications [2–35]. This would seem to indicate slow adoption of needlescopic techniques by the minimally invasive community and the surgical community at large.

It seems that many aspects of needlescopic surgery are still controversial, starting with its definition.

9.2
Discussion

9.2.1
The Definition of Needlescopic Surgery

The first point of controversy arises from any attempt at a definition of needlescopic surgery. Many surgeons who want to study needlescopic techniques with clinical randomized trials have been challenged by the difficulty of defining what is an ideal or even an acceptable definition of needlescopic surgery. Many have debated whether the substitution of a single 3-mm trocar with a 5-mm trocar disqualifies the procedure from being a true needlescopic operation even if the trocar is situated in a cosmetically hidden location like the umbilicus. The elements of this definition are worthy of discussion.

The *strict definition* directs that a needlescopic procedure is a procedure where all ports, instruments and laparoscopes are 3 mm or smaller. This limits the application of needlescopic surgery to a few procedures where organ excision is not a significant barrier or where control of named blood vessels is not required, i.e., diagnostic needleoscopy, thoracic needleoscopic symphatectomy, etc.

The *practical and most-used definition* specifies that a needlescopic procedure is one performed with as many port sites, instruments or laparoscopes <3 mm in size as possible, allowing placement of a 5-mm or 10- to 12-mm trocar in the umbilicus for control of blood supply, use of a linear stapler or specimen extraction. This allows for the important concept of the escape hatch as a necessary adjuvant in needlescopic surgery. The main limitations for performing significant procedures in a needlescopic fashion are that the smallest available clip appliers are 5 mm in diameter and the smallest linear staplers are 12 mm in diameter. If a procedure requires significant control of blood supply or organ extraction, a cosmetically acceptable 5-mm or 12-mm escape hatch is necessary. An escape hatch of 5 mm or 12 mm placed in the umbilicus fulfills the roles of hemostatic control and specimen extraction while maintaining impeccable cosmetic goals. It gives more leeway to the surgeon and provides for a more secure operative environment. The presence of an escape hatch allows needlescopic surgery for a broader category of procedures (Table 9.1). Whether this negatively affects outcomes is still debated.

Table 9.1. Reported needlescopic procedures

Strict needlescopic technique (all ports <3 mm)

Thoracic sympathetic chain cauterization

Diagnostic needleoscopy

Practical needlescopic technique (one 5- to 12-mm port for vascular control, specimen transection or extraction)

Cholecystectomy

Appendectomy

Extra peritoneal hernia repair

Nissen fundoplication

Heller myotomy

Sigmoid resection

Ventral hernia repair

Intra gastric resection of gastric stromal tumor

Splenectomy

Axillary lymphadenectomy

Placement of ventriculoperitoneal shunt

Adrenalectomy

Excision of urachal anomalies

Decapsulation of splenic cyst

Excision of adrenal cyst

Excision of retroperitoneal cyst

Thoracic sympathectomy

9.2.2
Equipment Limitations

Needlescopic surgery requires the use of smaller instruments and laparoscopes, and many feel that the performance debt of these instruments severely limits the applicability of the technique [2].

The Instruments. Instruments of <3 mm, and even more so if they are <2 mm, are fragile. They bend easily around a fixed fulcrum at their point of entry into the abdominal cavity. Their resistance to bending, in large part, depends on the rigidity of the small metallic trocars through which they are inserted. Therefore, they have limited ability to be used for retraction of large solid organs. The smaller jaws of these small instruments make it more difficult to grasp any tissue with inflammation. Iatrogenic trauma is produced more easily, requiring added caution during surgery. The insulation on the hook cautery may be thinner and require more care. There are currently no 3-mm clip applicators or linear staplers, and with the technical limitations of size, it is doubtful that they will ever be developed.

Most surgeons feel that instruments of <2 mm are unusable for any significant surgery. Others feel that these limitations create an atmosphere of a high-wire act in performing needlescopic procedures, making it difficult to justify their use in carrying out safe and efficient surgery.

The Laparoscopes. Despite the fact that the quality of laparoscopes is still improving, the truth remains that the quality of intracavitary vision is determined by the quantity of light reaching the body cavity. This is a factor of the diameter of the laparoscope and of the fiber optic cable. With smaller scopes, this becomes even more evident when blood contaminates the operative field. The focal size of smaller scopes can also become a limiting factor. The optical quality is acceptable but inferior in terms of brightness and resolution. For these reasons, during more complicated procedures, many surgeons alternate between 3-mm scopes and 5- or 10-mm scopes. Many use a double camera set up or just change scopes as needed. A larger scope is used in the larger umbilical (escape hatch) trocar for most of the dissection. For vessel control or specimen extraction, they switch to a 3-mm scope through a 3-mm port using the umbilical port for clip applier or linear stapler. All of this makes for a more complicated flow of instruments and laparoscopes.

9.2.3
Limited Applications

Despite the obvious limitations, the list of procedures successfully completed using a needlescopic technique is nothing short of amazing [2–35] (Table 9.1).

However, most authors agree that needlescopic surgery is not for everybody. Appropriate selection of patients is necessary. The poster-child for needlescopic surgery would be a young thin patient, like a woman working in the fashion industry where any scar represents a negative outcome. Relative contraindications include the obese, the patient with previous vertical scars from open surgery, and the septic patient (Table 9.2).

9.2.4
Objective Outcomes are Not Better

Many surgeons are reluctant to endure the difficulties of needlescopic surgery because few have been able to demonstrate clear advantages. Since part of the demand for needlescopic procedures is patient-driven, there is a concern that any proclaimed advantage may be only perceptual. There have been four randomized clinical trials comparing various aspects of needlescopic surgery.

Table 9.2. Current favorable conditions for needlescopic surgery

You are a thin individual
A thick abdominal wall makes these procedures difficult if not impossible with these fragile instruments
Cosmesis is an important value for you
You are probably younger, athletic, conscious of your body image, and view any scars as a negative outcome. You could be a woman working in the fashion industry. However, pudgy middle-aged men can also wish for similar outcomes...
You have not had previous surgery
The needlescopic procedure will not make your previous scar disappear, but will eliminate further disfigurement
No sepsis
Not impossible, but better suited for an elective setting

Schwenk et al. [4] randomized 50 patients to undergo laparoscopic (LC) or needlescopic cholecystectomy (NC). They could not find major differences between groups in postoperative pulmonary function, analgesic consumption during patient-controlled analgesia, or pain perception by visual analog scale. The overall visual analog scores for pain while coughing were higher in the LC group. The cosmetic results as judged by the patient were slightly superior in the NC patients. Bisgaard et al. [5] conducted a similar study with the main endpoint being pain control during the first week postoperatively. Their multimodal analgesic regimen consisted of incisional local anesthetic at the beginning of surgery, non-steroidal antiinflammatory drugs, and paracetamol. The study was stopped after the randomization because of a high conversion rate to LC of 38%. They attributed this to the technical limitations of 2-mm instruments for dissection and grasping power, and the narrow vision field of the 2-mm laparoscope. This was particularly evident in patients with dense adhesions. In the remaining patients the only advantage for NC was in the first 3 h after surgery. They concluded that further technical developments were required before needlescopic techniques could be used on a routine basis for laparoscopic cholecystectomy. Look et al. [6] studied 64 randomized patients and essentially found no difference between LC and NC in terms of operative time, postoperative pain or recovery. However, their conversion to LC and even open cholecystectomy, mostly for technical reasons, was high.

A fourth clinical trial by Huang et al. [7] involved the randomization of 75 patients with uncomplicated appendicitis into three groups: open appendectomy (OA), laparoscopic appendectomy (LA), and needlescopic appendectomy (NA). Outcomes studied included duration of surgery, length of hospital stay, analgesic dosage, and surgery-associated complications. Most advantages found favored the minimally invasive procedures over OA. However, there was no clear advantage for NA.

There have been many non-randomized cohort studies with matched controls. In one of the larger ones with 101 patients, Mamazza et al. [8] showed modest advantages for various needlescopic procedures. A higher proportion of patients were in hospital for <24 h for needlescopic versus laparoscopic splenectomies (40% vs 0%, p=0.087), fundoplications (68% vs 42%, p=0.107), and Heller myotomies (90% vs 30%, p=0.022). This advantage only reached statistical significance in the Heller group. In a trial comparing 60 needlescopic cholecystectomies with a matched group of laparoscopic cholecystectomies, Gagner and Garcia-Ruiz [2] showed lower analgesic requirements and better cosmesis scores for the needlescopic group. In the needlescopic group, 47% did not have to use narcotics for postoperative pain control compared with 9% in the laparoscopic group. Lau and Lee [9] compared 30 needlescopic extraperitoneal hernioplasties (TEP) with an age-matched cohort. They concluded that postoperative outcomes following needlescopic and conventional

TEP were similar. In a small trial of 15 needlescopic appendectomies and 21 laparoscopic appendectomies, where the patients demographics and operative findings were similar, Mostafa et al. [10] showed that the needlescopic group had a significantly shorter operative time (p=0.02), reduced postoperative narcotics requirements (p=0.05), shorter hospital stay (p=0.04), and quicker return to work (p=0.03) when compared with the laparoscopic group. Whether the results of these trials would resist blinded randomization is debatable. Most other authors advocate for the technique from the perspective of case series or case reports [11–35].

Some have postulated that the requirement for a 10- to 12-mm umbilical port for retrieval of the gallbladder or other organ may negate whatever benefit is obtained by the use of smaller instrument ports elsewhere. It may be that much of the pain is due to the 10- to 12-mm ports and that there is not much difference in pain production between the smaller 3- and 5-mm ports. So far not a resounding endorsement...

On the other hand, most authors agree that the cosmetic results of needlescopic procedures are far superior, and it alone can justify the technique. However, this has not been demonstrated in well-designed trials. When patients are asked to rate the cosmetic result of their procedure, there is no appreciable difference between laparoscopic and needlescopic procedures, except in Gagner and Garcia-Ruiz's trial [2]. The problem is that in most studies where this was looked at, the patients did not have the ability to compare both procedures for cosmetic outcomes. They only expressed their satisfaction with their own results. Furthermore, appreciation of cosmesis is highly subjective and difficult to score. It may well be that the best judge is a non-involved external observer using a global rating system. This has not yet been done frequently as part of a randomized trial. However, there is no doubt that cosmesis as a desirable patient-derived outcome in general surgery patients is here to stay, provided all other accepted outcomes are protected. This is in stark contrast with the teachings of past generations of professors who proclaimed: "Big Incisions...Big Surgeons..." For the modern surgeon, the bar has been raised again.

Finally, the difficulty in demonstrating advantages for needlescopic surgery may reside in the fact that a proper assessment methodology for subtle refinements of surgical technique where the advantages are mainly in patient-driven outcomes is not available. This could lead to an underestimation of the value of needlescopic surgery. Appropriately validated tools to service the potential advantages of such techniques have not yet appeared.

9.3
Summary

— The principle of reducing the trauma of surgery to its maximum and creating very small almost invisible scars is appealing to many patients. Although the current literature is hard pressed to demonstrate clear benefits with the usual outcomes of intraoperative and postoperative morbidity, postoperative pain, length of hospital stay and return to daily activities, a trend in improvement of selected outcomes is shown by some.
— A case can be made for needlescopic techniques in selected patients for selected procedures.
— All authors agree about the fact that 2-mm and 3-mm punctures become almost undetectable scars and that the cosmetic results following a needlescopic procedure are stunning.
— Abdominal wall layers do not need to be closed with small trocar sites, which may serve to explain the shorter operating times reported by some for certain procedures.
— No infection or incisional hernias have been reported in port sites of this size.
— All also agree that mature laparoscopic skills are required to perform safe needlescopic surgery.

References

1. Hackam DJ, Rotstein OD. Host response to laparoscopic surgery: mechanisms and clinical correlates. Can J Surg 1998;41:103–11.
2. Gagner M, Garcia-Ruiz A. Technical aspect of minimally invasive abdominal surgery performed with needlescopic instruments. Surg Laparosc Endosc 1998;3:171–9.
3. Schauer PR, Ikramuddin S, Luketich JD. Minilaparoscopy. Semin Laparosc Surg 1999;6:21–31.
4. Schwenk W, Neudecker J, Mall B, Bohm J, Muller JM. Prospective randomized blinded trial of pulmonary function, pain, and cosmetic results after laparoscopic vs microlaparoscopic cholecystectomy. Surg Endosc 2000;14:345–8.
5. Bisgaard T, Klarskov B, Trap R, Kehlet H, Rosenberg J. Pain after microlaparoscopic cholecystectomy. A randomized double blind controlled study. Surg Endosc 2000;14:340–4.
6. Look M, Chew SP, Tan YC, Liew SE, Cheong DM, Tan JC, Wee SB, The CH, Low CH. Post-operative pain in needlescopic versus conventional laparoscopic cholecystectomy: a prospective randomized trial. J R Coll Surg Edinb 2001;46:138–42.
7. Huang MT, Wei PL, Wu CC, Lai IR, Cher RJ, Lee WJ. Needlescopic, laparoscopic, and open appendectomy: a comparative study. Surg Laparosc Endosc 2001;11:306–12.
8. Mamazza J, Schlachta CM, Seshadri PA, Caddedu MO, Poulin EC. Needlescopic surgery. Surg Endosc 2001;15:1208–12.

9. Lau H, Lee F. A prospective comparative study of needlescopic and conventional endoscopic extraperitoneal inguinal hernioplasty. Surg Endosc 2002;16:1737–40.

10. Mostafa G, Matthews BD, Sing RF, Kercher KW, Heniford BT. Mini-laparoscopic versus laparoscopic approach to appendectomy. BMC Surg 2001;1:4.

11. Cheah WK, Goh P, Gagner M, et al. Needlescopic retrograde cholecystectomy. Surg Laparosc Endosc 1998;8:237–8.

12. Yuan RH, Lee WJ, Yu SC. Mini-laparoscopic cholecystectomy. J Laparoendosc 1997;7:205–11.

13. Rozsos I, Rozsos T. Micro and modern minilaparotomy cholecystectomy. Acta Chir Hung 1994;34:11–6.

14. Kimura T, Sakuramachi S, Yoshida M, Kobayashi T, Takeuchi Y. Laparoscopic cholecystectomy using fine-caliber instruments. Surg Endosc 1998;12:283–6.

15. Tanaka J, Andoh H, Koyama K. Minimally invasive needlescopic cholecystectomy. Surg Today 1998;28:111–3.

16. Watanabe Y, Sato M, Ueda S, Abe Y, Horiuchi A, Doi T, Kawachi K. Microlaparoscopic cholecystectomy – the first 20 cases: is it an alternative to conventional LC? Eur J Surg 1998;164:623–5.

17. Seshadri PA, Poulin EC, Mamazza J, Schlachta CM. Needlescopic splenic decapsulation of an epithelial cyst. Can J Surg 2000;43:303–5.

18. Tagaya N, Rokkaku K, Kubota K. Splenectomy using a completely needlescopic procedure: report of three cases. J Laparoendosc Adv Surg Tech A 2002;12:213–6.

19. Seshadri PA, Carr LK, Mamazza J, Schlachta CM, Cadeddu MO, Poulin EC. Laparoscopic excision of urachal anomalies: a review. Can J Urol 1999;6:906–10.

20. Chiasson PM, Pace DE, Schlachta CM, Poulin EC, Mamazza J. «Needlescopic» Heller myotomy. Surg Laparosc Endosc Percutan Tech 2003;13:67–70.

21. Chiasson PM, Pace DE, Mustard RA, Mamazza J, Poulin EC, Schlachta CM. "Needlescopic" sigmoid resection. Surg Endosc 2002;16:715.

22. Tagaya N, Kubota K. Experience with endoscopic axillary lymphadenectomy using needlescopic instruments in patients with breast cancer: a preliminary report. Surg Endosc 2002;16:307–9.

23. Shalaby R, Desoky A. Needlescopic inguinal hernia repair in children. Pediatr Surg Int 2002;18:153–6.

24. Tagaya N, Aoki H, Mikami H, Kogure H, Kubota K. The use of needlescopic instruments in laparoscopic ventral hernia repair. Surg Today 2001;31:945–7.

25. Chueh SC, Chen J, Chen SC, Lai MK. Clipless laparoscopic adrenalectomy with needlescopic instruments. J Urol 2002;167:39–42

26. Gaur DD, Gopichand M, Dubey, Jhunjhunwala V. Mini-access for retroperitoneal laparoscopy. J Laparoendosc Adv Surg Tech A 2002;12:313–5.

27. Lin TS, Chou MC. Needlescopic thoracic sympathetic block by clipping for craniofacial hyperhidrosis: an analysis of 28 cases. Surg Endosc 2002;16:1055–58.

28. Pace DE, Chiasson PM, Schlachta CM, Poulin EC, Boutros Y, Mamazza J. Needlescopic fundoplication. Surg Endosc 2002;16:578–80.

29. Kao MC. Needlescopic surgery for palmar hyperhidrosis. J Thorac Cardiovasc Surg 2001;122:633–4.

30. Tagaya N, Kita J, Kogure H, Kubota K. Laparoscopic intragastric resection of gastric leiomyoma using needlascopic instruments. Case report. Surg Endosc 2001;15:414.

31. Matthews BD, Mostafa G, Harold KL, Kercher KW, Reardon PR, Heniford BT. Mini-laparoscopic appendectomy. Surg Laparosc Endosc Percutan Tech 2001;11:351–5.
32. Roth JS, Park AE, Gerwirtz R. Minilaparoscopically assisted placement of ventriculo-peritoneal shunts. Surg Endosc 2000;14:461–3.
33. Croce E, Olmi S, Azzola M, Russo R. Laparoscopic appendectomy and minilaparo-scopic approach: a retrospective review after 8-years experience. JSLS 1999;3:285–92.
34. Reardon PR, Kamelgard JI, Applebaum B, Rossman L, Brunicardi FC. Feasibility of laparoscopic cholecystectomy with miniaturized instrumentation in 50 consecutive cases. World J Surg 1999;23:128–31.
35. Yuan RH, Yu SC. Minilaparoscopic splenectomy: a new minimally invasive approach. J Laparoendosc Adv Tech A 1998;8:269–72.

Commentary

Sen-Chang Yu

Definition of Needlescopic Surgery

There are no controversies over the definition of needlescope, minilaparo-scope or microlaparoscope, which cover all scopes that are 3 mm in diameter or smaller [1–4]. For the definition of needlescopic surgery, I would recom-mend that all scopes should be 3 mm or less with the exception of a 5- to 12-mm umbilical port [4]. When a second 5- to12-mm port is added, it becomes a "conversion". I have applied one 10-mm and three 2-mm ports to complete more than 1,500 cases of the so-called minilaparoscopic cholecystectomy. It became a "conversion" when I had to use a 5-mm epigastric port for dense tis-sue or bleeding. For minilaparoscopic splenectomy, I apply one 5- to 12-mm umbilical port and three 2-mm ports [5]. After the application of the Ligasure vessel-sealing system, I have changed the procedure to two 5- to 12-mm and two 2-mm ports. I call this modification the mini-instrument-assisted laparo-scopic splenectomy.

Limitations of Needlescopes

For scopes of 3 or 2 mm in diameter, the removal of the trocar will not re-sult in air leakage, prominent scars or prolonged postoperative pain. However, as Dr. Poulin states in his assessment, instruments of 3 mm in diameter, and especially the 2-mm scopes, are flexible and fragile [6]. Furthermore, there is a limited number of needlescopes available from which to choose to meet sur-geons' personal preferences. Unless a surgeon is experienced in conventional laparoscopic surgery and strives to achieve higher quality of surgeries and better outcomes, it is not easy to overcome the learning curve to practice the technically more demanding needlescopic surgeries.

The limited choice of scopes make it essential that port locations be carefully selected. An example is the minilaparoscopic cholecystectomy. If the ports are placed at the sites of conventional laparoscopic cholecystectomy, the minigrasper may not be able to displace the gall bladder and liver upward or expose the liver hilum clearly for dissection of the cystic artery and the cystic duct. As soon as the surgeon finds that a port site does not work, prompt relocation to another suitable area is needed in order to get the operation proceeding in an uneventful manner.

Dr. Poulin has referred to the limited visual field, resolution and brightness of the needlescopes. I have combined the 2-mm needlescope and a 10-mm laparoscope to conduct minilaparoscopic cholecystectomy [4]. Under the assistance of a 10-mm laparoscope, the 2-mm instruments can be used to dissect the cystic artery, cystic duct and the bladder tissues that adhere to the liver. The 2-mm bipolar forceps are used to cauterize the cystic artery. The needlescopes are mainly employed for endoclipping and dissection of the cystic duct and removal of the specimens. The same protocols apply to minlaparoscopic appendectomy and splenectomy [4, 5].

Limited Use of Needlescopes

I do not believe needlescopes and mini-instruments are indicated for every laparoscopic surgery or every patient. Careful selection of patients and the flexible combination of conventional laparoscopes and needlescopes as well as the interchangeable uses of mini-instruments and conventional instruments will lead to better surgical outcomes (reduced postoperative pain, less trauma and scars, and shorter hospital stay and recovery time) [4, 7–9].

Uncertain Advantages of Needlescopic Surgeries

As reviewed by Dr. Poulin, a limited number of randomized trials suggest that needlescopic cholecystectomy is not convincingly superior to the conventional procedure. The conversion rate was as high as 38% in these trials [10]. The procedures used in conventional laparoscopic cholecystectomy have been well developed and practiced by many surgeons. The instruments are larger in size and more rigid, making it easier to manipulate especially for separating dense adhesions or for handling acute cholecystitis. Needlescopic cholecystectomy is new to many surgeons who may not be experienced in using the delicate and fragile instruments, particularly in difficult cases. The conversion rate is expected to be high for the newcomers. My own record with 1,200 cases between November 1996 and October 2001 shows a conversion rate of 3.6% (43 cases). Among these 43 cases, 40 cases (3.33%) involved the conversion of a 2-mm to 5-mm epigastric port for cystic artery bleeding (two cases), severe adhesion (28 cases), thick wall (five cases), contracted gall bladder (one case) and cystic duct stone impaction (four cases). Another one case (0.08%) was converted to conventional laparoscopic procedures because of unclear anatomy. Two cases (0.17%) were resorted to open cholecystectomy due to common bile duct injuries.

Summary

— Needlescopic surgeries are appropriate for cholecystectomy with the exception of acute cholecystitis. It is also suitable for splenectomy in patients with idiopathic thrombocytopenic purpura. A third indication is appendectomy [1, 2].
— Needlescopic surgeries are technically demanding procedures. Anticipated advantages over the conventional laparoscopic surgeries include better cosmetic appearance, reduced postoperative pains, shortened operation time, faster recovery period, reduced hospital stay, no incisional hernia and lack of infection [1–5, 8, 9].
— Combined uses of needlescopes and a 10-mm laparoscope and the interchangeable applications of mini-instruments and conventional instruments are appropriate [4]. A recommended protocol is to apply mini-instruments for dissection under the 10-mm scope and endoclip and linear stapler under a 2- or 3-mm scope via the umbilical port.
— Results from the limited randomized trials suggest that appropriate selections of patients and disease conditions are important in order to achieve surgical outcomes that are better than the conventional laparoscopic surgeries [2, 10].

References

1. Gagner M, Garcia-Ruiz A. Technical aspect of minimally invasive abdominal surgery performed with needlescopic instruments. Surg Laparosc Endosc 1998;3:171–9.
2. Huang MT, Wei PL, Wu CC, Lai IR, Chen RJ, Lee WJ. Needlescopic, laparoscopic, and open appendectomy: a comparative study. Surg Laparosc Endosc 2001;11:306–12.
3. Yuan RH, Lee WJ, Yu SC. Mini-laparoscopic cholecystectomy: a cosmetically better, almost scarless procedure. J Laparoendosc Adv Surg Tech A 1997;7:205–11.

4. Yu SC, Yuan RH, Chen SC, Lee WJ. Combined use of mini-laparoscope and conventional laparoscope in laparoscopic cholecystectomy: preservation of minimal invasiveness. J Laparoendosc Adv Surg Tech A 1999;9:57–62.
5. Yuan RH, Yu SC. Minilaparoscopic splenectomy: a new minimally invasive approach. J Laparoendosc Adv Surg Tech A 1998;8:269–72.
6. Mamazza J, Schlachta CM, Seshadri PA, Caddedu MD, Poulin EC. Needlescopic surgery. A logical evolution from conventional laparoscopic surgery. Surg Endosc 2001;15:1208–12.
7. Chueh SC, Chen J, Chen SC, Lai MK. Clipless laparoscopic adrenalectomy with needlescopic instruments. J Urol 2002;167:39–42.
8. Tagaya N, Rokkaku K, Kubota K. Splenectomy using a completely needlescopic procedure: report of these cases. J Laparoendosc Adv Surg Tech A 2002;12:213–6.
9. Watanabe Y, Sato M, Ueda S, Abe Y, Horiuchi A, Doi T, Kawachi K. Microlaparoscopic cholecystectomy – the first 20 cases: is it an alternative to conventional LC? Eur J Surg 1998;164:623–5; discussion 626.
10. Bisgaard T, Klarskov B, Trap R, Kehlet H, Rosenberg J. Pain after microlaparoscopic cholecystectomy – a randomized double-blind controlled study. Surg Endosc 2000;14:340–4.

Robotic Surgery

Mark A. Talamini

> ▶ **Key Controversies**
>
> A. The cost of robotic surgery
> B. Operating room time
> C. Technology issues: loss of tactile feedback
> D. Telesurgery and teleconsultation
> E. Who should use robotics?

10.1
Introduction

Research activity into the use of robotics in surgery is considered by virtually all to be important. Most agree that sometime in the future robotics will be an important part of surgical care. However, the issue has recently emerged from the research lab. Robotic devices are now available for clinical use in the USA following FDA approval. But their use is indeed controversial.

The controversy revolves around a few key issues. The biggest of these is cost. Since we are currently in an economic contraction in the world of professional medical care, we have all become accustomed to thinking about how to save money rather than how to spend it. Since the surgical systems currently available are quite expensive, the cost of the systems themselves is controversial. The current systems are also cumbersome. They were created by modifying robotic devices used commonly in industry for medical applications. Therefore they are big and take up a large amount of room in the operating theatre. Another area of controversy is the additional time that robotic operations are perceived to consume. With respect to the technology itself, the absence of tactile feedback raises great controversy for many surgeons. Finally, whether laparoscopic surgeons should use such machines or surgeons who have not previously had laparoscopic experience is also an area of some debate.

10.2
Discussion

10.2.1
Costs

The cost of the currently available robotic system, the daVinci System from Intuitive Surgical, is somewhere around 1-million dollars per unit. Obviously, this is a lot of money. Additional expenses that are less obvious are training costs, cost of limited multi-use instruments, and the cost of any incremental operating room time. These costs vary from situation to situation. By any account, the cost is high.

General surgeons are not accustomed to spending these amounts of money on capital equipment in their operating rooms. Other specialties are accustomed to spending at this level. Neurosurgeons use expensive operating microscopes and surgical directional units (the operative "wand" for instance). Our invasive radiology colleagues spend this much and more to fit out an appropriately equipped invasive radiology suite. Even diagnostic radiologists are now commonly spending these amounts for real time computed tomography (CT) units, 3-D CT units, positron emission tomography scanners, and magnetic resonance angiography scanners. The current economics of these other specialties more easily take into account the start-up costs of high ticket price equipment. General surgery does not.

The question of cost is unfortunately a new one in the world of surgery. Leapfrog advances in surgery that occurred over the last centuries did not need to take cost into account as a significant factor. When Dr. Alfred Blalock conceived of and executed the Blalock-Taussig shunt, expense was not a factor. As the entire discipline of cardiac surgery and open heart cardiopulmonary bypass evolved, cost was not a limiting factor. Yet now in the twenty-first century, advances often must await a favorable financial argument to be considered or approved. One cannot help but wonder whether some of the great advances in medicine and surgery would have ever taken place had the overwhelming concerns for cost been laid as a burden upon the previous generations of incredibly creative surgeons. Yet we in the current generation clearly must address this issue.

How can we prove that a robotic system is "cost effective"? It is going to be difficult. There are certain types of operations where the enhanced visibility and improved tissue manipulation should be measurable in outcomes studies. Two possible examples come to mind. One is that of the Heller myotomy. In this operation, the ability to clearly identify muscle fibers as being different from mucosa and sub-mucosa is a terrific advantage. Similarly, the ability to pick up one strand of muscle at a time and divide it is a clear advantage relative to standard laparoscopy. Hopefully randomized series, or even retrospective comparative series will provide data addressing these potential advantages. Similarly, the laparoscopic repair of giant hiatal hernia defects has been documented to have a significant recurrence rate. We can optimistically hope that the improved suturing capability of robotic systems will also improve the outcome of this operation. This is a question that certainly can be put to a randomized prospective trial.

In a more general sense, it seems empirically obvious that the advantages of a robotic system should eventually lead to improved outcomes. If the surgeon can see better and manipulate tissue better, both the patient and the surgeon should be better off. By way of illustration, if a talented experienced surgeon had their normal tools taken away during an open operation and had them replaced with foot-and-a-half-long laparoscopic tools, and if one rubbed Crisco on the surgeon's glasses making their eye sight less clear, such a surgeon would be able to accomplish the intended operation. Given enough repetitions in time, they would even become good at accomplishing that operation. However, they would greatly prefer their clear vision and their familiar and effective instruments. How would one go about proving that the outcomes are better with clear glasses and normal instruments as opposed to Crisco glasses and chopstick instruments? Well, it would be hard. But it is intuitively obvious that if the surgeon is seeing better and manipulating tissue better, the patient will be better off.

10.2.2
Operating Room Time

Time is another area of controversy with respect to the use of robotics in surgery. There are two aspects to time with respect to robotics. The first is the additional time that might be necessary within the framework of a minimally invasive robotic operation. The second is the amount of time required for preparation and take-down before and after an operation.

With respect to the operation itself, the robotic device has to be moved or clamped into place after trocars for abdominal access have been inserted into the patient. If the patient's table position needs to be altered, or the robotic positioning needs to be changed during the case, this takes additional time. The time taken to set the machine up and move it into place is initially significant, but the learning curve is short. After only a very few cases this takes just a matter of minutes. During the procedure, time also must be taken for instrument exchanges. These exchanges are more complex and time consuming than standard laparoscopic surgery. It is not unreasonable to think that the additional ease of suturing and tissue dissection that the robotic device provides might more than compensate for instrument exchange time losses. Ongoing studies should answer this question.

The more significant and irreducible time issues relate to preparing and cleaning instruments and preparing and taking down the operating room after a robotic procedure. Once the robotic device is brought into the operating room, it must go through a start-up and safety check procedure that is automatic, but fairly extensive. Usually the operating room team can be about other work while this is occurring. However, it does take additional time to move all of the equipment from its stored spot into the room. It also takes time to render the machines sterile with bags, and to attach all of the cords and set up the telescopes and electronics. These time inefficiencies can be minimized if a consistent team does this work for each case. Future robotic designs may not have as many of these time inefficiencies. But for the current situation, some additional time for the robotic system is inevitable.

10.2.3
Technological Issues: Loss of Tactile Feedback

Current robotic systems do not provide any force feedback or haptic information to the surgeon. For some surgeons, this is simply unacceptable. The current systems make up for this by providing vivid visualization and therefore providing more information through visual cues than standard laparoscopic surgery. For many surgeons, this more than compensates for the loss of tactile feedback. The difficulty is even more pronounced for surgeons who need to use fine sutures such as cardiovascular and thoracic surgeons. Tying an 8-0 polypropylene suture without breaking it or making it weak by grabbing with metal instruments can be a challenge. This does not appear to be as big an issue for laparoscopic surgeons as for those attempting to move directly from open surgery to robotic surgery. Laparoscopic surgeons lost some of their proprioception when they went from having a hand in the belly and using short instruments to using foot-and-a-half-long chopsticks in laparoscopic surgery. Indeed, the laparoscopic instruments do provide some force feedback and tissue distensibility information, but it is certainly less than that of open surgery. The detection occurs at a significant distance, and is transmitted via the fulcrum of the abdominal wall trocar point. For laparoscopic surgeons, moving to robotic surgery means losing the remainder of what they had already become accustomed to doing without. However, for surgeons who have not made the transition from open surgery to laparoscopic surgery, this can be quite a challenge. It is best answered through training and experience with the individual robotic system.

Engineers both in industry and in academia are in hot pursuit of answers to this problem. Actually providing force feedback with the current generation of robotics devices is going to be extremely difficulty because of the large forces involved and the configurations of the current machines. The more immediate strategies being pursued seek to give the surgeon other data streams that can act as a surrogate for normal force feedback information. Such systems are in development and early data suggest that they are indeed helpful.

10.2.4
Telesurgery and Teleconsultation

Since the current robotic computer-assisted devices separate the surgeon from the immediate vicinity of the patient, they open up all of the possibilities of telesurgery and teleconsultation.

The possibilities surrounding this capability are incredibly exciting. This has been beautifully demonstrated by Dr. Gagner and team with the first transcontinental laparoscopic cholecystectomy. At the current time, the average American patient has only one location in mind for their responsible primary surgeon: right next to them in the operating room. However, there are many situations in which telesurgery and teleconsultation may have tremendous advantages for our patients. The most obvious is that of the military. The ability to project a single surgeon's capabilities and talents to multiple receiving robotic units in the field close to the soldier has been enticing to the military for years. For that reason, many of these technologies have in fact been developed and pursued either within the military or with support from military programs. Telementoring or teleassisting presents far fewer logistical and legal challenges. Consider a surgeon in a rural setting who finds himself performing an operation he did not expect and does not feel fully prepared to carry out. For instance, a trauma patient with an unexpected pancreatic injury requiring a distal pancreatectomy. There would be great power and advantage in being able to wheel up a robotic device to assist such a surgeon. A pancreatic surgery expert many miles away could actually participate in the operation seeing what the primary surgeon sees and actually assisting.

There are many areas of intense controversy in these considerations. For instance, who is responsible legally if the patient is in another county or state? Must the surgeon operating or assisting at a distance be licensed within the state or judicial locality in which the patient resides? Who reimburses the surgeon for their time in this effort? These are all important issues. But sure to override these issues is the simple fact that this capability now exists. It is up to the surgical community and society to determine how to best use such powerful tools.

10.2.5
Who Should Use Robotics?

How will these newly approved and available robotic devices fit in to the current surgical world? There are two groups of surgeons who stand to gain from the significant benefits of these machines and the devices that will follow them. The first group are those surgeons who gained enough laparoscopic skill for non-complicated procedures, such as laparoscopic cholecystectomy. It takes significant training to move beyond easy procedures to more complicated dissection and suturing tasks with standard laparoscopic instruments. Many surgeons, because of the shape of their practice and other surgical priorities, have not taken the time and energy to further develop their laparoscopic skills to those ends. Robotic surgical systems, because of their additional capabilities, have the potential to allow these surgeons to move to the next level of tissue dissection and suturing.

The second group that stands to gain are those who consider themselves "cutting edge" surgeons. The majority of these surgeons have become quite skilled with minimally invasive instruments. However, they still have roadblocks to performing increasingly complex operations in terms of tissue dissection and complex suturing. These machines have the capability of allowing the "cutting edge" group to move on to spectacular accomplishments in the minimally invasive environment. The laparoscopic Whipple is possible using standard minimally invasive instruments, but it is a daunting technical challenge. These instruments have the potential of making such complex operations more possible.

A third group of surgeons is already enjoying a huge advantage from these machines. These are specialty surgeons for whom standard minimally invasive approaches have had little benefit. This group, in many cases, has jumped directly from open surgery to a robotic approach. A clear example of this group is the robotic prostatectomy. This operation requires complex suturing of the urethra, and complex, and potentially bloody, tissue dissection. In at least some centers, what was extremely difficult or impossible laparoscopically is now being done rather routinely robotically.

10.3
Summary

While this general field is indeed a current focus of controversy, most, if not all, would agree that the surgery performed in the next 10 to 20 years will be vastly different than surgery being performed today. Most would also agree that robotics and computer-assisted technology will play a major role in that evolution. What will surgery look like, and what will the robotics devices look like in that future? That nobody knows. The current devices available clinically and those being developed in the research lab are strong starting points on the journey toward robotic surgery.

References

1. Jacobsen G, Berger R, Horgan S. The role of robotic surgery in morbid obesity. J Laparoendosc Adv Surg Tech A 2003;13:279–83.
2. Boyd WD, Stahl KD. The Janus syndrome: a perspective on a new era of computer-enhanced robotic cardiac surgery. J Thorac Cardiovasc Surg. 2003;126:625–30.
3. Chang L, Satava RM, Pellegrini CA, Sinanan MN. Robotic surgery: identifying the learning curve through objective measurement of skill. Surg Endosc 2003;17:1744–8
4. Melvin WS. Minimally invasive pancreatic surgery. Am J Surg 2003;186:274–8.
5. Honl M, Dierk O, Gauck C, Carrero V, Lampe F, Dries S, Quante M, Schwieger K, Hille E, Morlock MM. Comparison of robotic-assisted and manual implantation of a primary total hip replacement. A prospective study. J Bone Joint Surg Am 2003;85-A:1470–8.
6. Talamini MA, Chapman S, Horgan S, Melvin WS. A prospective analysis of 211 robotic-assisted surgical procedures. Surg Endosc 2003;17:1521–4.
7. Horgan S, Berger RA, Elli EF, Espat NJ. Robotic-assisted minimally invasive transhiatal esophagectomy. Am Surg 2003;69:624–6.
8. Patel YR, Donias HW, Boyd DW, Pande RU, Amodeo JL, Karamanoukian RL, D'Ancona G, Karamanoukian HL. Are you ready to become a robo-surgeon? Am Surg 2003;69:599–603.
9. Gettman MT, Hoznek A, Salomon L, Katz R, Borkowski T, Antiphon P, Lobontiu A, Abbou CC. Laparoscopic radical prostatectomy: description of the extraperitoneal approach using the da Vinci robotic system. J Urol 2003;170:416–9.
10. Kypson AP, Nifong LW, Chitwood WR Jr. Robotic mitral valve surgery. Semin Thorac Cardiovasc Surg 2003;15:121–9.
11. Talamini MA. Overview – current clinical and preclinical use of robotics for surgery. J Gastrointest Surg. 2003;7:479–80.
12. Talamini MA. Robotic surgery: is it for you? Adv Surg 2002;36:1–13.
13. Parr KG, Talamini MA. Anesthetic implications of the addition of an operative robot for endoscopic surgery: a case report. J Clin Anesth 2002;14:228–33.
14. Talamini MA. Surgery of the 21st century. Ann Surg 2001;234:8–9.

Commentary

Andres Castellanos, William C Meyers

There is no controversy that we are just barely scratching the surface of the field of robotic surgery. We do not know about other surgeons, but we feel that we are presently at a standstill with respect to the development of this field. With the struggles on the business side of medicine all around us, we, as surgeons, have become much more insular than we were just 10 years ago. Have we lost our energy already about new advances? Come on, guys and gals – it is time for us to more actively promote this new field of robotic surgery!

The advantages of minimally invasive surgery (MIS) over open surgery include: smaller incisions, shorter hospital stay, rapid recovery and less pain. These advantages outweigh the inherent technical disadvantages of MIS such as inferior depth perception, less tactile feedback (haptic), instrument limitations, and prolonged learning curve. Robotic surgery can correct the lack of depth perception. Current research in haptic will develop a whole new world of tactile feedback. The instruments are going to get better, and for those of us who still feel a little nervous about doing certain kinds of MIS, the new robotic surgery is the answer! Robotic surgery will remove these limitations plus it will provide all the other advantages of the MIS. All we need is to keep doing it and studying it!

Dr. Talamini has nicely reviewed the controversies of robotic surgery. One important controversy, however, needs to be emphasized – does robotic surgery really benefit the patient? The answer right now in certain specific areas is definitely yes, even though most current data focuses on technical feasibility rather than patient benefit. Robotics will add important improvements in surgeon capabilities, such as increasing dexterity and decreasing fatigue, tremor, and steepness of the learning curve, and we believe strongly that some of these improvements do and will have impacts on patient safety. We currently need more measuring sticks that insurance companies and other doctors will understand in order to advance this field that way.

There is no question that cardiothoracic surgery, urology and gynecology are indeed using the surgical robot to maneuver in small spaces where they have never been before. The world of surgery and medicine still awaits more demonstration of real benefits for patients from those particular specialties. Zealots like ourselves believe we are doing good with these machines, but we are foolish to think that we have proved to others that this is so. It is time to get out and show the data.

The million-dollar cost of these systems is still prohibitive for many medical centers. So far, we, robotic/MIS physicians and hospitals, have been absorbing this cost. This is not a sustainable business model! We need the insurance companies to start to kick in. We need the federal government to kick in. We also need the industry to survive because we know this instrumentation is good. We know that the only question now is – how good? Right now the insurance companies are giving us a hard time since the benefits have not been clearly proved. We need this field. We also need to support the company in any way that we can since a one-huge-product company is also not a sustainable business model. The company needs a few more certain revenue streams.

Let us start acting like the zealots that we say we are. It is time to put more pressure on our systems to support robotics. With all the other pressures in medicine right now, robotics will die if we don't do this. Robotics is sort of like NASA. We, as a society, will get more out of the development of this field than just going to the moon.

A great example of what will happen if more support happens is haptic. There is no doubt that haptic feedback will make robotic systems safer and more user-friendly. As Dr. Talamini's says, haptic feedback combined with visual augmentation will greatly augment surgeon capabilities. But there are greater capabilities that will occur as we develop the know-how of haptic. Haptic feedback research will provide the smart tools that will improve intra-operative recognition and other diagnostic capabilities. Just think if our present imaging capabilities could be combined with haptic. We have the technical capabilities right now for such imaging to develop. But not if the field or company is dead!

We are living through very exciting innovation in surgery – since the introduction of laparoscopic surgery in the mid 1980s. Technology has become an integral part of the future of surgery. To deny this would be to push surgery back to the Dark Ages. It takes only a little bit of imagination, but a strong sense of the importance of innovation to really produce advances. With the mess that the business side of medicine is in these days, these advances will not continue easily. These will not just happen magically. We need to put pressure in the right places to advance our field. There is no question that advances in robotics will pave the road to more success. There is no question that better robots will follow. Maybe, like the space program, we need a lot more federal support for this project. Whatever the case, it is time for us surgeons to become more out-spoken about robotics.

Hiatal Hernia

CLAUDE DESCHAMPS

> ▶ **Key Controversies**
>
> A. Which approach for which patient?
> B. Surgical technique
> C. Addressing the shortened esophagus

11.1
Introduction

Gastroesophageal reflux disease (GERD) and diaphragmatic hernia (DH) at the esophageal hiatus are common abnormalities affecting millions of people on a daily basis. In paraesophageal hernias, the gastroesophageal junction remains below the diaphragm, but the fundus and successively larger portions of the greater curvature of the stomach herniate through the hiatus alongside the esophagus, into the thorax. Eventually the entire stomach is displaced into the thorax in an inverted position. In this advanced stage many of these hernias display characteristics of both sliding and paraesophageal hernias. A large diaphragmatic hernia or complete intrathoracic stomach can cause obstructive symptoms including nausea, vomiting, bloating, substernal pain, and less commonly, chronic anemia. It may or may not be associated with GERD. Over the years numerous surgical procedures have been developed to correct these problems. The surgical treatment of diaphragmatic hernia repair, whether it be for GERD from an incompetent lower esophageal sphincter or for obstruction due to a large diaphragmatic hernia, has evolved over time. Initially, the reduction of the hernia was thought to be sufficient, but because it did not adequately address the incompetent lower esophageal sphincter, it frequently did not correct the problem.

11.2
Discussion

11.2.1
Which Approach for Which Patient?

Although no ideal operation exists, the goal of repair remains anatomic reduction of the hernia and a competent lower esophageal sphincter. The choice of which procedure to perform can be difficult. While currently the three major techniques for creation of an antireflux valve include the Nissen fundoplication, the Belsey-Mark IV repair, and the Hill repair, partial transabdominal fundoplication like the Toupet (partial posterior fundoplication) and the Dor (partial anterior fundoplication) have gained popularity in recent times [1–12]. This can be accomplished either transabdominally or transthoracically [1]. While traditionally, we have favored a transthoracic approach because of improved exposure, especially in obese patients or patients with large hernias or previous repairs, the laparoscopic approach has been applied to a widening spectrum of patients, partly because of increased comfort with the procedure and improved short- and long-term results.

Successful reduction of the hernia may require extensive dissection with mobilization of both the esophagus and stomach and the hernia sac must be completely resected from the mediastinum. Crural approximation and fundoplication should be inherent part of the repair to prevent anatomical recurrence and postoperative GERD [1, 4, 9, 11, 12]. Gastrostomy and gastropexy have also been used to anchor the stomach in the abdomen [4, 13, 14]. More recently, closure of the diaphragmatic defect with prosthetic material has been proposed [15–17].

While the success of laparoscopy for achalasia and GERD had made it tempting to offer laparoscopic approach to an increasing number of patients, several factors make the laparoscopic repair of large DH more difficult, which include preoperative comorbidities, body habitus, the propensity for some hernias to incarcerate and strangulate, the necessity of excising the sac without damage to neighboring structures and adequate closure of a large hiatus [4, 14, 18, 19].

Like others at the beginning of our experience, we have identified a high prevalence of recurrent hernia on early radiographic investigation of patients [20, 21]. Inadequate crural closure and sac excision are the technical factors most often associated with recurrent herniation [22]. Other factors include slippage of the fundoplication or a fundoplication that is too tight [23]. In our series, acute recurrent herniation was believed to result from breakdown of the crural closure.

11.2.2   Surgical Technique

The optimal technique for closure of a large crural defect is also controversial. Some authors have cited excessive tension of the crural closure as the cause of breakdown and modified their closure to include posterior placement of polypropylene mesh [24, 25]. Others have advocated the use of polytetrafluoroethylene because it may a allow tissue ingrowth without stimulating excessive adhesion formation [26]. Yet others have cautioned against using prosthetic material because of concerns of excessive adhesion formation and erosion into esophagus with respiratory motions [27]. In addition, authors who examined early recurrences following laparoscopic repair have attributed recurrence to inadequate excision of the hernia sac [22]. We have found, however, that lowering intraperitoneal gas pressure or creating an iatrogenic pneumothorax intraoperatively does decrease tension on the crura and facilitates closure. If a secure closure of the crura cannot be performed laparoscopically, the operation should be converted to an open procedure.

11.2.3
Addressing the Shortened Esophagus

Equally as important, failure to recognize and manage a shortened esophagus is associated with an increased risk of postoperative herniation [6]. The esophagogastric junction must be reduced to below the diaphragm without tension. Several authors have now reported that a laparoscopic gastroplasty be added to an antireflux procedure if the repair alone results in tension on the fundoplication [28, 29]. The easy performance of a wedge gastroplasty as a lengthening procedure have made the laparoscopic approach of the shortened esophagus a potentially more successful operation.[30]

A majority of our patients had either excellent or good functional outcome after laparoscopic repair of large DH [20]. Those results are similar to that reported by others (Table 11.1). But, as with other surgical procedures, a period of learning is required [2]. We believe that as experience is gained, morbidity will be less and a higher percentage of patients will have good to excellent results.

Table 11.1. Other reported series on laparoscopic repair of diaphragmatic hernia

Authors [ref.]	Year	No. of patients	Conversion number (%)	Type of repair	Mortality no. (%)	Follow-up (months)	Recurrent hernia (%)	Results[a]
Oddsdottir et al. [14]	1995	10	0	Nissen[b]	0	9	10%	89%
Huntington [33]	1997	58	1 (1.7%)	Nissen/Toupet	1(1.7%)	12	0%[f]	100%
Willekes et al. [37]	1997	30	0	Nissen/Toupet[c]	0	–	0%	100%
Perdikis et al. [35]	1997	65	2 (3.0%)	Nissen/Toupet	0	18	15%	93%
Krahenbuhl et al. [34]	1998	12	1 (8%)	Nissen[d]	0	21	–	92%
Edye et al. [31]	1998	55	–	Nissen/Toupet	0	29	14.5%	85%
Schauer et al. [36]	1998	67	3 (4%)	Nissen/Toupet	1 (1.5%)	13	–	94%
Gantert et al. [13]	1998	55	5 (9%)	Various[e]	1 (1.8%)	11	4%	89%
Wu et al. [38]	1999	38	1 (2.6%)	Nissen/Toupet	2 (5%)	24	15%[g]	95%
Horgan et al. [32]	1999	41	2 (5%)	Nissen/Toupet	1 (2.5%)	36	5%	100%
Hashemi et al. [21]	2000	27	–	Nissen	0	17	42%	77%
Dahlberg et al. [20]	2001	37	2 (5.4%)	Nissen	2 (5.4%)	13	12%	84%

[a] Excellent and good, [b] One patient had a gastropexy, [c] Two patients had gastropexy, [d] Gastropexy added in all patients, [e] Nissen, 270° wrap, gastropexy, [f] Based on symptoms only, [g] Three other patients had intrathoracic wraps

11.3
Summary

— Laparoscopic repair of large DH is a challenging operation associated with a higher early recurrence rate.
— As experience is gained and further refinement of the operative technique occur, laparoscopic approach for treatment of large DH is becoming a viable alternative to the standard open approach.

References

1. Allen MS, Trastek VF, Deschamps C, Pairolero PC. Intrathoracic stomach. Presentation and results of operation. J Thorac Cardiovasc Surg 1993;105:253–9.
2. Deschamps C, Allen MS, Trastek VF, Johnson JO, Pairolero PC. Early experience and learning curve associated with laparoscopic Nissen fundoplication. J Thorac Cardiovasc Surg 1998;115:281–5.
3. Skinner DB. Esophageal hiatal hernia. The condition: clinical manifestations and diagnosis. In: Sabiston DC Jr, Spencer FC, eds. Surgery of the chest, 5th edn. Philadelphia: W.B. Saunders; 1990. pp. 890–902.
4. Soper NJ. Laparoscopic management of hiatal hernia and gastroesophageal reflux. Curr Probl Surg 1999;36:767–838.
5. Valiati W, Fuchs KH, Valiati L, Freys SM, Fein M, Maroske J, et al. Laparoscopic fundoplication – short- and long-term outcome. Langenbecks Arch Surg 2000;385:324–8.
6. Darling G, Mackay M. The Belsey Mark IV and Collis-Belsey fundoplications. In: Deschamps C, guest ed. Operative techniques in general surgery. Repair of esophageal hiatal hernias. Philadelphia: W.B. Saunders; 2000. pp. 60–81.
7. Deschamps C, guest ed. Repair of esophageal hiatal hernias. In: JA van Heerden, DR Farley, eds. Operative techniques in general surgery, vol. 2, no. 1, Philadelphia: W.B. Saunders; 2000.
8. Fernando HC. Luketich JD. Christie NA. Ikramuddin S. Schauer PR. Outcomes of laparoscopic Toupet compared to laparoscopic Nissen fundoplication. Surg Endosc 2002;16:905–8.
9. Maziak DE, Todd TR, Pearson FG. Massive hiatus hernia: evaluation and surgical management. J Thorac Cardiovasc Surg 1998;115:53–60.
10. Pera M, Deschamps C, Taillefer R, Duranceau A. The uncut Collis-Nissen gastroplasty: early functional results. Ann Thorac Surg 1995;60:915–21.
11. Trastek VF, Allen MS, Deschamps C, Pairolero PC, Thompson A. Diaphragmatic hernia and associated anemia: response to surgical treatment. J Thorac Cardiovasc Surg 1996;112:1340–5.
12. Trastek VF, Deschamps C, Allen MS, Miller DL, Pairolero PC, Thompson AM. Uncut Collis-Nissen fundoplication: learning curve and long-term results. Ann Thorac Surg 1998;66:1739–44.
13. Gantert WA, Patti MG, Arcerito M, et al. Laparoscopic repair of paraesophageal hiatal hernias. J Am Coll Surg 1998;186:428–33.

14. Oddsdottir M, Franco AL, Laycock WS, Waring JP, Hunter JG. Laparoscopic repair of paraesophageal hernia. New access, old technique. Surg Endosc 1995;9:164–8.
15. Carlson MA, Richards CG, Frantzides CT. Laparoscopic prosthetic reinforcement of hiatal herniorrhaphy. Dig Surg 1999;16:407–10.
16. Frantzides CT, Carlson MA. Prosthetic reinforcement of posterior cruroplasty during laparoscopic hiatal herniorrhaphy. Surg Endosc 1997;11:769–71.
17. Koger KE, Stone JM. Laparoscopic reduction of acute gastric volvulus. Am Surg 1993;59:325–8.
18. Cuschieri A, Shimi S, Nathanson LK. Laparoscopic reduction, crural repair and fundoplication of large hiatal hernia. Am J Surg 1992;163:425–30.
19. Watson DI, Davies N, Devitt PG, Jamieson GG. Importance of dissection of the hernia sac in laparoscopic surgery for large hiatal hernias. Arch Surg 1999;134:1069–71.
20. Dahlberg PS, Deschamps C, Miller DL, Allen MS, Nichols FC, Pairolero PC. Laparoscopic repair of large paraesophageal hiatal hernia. Ann Thorac Surg 2001;72:1125–9.
21. Hashemi M, Peters JH, DeMeester TR, et al. Laparoscopic repair of large type III hiatal hernia: objective follow-up reveals high recurrence rate. J Am Coll Surg 2000;190:553–61.
22. Edye M, Salky B, Posner A, Fierer A. Sac excision is essential to adequate laparoscopic repair of paraesophageal hernia. Surg Endosc 1998;12:1259–63.
23. Hunter JG, Smith CD, Branum GD et al. Laparoscopic fundoplication failures; patterns of failure and response to fundoplication revision. Ann Surg 1999;230:595–606.
24. Basso N, De Leo A, Genco A, et al. 360° Laparoscopic fundoplication with tension-free hiatoplasty in the treatment of symptomatic gastroesophageal reflux disease. Surg Endosc 2000;14:164–9.
25. Basso N, Rosato P, De Leo A, Genco A, Rea S, Neri T. Tension-free hiatoplasty, gastrophrenic anchorage, and 360° fundoplication in the laparoscopic treatment of paraesophageal hernia. Surg Laparosc Endosc 1999;9:257–62.
26. Paul MG, DeRosa RP, Petrucci PE, Palmer ML, Danovitch SH. Laparoscopic tension-free repair of large paraesophageal hernias. Surg Endosc 1997;11:303–7.
27. Trus TL, Hunter JG. Minimally invasive surgery of the esophagus and stomach. Am J Surg 1997;173:242–55.
28. Jobe BA, Hovath KD, Swanstrom LL. Postoperative function following laparoscopic Collis gastroplasty for shortened esophagus. Arch Surg 1998;133:867–74.
29. Pierre AF. Luketich JD. Fernando HC. Christie NA. Buenaventura PO. Litle VR. Schauer PR. Results of laparoscopic repair of giant paraesophageal hernias: 200 consecutive patients. Ann Thorac Surg 2002;74:1909–15.
30. Champion JK. Laparoscopic vertical banded gastroplasty with wedge resection of gastric fundus. Obes Surg 2003;13:465.
31. Edye M, Canin-Endres J, Gattorno F, Salky BA. Durability of laparoscopic repair of paraesophageal hernia. Ann Surg 1998;118:528–35.
32. Horgan S, Eubanks TR, Jacobsen G, Omelanczuk, Pellegrini CA. Repair of paraesophageal hernias. Am J Surg 1999;177:354–8.
33. Huntington TR. Short-term outcome of laparoscopic paraesophageal hernia repair. Surg Endosc 1997;11:894–8.
34. Krahenbuhl L, Schafer M, Farhadi J, Renzulli P, Seiler CA, Buchler MW. Laparoscopic treatment of large paraesophageal hernia with totally intrathoracic stomach. J Am Coll Surg 1998;187:231–7.

35. Perdikis G, Hinder RA, Filipi CJ, et al. Laparoscopic paraesophaegal hernia repair. Arch Surg 1997;132:586–90.
36. Schauer PR, Ikramuddin S, McLaughlin RH, et al. Comparison of laparoscopic versus open repair of paraesophageal hernia. Am J Surg 1998;176:659–65.
37. Willekes CL, Edoga JK, Frezza E. Laparoscopic repair of paraesophageal hernia. Ann Surg 1997;225:31–8.
38. Wu JS, Dunnegan DL, Soper NJ. Clinical and radiologic assessment of laparoscopic paraesophageal hernia repair. Surg Endosc 1999;13:497–502.

Commentary

J. David Richardson

Dr. Deschamps properly notes the importance of diaphragmatic hernias as a problem that requires surgical correction. While mild GERD is probably overtreated by many physicians in the USA, large hiatal hernias are often undertreated because surgical referral is required. Many of the patients with large DH or paraesophageal hernias treated in our unit are elderly. Interestingly, many have had large DH diagnosed for many years and have been allowed to become increasingly symptomatic prior to referral for operative treatment.

I perform repairs of DH and antireflux operations using one of three approaches: laparoscopic, open transabdominal, and transthoracically, depending on patient factors. I reserve the transthoracic approach for patients with re-do operations or with very short esophagus usually associated with stricture formation. The use of a laparoscopic lengthening procedure, as noted by the author, obviates the need for a transthoracic approach to this problem in some patients. However, in the past, I have encountered patients with severe transmural scarring that could not have been properly addressed without a transthoracic approach and a thorough mobilization of the esophagus prior to the lengthening procedure. In my mind, obesity is only a relative indication for a thoracotomy. Since most Americans are overweight, obesity should not be used as a reason for a transthoracic approach in a patient who could be treated transabdominally. Clearly, the incisional morbidity of thoracotomy is much higher.

On the other hand, the pendulum may occasionally swing too far, vis-à-vis, the laparoscopic approach. I have seen several patients with laparoscopic failures following treatment of large DH. The common denominator appears to be disruption of the crural repair. It is undoubtedly easier, in some patients, to assess crural strength and integrity using an open abdominal approach rather than a laparoscopic approach. Therefore, the trade-off of decreased postoperative morbidity with a laparoscopic operation should be balanced against the ability to do a better operation with an open procedure. The surgeon's mindset should not be one that considers the need to convert to an open procedure a failure.

Dr. Deschamps correctly notes the learning curve for repair of large DH. These procedures are more technically demanding than a straightforward anti-reflux operation. The important features, as he notes, are adequate dissection of the sac and good crural closure. The sac often tethers the stomach in the mediastinum, and failure to release these attachments creates tension on the closure even though the stomach can be reduced to the abdomen at the time of operation.

I believe every stomach that is inverted in the chest should have a gastropexy (or gastrostomy). Even with facile gastric reduction into the abdomen, the stomach that has been inverted for years tends to rotate even in the abdomen. Gastropexy combats these rotational forces and allows the repair to heal in a more normal anatomic position.

I was not sure where the author stood on the issue of prosthetics. I am a non-believer except in very unusual circumstances. The problems I have with buttressing with mesh are the following: many patients do not need prosthetic use, and in those patients in whom prosthetics would be most useful, i.e., a large patulous hiatus with flimsy crura, there is often little good tissue in which to secure the mesh. Clearly, prosthetics have some risk of gastointestinal erosion that is real, albeit low. Thus, I use a prosthetic when I am very concerned about the repair, but always question what benefit this maneuver has.

Most patients with repair of a paraesophageal hernia should have an anti-reflux procedure added. In our practice this is a total fundoplication. The natural history of partial wraps has been a high incidence of failure. Therefore, we reserve partial fundoplication only for those with clearly demonstrated esophageal motility issues.

Gastroesophageal Reflux Disease

J. Andrew Isch, Brant K. Oelschlager, Carlos A. Pellegrini

> ▶ **Key Controversies**
>
> A. Which antireflux operation is appropriate for ineffective esophageal motility?
> B. Laparoscopic surgery and Barrett's esophagus
> C. Laparoscopy and the short esophagus
> D. Antireflux surgery in patients with respiratory symptoms

12.1
Introduction

Gastroesophageal reflux disease (GERD) is the leading gastrointestinal disorder in the United States and multiple therapies are available to treat it. With the advent of minimally invasive surgical techniques, the number of operations being performed to treat GERD has increased significantly. This increase has raised a number of controversies related to surgical management. This chapter aims to examine several of these controversies and to discuss the rationale for our approach to them.

12.2
Discussion

12.2.1
Which Antireflux Operation is Appropriate for Ineffective Esophageal Motility?

Dysphagia is a feared complication of antireflux surgery. Its reported incidence varies from 2–20% [1–4]. Concern that postoperative dysphagia will be induced or made worse as a result of a full wrap has led many surgeons to prefer a partial wrap when there is dysphagia preoperatively or when manometric data reveal ineffective esophageal motility [4, 5]. Since manometric evaluation of esophageal peristalsis is an integral component of the preoperative work-up to rule out other motility disorders, some have recommended "tailoring" the antireflux procedure based on the effectiveness of peristalsis on manometry.

When ineffective esophageal motility (IEM) is discovered (average distal esophageal contraction amplitude less than 30 mmHg, and/or a lack of peristalsis in 30% or more wet swallows), many surgeons perform a partial wrap. Lund et al performed Toupet fundoplications on 46 patients with reflux and distal esophageal amplitudes of <30 mmHg and 10% simultaneous or interrupted waves [4]. Compared with a similar group of patients undergoing a Nissen fundoplication, the Toupet group had significantly less dysphagia (9 vs 44%) with effective reflux control. Wetscher et al. reported on 32 patients undergoing Toupet fundoplication with similar manometric parameters [1]. The incidence of postoperative dysphagia was low and many patients demonstrated improvement in esophageal motility after surgery.

Other authors favor a partial wrap, regardless of esophageal function, believing it to be an equivalent operation for GERD [6–8]. Holzinter et al. have demonstrated normalization in the DeMeester score and esophageal acid exposure after Toupet fundoplication [6]. Although the follow-up was limited to only 1 year, the incidence of dysphagia requiring dilation was 5%. Hill and colleagues perform a partial wrap with a posterior gastropexy (Hill procedure) as their operation of choice. In this technique, the fundus is brought anterior to the esophagus and secured to the pre-aortic fascia. Proponents of this approach believe that it provides equivalent outcomes but avoids many of the complications of a total fundoplication [9]. Hill has argued that a "classic" Nissen produces a blind, acid-producing parietal cells mass, which drains poorly and can result in gastric ulceration. While there is some limited data to suggest that this technique results in good or equivalent outcomes, mostly from Hill himself, no study demonstrates it to be superior then other techniques. Outcomes have been difficult to reproduce and success may depend on calibration of the cardia with intraoperative manometery [10].

There is an increasing number of studies, which refutes the need to "tailor" an operation, observing no increase in postoperative dysphagia among those with a total wrap [11–14]. Puhalla et al. demonstrated no increase in post-operative dyshagia in patients with impaired distal esophageal motility undergoing a Nissen when compared with those undergoing a Toupet fundoplication [11]. Rydgerg and colleagues reported similar findings [12]. Heider et al. found no difference in post-operative dysphagia rates between those undergoing Nissen vs. Toupet, regardless of baseline esophageal motility status [15]. In a follow-up study, these authors demonstrated an actual improvement in peristaltic amplitudes and frequencies after surgery in those with disordered motility pre-operatively [16]. They concluded that complete fundoplication should be applied liberally, even in those with disordered motility.

Of approximately 750 patients undergoing laparoscopic antireflux surgery at the University of Washington between 1994 and 2000, 30% had some amount of dysphasia during the first postoperative week. Only ten patients (2%) required dilation with none of the last 200 requiring dilation. In a subset of 96 patients with defective peristalsis identified preoperatively, 39 patients had a partial wrap (our initial approach for IEM) and 53 had a full wrap (our latter approach) [17]. While both procedures were effective at controlling symptoms of GERD, dysphagia was actually improved significantly after total fundoplication. This did not occur in patients with partial fundoplication and may be a result of less effective reflux control in this subset of patients. These findings would seem to corroborate Heider's report [15] discussed above. Of note, we also observed no new dysphasia in any patients who did not have this complaint preoperatively.

If a total fundoplication does not result in higher rates of dysphagia, it would be preferred if it provided superior control of reflux. Schauer and colleagues have shown that short-term outcomes after Nissen and Toupet fundoplications are similar [18]. Over time, however, a significantly greater percentage of patients who underwent a Toupet fundoplication required resumption of proton pump inhibitor medication and became less satisfied with their operation. Inferior results from partial fundoplication have been seen by many others [19–24]. Hunter and colleagues demonstrated a re-emergence in heartburn and regurgitation in patients at one year following a Toupet as compared to those undergoing a Nissen [23].

It has been our experience that a 360° wrap results in normalization or improvement of esophageal acid exposure, reestablishes normal lower esophageal sphincter (LES) pressure, and relieves typical symptoms (heartburn and regurgitation). The critical steps in the operation can be taught and reproduced fairly easily and require no routine intraoperative tests. Manometric results prior to surgery do not alter this approach unless the patient suffers from a complete lack of peristalsis. In this instance, a partial wrap is performed. If dysphasia does occur in the postoperative period, it is usually short lived and managed expectantly for the first several months. If the wrap is constructed loosely using appropriate gastric and esophageal geometry, reflux is controlled, symptoms are relieved, and long-term dysphagia is a rare problem.

12.2.2
Laparoscopic Surgery and Barrett's Esophagus

Barrett's disease of the esophagus represents a severe form of GERD. It is believed that chronic exposure of the esophageal muscosa to gastric contents can lead to intestinal metaplasia. Barrett's esophagus can subsequently progress to dysplasia and eventually adenocarcinoma. Two primary controversies surround the surgical treatment of Barrett's disease: (1) the effectiveness of surgery to control GERD symptoms compared with uncomplicated GERD patients, and (2) the impact of laparoscopic antireflux surgery upon the risk of malignancy and/or the state of the epithelium.

Surgical therapy is effective in controlling the symptoms of reflux in patients with Barrett's. Surgery is often reserved for the symptomatic failures. Atwood et al. showed a higher chance to develop recurrence of esophagitis and strictures for patients in medical therapy than for those treated surgically [25]. Farrell et al. demonstrated that the excellent results observed at one year after surgery persisted in longer follow-up (2–5 years) [26]. Hofstetter et al. have shown that after antireflux surgery patients with Barrett's disease have long-lasting relief of symptoms and nearly all consider themselves cured or improved after surgery [27]. While medical therapy is effective, patients often require increasing doses for control with many experiencing breakthrough symptoms even on the best of regimens. In a young patient, the diagnosis of Barrett's esophagus may amount to lifelong medical therapy that is both inconvenient and expensive. Lifestyle modifications may become too taxing, and compliance may become an issue as many patients may discontinue medical therapy when their symptoms improve or resolve [28].

We studied the course of 106 patients undergoing laparoscopic antireflux surgery at the University of Washington between 1994 and 2000. We found that surgery was effective in controlling symptoms and reducing acid exposure with no patients requiring reoperation to date. Resolution was found in 79% of patients and 93% had improvement in their heartburn after laparoscopic surgery; 94% had improvement in their regurgitation and 83% in their dysphagia. There was a statistically significant decrease in DeMeester score and proximal and distal esophageal acid exposure as well as an increase in the mean lower esophageal sphincter pressure after surgery. While surgery in patients with Barrett's esophagus is often more difficult (secondary to higher incidence of large hiatal hernias, esophageal inflammation, and shortened esophagus) these findings would suggest that surgery is equally effective for controlling symptoms in Barrett's patients as for those with uncomplicated reflux.

Secondly, antireflux surgery is more likely to be associated with control, and even regression of Barrett's mucosa when compared to medical therapy. In our own series of 54 patients with short segment Barrett's esophagus (<3 cm) undergoing a laparoscopic antireflux operation, 30 (55%) had complete regression of their disease at a mean follow-up of 43 months. While we did observe the resolution of dysplasia in many cases, complete regression of long segment Barrett's (>3 cm) did not occur after LARS. The regression of dysplasia is reported by other authors [27, 29, 30]. An increase in apoptosis in metaplastic cells and stabilization of cellular proliferation after surgery have also been described, and may be at least one explanation for the superiority of surgical therapy [31, 32]. There is little data to support significant regression rates in patients being treated with medical therapy. Hameeteman and colleagues demonstrated that at 5 years, 5 of 50 patients treated medically developed cancer; four developed low-grade dysplasia and two high-grade dysplasia [33].

These observations may be the result of more effective control of regurgitation after an operation. Many patients on medical therapy will experience symptom control, but most will continue to have abnormal esophageal acid exposure [34]. In addition, medical therapy does not control or prevent bile reflux. Bile salts can induce the development of intestinal metaplasia when exposed to the esophageal mucosa. In the only randomized study comparing medical and. surgical therapy for GERD with long-term follow-up, roughly a third of patients enrolled had Barrett's esophagus [35]. At 10-year follow-up, no patient in the surgical arm died of esophageal caner, while 4% of patients in the medical arm succumbed to the disease.

While regression of Barrett's esophagus is possible after operation, surgery does not alleviate or replace the need for ongoing surveillance, as our series and others demonstrate. We believe, however, that surgery should be considered in young patients, those desiring cessation of medical therapy and/or those with breakthrough symptom, older patients with good functional status and life expectancy, those with indeterminate or low-grade dysplasia, and those with large hiatal hernias. A laparoscopic approach is appropriate in these patients and results in excellent patient satisfaction [27, 36]. It controls symptoms, allows for the discontinuation of medicine, and gives the patient the best chance at regression of the disease.

12.2.3
Laparoscopy and the Short Esophagus

Various disease processes (peptic stricture, Barrett's esophagus, hiatal hernia) can foreshorten the esophagus resulting in migration of the gastroesophageal junction (GEJ) above the diaphragm. Critical to achieving good outcomes after antireflux surgery is ensuring adequate esophageal length. If the esophagus is left foreshortened at the time of surgery, the repair may be left under tension increasing the risk of a post-operative hiatal hernia and ultimate failure of the operation to control the patient's symptoms. Thus, how can the short esophagus be identified, either pre-operatively or at the time of surgery, and what is the best way to correct the problem when it is discovered?

Various studies have attempted to identify risk factors associated with the short esophagus. DeMeester and colleagues found that while a short esophageal length could be identified with preoperative manometry, only the presence esophageal stricture predicted the need for a lengthening procedure at the time of surgery [37]. In this same study, patients with Barrett's of 3 cm or greater had shortened esophagus, but could be managed with esophageal mobilization alone. Urbach et al. used logistic regression to demonstrate that a patient's clinical characteristics alone were sufficient to predict who would need a lengthening procedure as a result of esophageal shortening [38]. These characteristics included the presence of a stricture, a paraesophageal hernia, Barrett's esophagus, and previous surgery. Filipi and colleges found endoscopy to be the most sensitive tool for preoperative screening [39]. The sensitivity could be increased when combined with esophagraphy and manometry. While we routinely obtain these studies as part of the patient's preoperative evaluation, they will never assure the presence or absence of this problem. They can, however, suggest when to discuss surgical options with the patent.

If a short esophagus is identified, the surgeon has several options. A Collis gastroplasty can be performed laparoscopically. While most series report the improvement or resolution of patient symptoms with this approach, this procedure is not without problems. The neoesophagus that is created has an acid-secreting gastric mucosa proximal to the fundoplication as well as a loss of distal esophageal motility [40]. Kleimann and Halbfass reported on a series of patients undergoing laparoscopic Collis gastroplasty at the time of antireflux surgery [41]. While the procedure was effective in obtaining esophageal length and controlling symptoms, acid production from the neoesophagus above the wrap lead to incomplete restitution of acid exposure. In Swanstrom and colleagues' series of 15 patients, 50% had abnormal 24-h pH studies postoperatively [40]. As a result, the authors recommended maintenance acid-suppression therapy after surgery.

In our experience, the need for creating a neoesophagus is unnecessary in the vast majority of patients, as adequate esophageal mobilization is usually possible since the dissection can be carried out with relative ease high up in the mediastinum. We place all patients in steep head-up position (reverse Trendelenberg) and use a 30° angled laparoscope. This allows for excellent visualization of the hiatus and distal thoracic esophagus. A Penrose drain placed around the esophagus enables the surgeon to apply gentle traction such that extensive mobilization into the chest can be safely performed. CO_2 peritoneum often facilitates this mobilization as gas dissects into the mediastinum enhancing exposure. If the GEJ does not clearly reach well into the abdomen, we advocate the use of endoscopy to assure adequate esophageal length. We prospectively studied 40 patients with intraoperative endoscopy to assess the accuracy of identifying the GEJ with laparoscopy [42]. In 90% of patients the "laparoscopic" GEJ was within 1 cm of the "endoscopic" GEJ. Of the remaining 10% the GEJ was always higher endoscopically; in other words, the esophagus was even shorter than the surgeon believed. This is an important finding, since all of these patients had complicated GERD (esophagitis, Barrett's esophagus, and/or hiatal hernia), the very patients at risk for a short esophagus and surgical failure.

12.2.4
Antireflux Surgery in Patients with Respiratory Symptoms

The association between GERD and typical symptoms (e.g., regurgitation, heartburn) is fairly clear. It is difficult, however, to link respiratory symptoms to reflux, and as such, it is even more difficult to provide appropriately directed therapy for these patients. This is secondary to the fact that respiratory symptoms (cough, hoarseness, etc.) are nonspecific in nature.

The exact mechanism by which reflux causes respiratory symptoms is unclear. Aspiration is one obvious, and likely common mechanism of airway injury. Studies have demonstrated that aspiration is often the result of GER and a motor dysfunction in the esophagus impairing esophageal clearance [43, 44]. Vagal nerve stimulation may induce brochospasm or potentiate the bronchomotor response to other triggers [45]. The volume of reflux may also have direct impact on patients' symptoms. Irwin et al. demonstrated that the mechanism by which GER causes cough is related to a critical number and/or duration of reflux episodes in the proximal and/or distal esophagus [46]. Varying amounts of aspiration may induce local irritation in the larynx and upper airways. While an acidic refluxate may cause mucosal irritation, it is possible that neutralized and/or alkaline gastric contents may cause symptoms. New diagnostic tools such as multichannel impedance, which measures all refluxate regardless of pH, may help to further clarify and understand this pathophysiology.

The most difficult problem in this disease is one of diagnosis. Symptoms alone are not sufficient for diagnosing reflux-induced respiratory disease. Respiratory symptoms have many etiologies, only one of which is GERD. The presence of typical symptoms of reflux (heartburn, regurgitation) does not mean that GERD is the cause (since they are present in up to 40% of the population), nor does their absence exclude GERD as the cause (as they are absent in many patients with proven microaspiration). This poor predictive value of symptoms has been clearly demonstrated [47]. In our own series of 518 patients evaluated for pharyngeal reflux (PR), a strong indicator of microaspiration, the presence of these symptoms were equally present between those with and without the disease.

We must, therefore, rely on more objective measures. The most common tests are 24-h pH monitoring (with at least proximal esophageal, if not pharyngeal, monitoring) and direct laryngoscopy. We have found the strongest correlation between GERD and respiratory symptoms can be made with a combination of these two studies which includes pharyngeal pH monitoring [48, 49]. While this combination is not as effective as endoscopy and pH monitoring in diagnosing typical GERD, they are currently the best link between respiratory symptoms and reflux. The technique used for pharyngeal pH monitoring will not be reviewed here, but we emphasize the importance of this test since it gives the strongest evidence for microaspiration. We have found it to be extremely helpful, and not equivalent to traditional pH monitoring. In fact, some patients with significant PR will have normal esophageal acid exposure, and thus would be missed by traditional monitoring [50].

Treatment options are the same as for those with typical symptoms. While medical therapy works in some patients, it is less effective for atypical GERD symptoms and less effective than surgery [51–54]. Larrain et al. demonstrated at long-term follow up (6 years) that patients treated with surgery for non-allergic asthma continued to have symptom improvement and a decrease in their medication requirement [55]. This was not the case in those treated with medicine or placebo. This is probably due the inability of medicine to adequately control regurgitation and aspiration. In addition to removing acid, surgery eliminates regurgitation and thus aspiration potential. This is critical, because even small amounts of regurgitation may result in the persistence of airway symptoms [56].

We have found that the presence of pharyngeal reflux on pH monitoring is an excellent predictor of respiratory symptom response after surgery [57]. We studied 21 patients with extraesophageal symptoms of reflux and found nine with PR. After operation, seven had resolution of PR on 24-h pH evaluation. Of the two with persistent PR, persistent esophageal reflux was demonstrated, thus indicating GEJ incompetence. If esophageal acid exposure normalized, PR was eliminated and respiratory symptoms improved. If pharyngeal reflux was absent preoperatively, however, respiratory symptoms were more likely to persist after surgery.

12.3
Summary

— We believe that surgery is an effective therapy for GERD. A Nissen fundoplication is the procedure of choice, as it provides the best control of reflux and uncommonly results in long-term dysphagia. Even in the face of clinical and/or manometric dysphagia, a floppy Nissen is effective and can actually improve swallowing in many patients.

— Surgery is the most effective therapy for Barrett's esophagus, as it controls symptoms and may lead to regression of the disease.

— The short esophagus rarely requires a lengthening procedure if appropriate mobilization of the esophagus is performed. Construction of a neoesophagus can be done laparoscopically if mobilization fails, but the surgeon should be aware of the potential problems associated with it.

— Surgery is effective in treating respiratory symptoms if patients are selected carefully using appropriate diagnostic techniques. Outcomes, however, are less predictable than for those in patients with typical GERD symptoms.

References

1. Wetscher GJ, Glaser K, Wieschemeyer T, Gadenstaetter M, Prommegger R, Profanter C. Tailored antireflux surgery for gastroesophageal reflux disease: effectiveness and risk of postoperative dysphagia. World J Surg 1997;21:605–610.

2. Patti MG, De Pinto M, de Bellis M, Arcerito M, Tong J, Wang A, et al. Comparison of laparoscopic total and partial fundoplication for gastroesophageal reflux. J. Gastrointest Surg 1997;1:309–15

3. DeMeester TR, Stein HJ. Minimizing the side effects of antireflux surgery. World J. Surg 1992;16:335–6.

4. Lund RJ, Wecher GJ, Raiser F, Glaser K, Perdikis G, Gadenstatter M, et al. Laparoscopic Toupet fundoplication for gastroesophageal reflux disease with poor esophageal body motility. J Gastrointest Surg 1997;1:301–8

5. Katzka DA. Motility abnormalities in gastroesophageal reflux disease. Gastroenterol Clin North Am 1999;28:905–15.

6. Holzinger F, Banz M, Tscharner GG, Merki H, Muller E, Klaiber C. Laparoscopic Toupet partial fundoplication as general surgical therapy of gastroesophageal reflux. 1-Year results of a 5-year prospective long-term study. [In German]. Chirurg 2001;72:6–13.

7. McKernan JB. Laparoscopic repair of gastroesophageal reflux disease. Toupet partial fundopliation versus Nissen fundoplication. Surg Endosc 1994;8:851–6.

8. Thor KB, Silander T. A long-term randomized prospective trial of the Nissen procedure versus a modified Toupet technique. Ann Surg 1989;210:719–24.

9. Low DE, Mercer CD, James EC, Hill LD. Post Nissen syndrome. Surg Gynecol Obstet 1988;167:1–5.

10. Csendes A, Burdiles P, Korn O, Braghetto I, Huertas C, Rojas J. Late results of a randomized clinical trial comparing total fundoplication versus calibration of the cardia with posterior gastropexy. Br J Surg 2000;87:289–97.

11. Puhalla H, Lenglinger J, Bischof G, Miholic J, Fugger R, Stacher G. Nissen and Toupet laparoscopic fundoplication in patients with gastroesophageal reflux and motility disorders of the distal esophagus. Chirurg 2002;73:230–4.

12. Rydberg L, Ruth M, Abrahamsson H, Lundell L. Tailoring antireflux surgery: a randomized clinical trial. World J Surg 1999;23:612–8.
13. Fibbe C, Layer P, Keller J, Strate U, Emmermann A, Zornig C. Esophageal motility in reflux disease before and after fundoplication: a prospective, randomized, clinical, and manometric study. Gastroenterology 2001;121:5–14.
14. Bessell JR, Finch R, Gotley DC, Smithers BM, Nathanson L, Menzies B. Chronic dysphagia following laparoscopic fundoplication Br J Surg 2000;87:1341–5.
15. Heider TR, Farrell TM, Kircher AP, Colliver CC, Koruda MJ, Behrns KE. Complete fundoplication is not associated with increased dysphagia in patients with abnormal esophageal motility. J Gastrointest Surg 2001;5:36–41.
16. Heider TR, Behrns KE, Koruda MJ, Shaheen NJ, Lucktong TA, Bradshaw B, et al. Fundopliation improves disordered esophageal motility. J Gastrointest Surg 2003;7:159–63.
17. Oleynikoiv, D, Eubanks TR, Oelschlager BK, Pellegrini CA. Total fundoplication is the operation of choice for patients with gastroesophageal reflux and defective peristalsis. Surg Endosc 2002;6:909–13.
18. Fernando HC, Luketich JD, Christie NA, Ikramuddin S, Schauer PR. Outcomes of laparoscopic Toupet compared to laparoscopic Nissen fundoplication. Surg Endosc 2002;6:905–8.
19. Jobe BA, Wallace J, Hansen PD, Sanstrom LL. Evaluation of laparoscopic Toupet fundoplication as a primary repair for all patients with medically resistant gastroesphageal reflux. Surg Endosc 1997;11:1080–3.
20. Ottignon Y, Pelissier EP, Mantion G, Clement C, Birgen C, Deschamps JP, et al. Gastroesophageal reflux. comparison of clinical, pH-metric and manometric results of Nissen's and of Toupet's procedures. Gastroenterol Clin Biol 1994;18:920–6.
21. Horvath KD, Jobe BA, Herron DM, Swanstrom LL. Laparoscopic Toupet fundoplication is an inadequate procedure for patients with severe reflux disease. J Gastrointest Surg 1999;3:583–91.
22. Farrell TM, Archer SB, Galloway KD, Branum GD, Smith CD, Hunter JG. Heartburn is more likely to recur after Toupet fundoplication than Nissen fundoplication. Am Surg 2000;66:229–36.
23. Klapow JC, Wilcox CM, Mallinger AP, Marks R, Heudebert GR, Centor RM, et al. Characterization of long-term outcomes after Toupet fundoplication: symptoms, medication use and health status. J Clin Gastroenterol 2002;34:509–15.
24. Bell RC, Hanna P, Mills MR, Bowrey D. Patterns of success and failure with laparoscopic Toupet fundoplication. Surg Endsoc 1999;13:1189–94.
25. Atwood SE, Barlow AP, Norris TL, Watson A. Barrett's oesophagus: effect of antireflux surgery on symptom control and development of complications. Br J Surg 1999;79:1050–3.
26. Farrell TM, Smith CD, Metreveli RE, Johnson AB, Galloway KD, Hunter JG. Fundoplication provides effective and durable symptom relief in patients with Barrett's esophagus. Am J Surg 1999;178:18–21.
27. Hofstetter WL, Peters JH, DeMeester TR, Hagen JA, DeMeeester SR, Crookes PF, et al. Long-term outcome of antireflux surgery in patients with Barrett's esophagus. Annal Surg 2001;4:532–9.
28. Klaus A, Hinder RA. Medical therapy versus antireflux surgery in Barrett's esophagus: what is the best therapeutic approach. Dig Dis 2000;234:224–31.

29. DeMeester SR, DeMeester TR. The diagnosis and management of Barrett's esophagus. Adv Surg 1999;33:29–68.
30. Low DE, Levine DS, Dail DH, Kozarek RA. Histological and anatomic changes in Barrett's esophagus after antireflux surgery. Am J Gastroenterol 1999;94:80–5.
31. Chen LQ, Hu CY, Der Sarkissian S, Ferraro P, Pera M, deBlois D, Gaboury L, Duranceau AC. Apoptosis in Barrett's oesophagus following antireflux surgery. Br J Surg 2002;89:1444–9.
32. Chen LQ, Hu CY, Gaboury L, Pera M, Ferraro P, Duranceau AC. Proliferative activity in Barrett's esophagus before and after antireflux surgery. Annal Surg 2001;234:172–80.
33. Hameeteman W, Tytgat GW, Houthoff HJ, van den Tweel JG. Barrett's esophagus: development of dysplasia and adenocarcinoma. Gastroenterology 1989;96:1249–56.
34. Kuo B, Castell DO. Optimal Dosing of Omeprazole 40 mg Daily: effects on gastric and esophageal pH and serum gastrin in healthy controls. Am J Gastroenterol 1996;91:1532–8.
35. Spechler SJ, Lee E, Ahnen D, Goyal RK, Hirano I, Ramirez F, et al. Long-term outcome of medical and surgical therapies for gastroesophageal reflux disease: follow-up of a randomized controlled trial. JAMA 2001;285:2331–8.
36. Yau P, Watson DI, Devitt PG, Game PA, Jamieson GG. Laparoscopic antireflux surgery in the treatment of gastroesophageal reflux in patients with Barrett esophagus. Arch Surg 200;135:801–5.
37. Gastal OL, Hagen JA, Peters JH, Campos GM, Hashemi M, Theisen J, et al. Short esophagus: analysis of predictors and clinical implications. Arch Surg 1999;134:633–6.
38. Urbach DR, Khajanchee YS, Glasgow RE, Hansen PD, Swanstrom LL. Preoperative determinants of an esophageal lengthening procedure in laparoscopic antireflux surgery. Surg Endosc 2001;15:1408–12.
39. Awad ZT, Mittal SK, Roth TA, Anderson PI, Wilfley WA Jr, Filipi CJ. Esophageal shortening during the era of laparoscopic surgery. World J Surg 2001;25:558–61.
40. Jobe BA, Horvath KD, Swanstrom LL. Postoperative function following laparoscopic collis gastroplasty for shortened esophagus. Arch Surg 1998;133:867–74.
41. Kleimann E, Halbfass HJ. The „short esophagus problem" in laparoscopic anti-reflux surgery. [In German]. Chirurg 2001;72:408–13.
42. Chang L, Oelschlager B, Barreca M, Pellegrini C. Improving accuracy in the identification of the gastroesophageal junction during laparoscopic antireflux surgery. Surg Endosc 2003;17:390–3.
43. Pellegrini CA, DeMeester TR, Johnson LF, Skinner DB. Gastroesophageal reflux and pulmonary aspiration: incidence, functional abnormality, and results of surgical therapy. Surgery 1979;86:110–9.
44. Patti MG, Debas HT, Pellegrini CA. Esophageal manometry and 24-hour pH monitoring in the diagnosis of pulmonary aspiration secondary to gastroesophageal reflux. Am J Surg 1992;163:401–6.
45. Simpson WG. Gastroesophageal reflux disease and astham. diagnosis and management. Arch Intern Med 1995;155:798–803.
46. Irwin RS, Zawacki JK, Curley FJ, French CL, Hoffman PJ. Chronic cough as the sole presenting manifestation of gastroesophageal reflux. Am Rev Respir Dis 1989;140:1294–3000.

47. Oelschlager BK, Chang L, Barreca M, Pope CE II, Pellegrini CA. Typical GERD symptoms and esophageal ph monitoring are not enough to diagnose pharyngeal reflux: analysis of 518 patients. Am J Gastroenterol 2004; (in press).

48. Oelschlager BK, Pellegrini CA. Surgical treatment of repiratory complications associated with gastroesophageal reflux disease. Am J Med 2003;115 Suppl 3A:72S–7S.

49. Oelschlager B, Eubanks TR, Maronian N, Hillel A, Oleynikov D, Pope CE, Pellegrini CA. Laryngoscopy and pharyngeal pH are complimentary in the diagnosis of gastroesophageal-laryngeal reflux. J Gastrointest Surg 2002;6:189–94.

50. Katz P. Ambulatory esophageal and hypopharyngeal pH monitoring in patients with hoarseness. Am J Gastroenterol 1990;85:38–40.

51. Gadenstatter M, Wykypiel H, Schwab GP, Profanter C, Wetscher GJ. Respiratory symptoms and dysphagia in patients with gastroesophageal reflux disease: a comparison of medical and surgical therapy. Langenbecks Arch Surg 1999;384:563–7.

52. Ours TM, Kavuru MS, Schilz RJ, Richter JE. A prospective evaluation of esophageal testing and a double-blind, randomized study of omeprazole in a diagnostic and therapeutic algorithm for chronic cough. Am J Gastroenterol 1999;94:3131–8.

53. Lundell L, Dalenback J, Hattlebakk J, Janatuinen E, Levander K, Miettinen P, et al.; Nordic GORD-Study Group. Outcome of open antireflux surgery as assessed in a Nordic multicentre prospective clinical trial. Eur J Surg 1998;164:751–7.

54. Bowrey DJ, Peters JH, DeMeester TR. Gastroesophageal reflux disease in asthma. effects of medical and surgical antireflux therapy on asthma control. Ann Surg 2000;231:161–72.

55. Larrain A, Carrasco E, Galleguillos F, Sepulveda R, Pope CE 2nd. Medical and surgical treatment of nonallergic asthma associated with gastroesophageal reflux. Chest 1991;99:1330–5.

56. Wetscher GJ, Glaser K, Hinder RA, P:erdikis G, Klinger P, Bammer T, et al. Respiratory symptoms in patients with gastroesophageal reflux disease following medical therapy and following antireflux surgery. Am J Surg 1997;174:639–43.

57. Oelschlager BK, Eubanks TR, Oleynikov D, Pope C, Pellegrini CA. Symptomatic and physiologic outcomes after operative treatment for extraesophageal reflux. Surg Endosc 2002;16:1032–6.

Commentary

Zygmunt H. Krukowski

This is an interesting assessment of four issues addressed on a regular basis by surgeons treating patients with GERD and its complications. Whilst these issues are only controversial because of a lack of high quality evidence, this is true for much of contemporary surgical practice.

Which Antireflux Operation for Ineffective Esophageal Motility?

Of the four controversies addressed, the first is the most contentious. The arguments about the optimal antireflux procedure are far from resolved and the weakness of the current fashion for evidence-based practice is exposed if clinical preference, even prejudice, is supported by selective reference to low-quality evidence. This section illustrates how, as surgeons, our practice is biased towards personal experience bolstered by reference to favorable reports especially when the "gold standard" of methodologically sound randomized clinical trials is lacking.

The question of tailoring the extent of the fundoplication to suit esophageal motility determined by preoperative manometry appears redundant. Numerous individual reports and a recent review [1] have confirmed that postoperative dysphagia that persists is not related to the extent of the fundoplication. Most cases of severe early dysphagia are due to technical errors and may be related to the institutional and surgical experience [2]. The motor disorder demonstrated preoperatively appears to be reversible in many patients, and the anxiety that dysphagia will be aggravated following total fundoplication is erroneous. Many patients experience improvement in dysphagia following successful fundoplication and those who develop it as a new feature postoperatively may be from a different subset.

A corollary, if preoperative motility testing is largely irrelevant in the routine assessment, is that the choice of operation may be equally irrelevant. The authors have a substantial practice in laparoscopic Nissen fundoplication. The satisfactory outcome for the treated population is such that they are convinced that this is the optimum procedure although their opinion is based on historical, sequential and nonrandomized data. This is scarcely a criticism in that possession of prospectively collected surgical outcome data is the exception rather than rule. However, if information from only randomized trials is selectively quoted there is not a single trial comparing partial with total fundoplication that shows a clear advantage for the Nissen procedure. Indeed when the trial does not show equivalence the preferred option is always for the partial wrap (Table 12.1).

If there is comparable control of reflux and less risk of dysphagia with a partial wrap, will they be of comparable durability. Unlike upper gastrointestinal surgery for malignancy, where a few years survival is an achievement, antireflux surgery is expected to last a lifetime, which may mean 50 years for many patients. Recurrent symptoms are often the trigger for surgical reassessment and for most surgeons long-term review is limited to these patients. Determining durability is a minefield. Firstly, one needs to define failure – is this clinical, which may be as insubstantial as the patient being prescribed a proton pump inhibitor again, or by rigorous physiological testing. If the lat-

Table 12.1. Preferred options of antireflux operation for ineffective esophageal motility

Authors [ref.]	Date	Comparison	Preference
Thor and Silander [3]	1989	Open Nissen vs open Toupet	Toupet
Lundell et al. [4]	1996	Open Nissen vs open Toupet	Toupet
Laws et al. [5]	1997	Lap Nissen vs lap Toupet	Equal / Toupet
Rydberg et al. [6]	1999	Open Nissen vs open Toupet	Equal / Toupet
Watson et al. [7]	1999	Lap Nissen vs lap anterior	Anterior
Csendes et al. [8]	2000	Open Nissen vs open Toupet	Equal
Fibbe et al. [9]	2001	Open Nissen vs open Toupet	Equal / Toupet

ter, it is hard to persuade the majority of patients to undergo repeat 24-h pH monitoring and, if an abnormal profile is produced in an asymptomatic patient, how is that to be classed? Equally a symptomatic patient with a normal profile can be counted as either an objective surgical success or a subjective patient failure depending on perspective.

Our experience includes a three center comparison between open Nissen, laparoscopic Nissen and laparoscopic anterior fundoplication. Outcomes assessed by quality of life and gastrointestinal symptom measures showed a similar cumulative recurrence of reflux symptoms with the passage of time with each procedure. One effect of the study was to contribute to a change to partial fundoplication in the laparoscopic Nissen centre. The authors state, and one cannot disagree, that with a well-fashioned floppy Nissen long-term dysphagia is a rare problem. In a consecutive personal series of 514 laparoscopic hiatal procedures, however, none of 447 laparoscopic anterior fundoplications for uncomplicated GERD have experienced serious long-term dysphagia although 18 (4.0%) have required reoperation to date for either recurrent reflux or a (small) para-esophageal hernia. Without large randomized trials these are issues that will keep this debate live for another 20 years unless, of course, antireflux surgery goes the way of elective duodenal ulcer surgery.

Laparoscopic Surgery and Barrett's Esophagus

The concept of a relationship between gastroesophageal reflux and esophagogastric cancer is innately attractive and supported by the increasing incidence of both in the Western World. Insofar as medical therapy may treat symptoms but does not prevent reflux, surgery is a more attractive option if the intent is to abolish the stimulus to metaplasia, dyplasia and, presumably, subsequent neoplasia. There is accumulating collateral and circumstantial evidence that supports this hypothesis. The overlap between short-segment Barrett's and a small hiatus hernia suggests that some of the regression noted in short-segment Barrett's esophagus after laparoscopic fundoplication may be a consequence of the reconstructed anatomy. The failure of surgery to completely reverse long-segment disease should be interpreted positively in view of the lack of any alternative therapy.

Laparoscopy and the Short Esophagus

One of the great benefits of the introduction of laparoscopic techniques to antireflux surgery was the dramatically improved visualization of the thoracic esophagus through the hiatus. This permits more accurate and extensive mobilization than was possible under direct vision and the problem of inadequate esophageal length has become vanishingly rare. This may well have been influenced by the advent of proton pump inhibitors and the reduced threshold for referral for surgery that accompanied laparoscopic surgery. Consequently patients with a chronically strictured esophagus requiring an esophageal lengthening procedure as a primary procedure are extremely uncommon and I have not encountered such a patient in 514 procedures – none of whom required conversion to a laparotomy.

Antireflux Surgery in Patients with Respiratory Symptoms

This is a relatively disappointing area in terms of outcome after laparoscopic fundoplication. The attractive concept that many respiratory symptoms may be caused or aggravated by overt or occult reflux and aspiration has proved an oversimplification, as the authors demonstrate. Measurement of pharyngeal reflux is a refinement to pH monitoring that is not universally available but appears to be more discriminating, albeit with a failure rate of 2 in 9 (22%) patients.

References

1. Wills V, Hunt DR. Dysphagia after antireflux surgery. Br J Surg 2001;88:486–99
2. Hunter JG, Smith CD, Branum GD, et al. Laparoscopic fundoplication failures: patterns of failure and response to fundoplication revision. Ann Surg 1999;230:595–606
3. Thor KB, Silander T. A long-term randomized prospective trial of the Nissen procedure versus a modified Toupet technique. Ann Surg 1989;210:719–24
4. Lundell L, Abrahamsson H, Ruth M, Rydberg L, Lonroth H, Olbe L. Long-term results of a prospective randomized comparison of total fundic wrap (Nissen-Rossetti) or semifundoplication (Toupet) for gastro-oesophageal reflux. Br J Surg 1996;83:830–5
5. Laws HL, Clements RH, Swillie CM. A randomized, prospective comparison of the Nissen fundoplication versus the Toupet fundoplication for gastroesophageal reflux disease. Ann Surg 1997;225:647–54
6. Rydberg L, Ruth M, Lundell L. Mechanism of action of antireflux procedures. Br J Surg 1999;86:405–10
7. Watson DI, Jamieson GG, Devitt PG. Prospective randomized double-blind trial between laparoscopic Nissen fundoplication and anterior partial fundoplication. Br J Surg 1999;86:971
8. Csendes A,. Burdiles P, Korn O, et al. Late results of a randomized clinical trial comparing total fundoplication versus calibration of the cardia with posterior gastropexy. Br J Surg 2000;87:289–97
9. Fibbe C, Layer P, Keller J, et al. Esophageal motility in reflux disease before and after fundoplication: a prospective, randomized, clinical, and manometric study. Gastroenterology 2001;121:5–14

Achalasia

Laurent Biertho, Bernard Dallemagne

> ► ## Key Controversies
>
> A. Therapeutic options: dilatation versus surgery
> B. Laparoscopic versus thoracoscopic approach
> C. Extent of myotomy
> D. Fundoplication versus no fundoplication
> E. Partial versus 360° fundoplication
> F. Management of patients with mega-esophagus

13.1
Introduction

The term "achalasia" is of Greek derivation and literally means "failure to relax", which describes one of the cardinal feature of this disorder: a lack of relaxation in the lower esophageal sphincter (LES). Associated with a poorly contracting esophageal body, this creates the classical symptoms associated with motor disorders of the esophagus: dysphagia, chest pain, regurgitation and eventually weight loss. Another potential risk with long-standing achalasia is esophageal cancer, which is increased about 140-fold over that of the general population [1].

Even if many factors have been advocated for the etiology of this disease (viral infection, genetic factors, auto-immune response, etc.), the cause of achalasia is still unknown and its treatment is thus directed at palliation of symptoms and prevention of complications instead of cure [2].

Heller, who first described the surgical management of achalasia in 1913 [3], performed an anterior and posterior esophageal myotomy. The technique was then modified by Zaaijer who described the classical anterior myotomy, and by Ellis who reported, in 1958, the left thoracic approach for the treatment of this disease. At the beginning of the 1990s, minimally invasive techniques were applied to achalasia and quickly superseded the open procedure.

We will discuss in this chapter the best therapeutic options for achalasia and controversies in its laparoscopic management.

13.2
Discussion

13.2.1
Therapeutic Options: Dilatation versus Surgery?

Four palliative treatments are currently available: medical treatment, botulinum toxin injections, endoscopic dilatation and myotomy. All are intended to reduce LES pressure and improve emptying by gravity, but none have an effect on esophageal aperistalsis. Each treatment has been advocated for the treatment of achalasia but the ideal treatment is still controversial.

Muscle relaxant medications and botulinum toxin injections seem to be best suited for patients with contraindications to pneumatic dilatation or surgery, or patients who would benefit from their short-term effects. Moreover, as botulinum toxin injection seems to make dissection of the submucosal plane more difficult and contributed to an increased number of mucosal perforations, some authors consider that it should be used only in patients who are not eligible for surgery [4].

Pneumatic dilatation and surgical myotomy seem to offer longer-lasting benefits for both symptoms and esophageal emptying and are considered as the two optimal treatments for this disease (Table 13.1) [5–7].

The only available prospective randomized control trial comparing open surgical myotomy and pneumatic dilatation supports the benefit of surgical treatment [8]. In this trial, 91% of the surgical group and 51% of the dilatation group had near-complete symptom resolution after 5 years of follow-up. In a meta-analysis examining the efficacy of the three major treatment options, Spiess et al. [9] concluded that laparoscopic myotomy was superior to pneumatic dilatation or botulinum toxin injections. They also found laparoscopic myotomy to be superior or equivalent to open approach. For the management

Table 13.1. Results of various management options in achalasia

	Botulinum toxin	Pneumatic dilatation	Surgical myotomy + fundoplication
Initial response	90% at 1 month	60–90% at 1 year	>90% at 1 year
Later response	60% at 1 year	60% at 5 years	85% at 5 years
Morbidity	Not available	25–35% reflux 0–5% perforation	10–15% reflux

of initial stage of megaesophagus, Felix et al. [7], comparing balloon dilatation with myotomy with esophagofundopexy, showed that both methods had similar results regarding ongoing suppression of dysphagia and development of reflux esophagitis but dilatation provoked a greater index of esophageal acid exposition time. Finally, long-term studies have shown that success rate of pneumatic dilatation decreases to about 50% after 10 years [10], while the effect of surgery tends to persist over time (>90% success rate with symptomatic gastroesophageal reflux disease in 10–15% of cases), as most of the failure manifests during the first postoperative year [8, 11, 12].

Pneumatic dilatation remains thus an acceptable option, with its brief period of discomfort, very short hospital stay and consequent low expenses. However, the non-negligible morbidity rate, with a perforation rate up to 5%, frequent need for redilation and high prevalence of recurrent dysphagia within the first several years limits its appeal [13].

These facts, coupled with the long-term success and safety of laparoscopic myotomy, are shifting the balance toward surgical therapy.

13.2.2
Laparoscopic versus Thoracoscopic Approach

Both procedures seem to be as affective as their open counterparts yet have the advantages of offering shorter hospital stays, less blood loss, less postoperative pain, less incisional hernia and better cosmetic results.

Thoracoscopic approach has an 85–90% very-good-to-excellent result, which is similar to laparoscopic technique [14–16]. However, in a study comparing 35 left thoracoscopic myotomy and 133 laparoscopic myotomy plus partial fundoplication, Patti and colleagues [16, 17] concluded that laparoscopic approach should be considered the primary approach for esophageal achalasia for different reasons: patients operated by laparoscopy had less postoperative gastroesophageal reflux (17% for laparoscopic myotomy versus 60% for thorascopic), dysphagia was completely relieved in a higher percentage of the patients (77% versus 70%, respectively), and patients were more comfortable and left the hospital earlier after laparoscopy. Ramacciato et al. [18] also compared a series of 16 thoracoscopic myotomies with another series of 17 laparoscopic myotomies with fundoplication. They found significant advantages in the laparoscopic group: a reduced operative time and hospital stay, reduced persistence of recurrent dysphagia and a diminished postoperative reflux. They also concluded that laparoscopic myotomy with fundoplication was associated with a lower LES pressure and mean esophageal diameter.

Interestingly, Cade [19] compared a series of 18 achalasia patients operated by thoracoscopy and a series of 18 patients operated by laparoscopy without fundoplication. In that study, laparoscopy failed to show any advantage over thoracoscopy. The advantages of laparoscopy could thus possibly result from fundoplication being performed in the laparoscopic group but not in the thoracoscopic group.

Other limitations of thoracoscopic approach are the poor exposure of the gastroesophageal junction when trying to extend the myotomy onto the gastric wall, intraoperative management is much more cumbersome (i.e., selective ventilation, lateral decubitus), postoperative discomfort due to the chest tube and difficulty to correct preexisting reflux from pneumatic dilatation.

Laparoscopic approach is thus considered by many authors the operation of choice for the treatment of achalasia, with main advantages being a reduced incidence of postoperative dysphagia and reflux when an antireflux procedure is added.

13.2.3
Extent of Myotomy

The extent of myotomy remains an unresolved technical question in the treatment of achalasia.

A complete exposition of the gastroesophageal junction is mandatory. A longitudinal incision is made on the gastroesophageal junction and the muscle fibers are split until the hypertrophied circular muscles fibers are exposed. The circular fibers are then divided until the epithelial tube spouts out. Separation of the muscularis from the submucosa at the margin of the incision is important to prevent the divided layers to reapproximate as healing occurs. Laparoscopic magnification allows this to be done with precision. The myotomy is extended proximally until reaching normal circular esophageal muscle.

Some surgeons advocate a short esophagomyotomy carried onto the stomach only far enough to ensure complete division of the distal esophageal musculature, but not far enough to induce incompetence of the LES mechanism. With this approach, several surgeons reported a late incidence of postoperative gastroesophageal reflux of about 8% [20].

Most authors however consider that complete relief of the obstruction caused by the uncoordinated LES can be achieved only by rendering the LES totally incompetent, i.e., by carrying the esophagomyotomy onto the stomach for 1–2 cm. Most esophageal surgeons now carry out a complete esophago-cardiomyotomy for achalasia, extending 4–6 cm above the gastroesophageal junction and 1–2 cm onto the stomach, with some type of fundoplication to prevent the subsequent development of gastroesophageal reflux. Excellent long-term results suggest that a distal esophagomyotomy combined with a partial fundoplication may be the surgical approach of choice in achalasia.

These results, however, need to be confirmed by prospective randomized trials.

13.2.4
Fundoplication versus No Fundoplication

Gastroesophageal reflux is the most common complication after Heller myotomy without fundoplication. However, the frequency of gastrointestinal reflux disease (GERD) after destruction of LES competency ranges from 0 to 50% [21]. This disparity contributes to the controversy regarding the interest for an antireflux procedure.

Reflux has been reported more frequently after transabdominal Heller than after transthoracic Heller myotomy [22]. A disruption of LES mechanism after abdominal approach is suspected as the reason for this difference. This would justify the addition of fundoplication after laparoscopic myotomy. It is Ellis's opinion [10] that an antireflux procedure is effectively mandatory after abdominal Heller myotomy, but is unnecessary after transthoracic Heller except when a hiatal hernia, reflux or both are present preoperatively.

Moreover, deterioration of results and increased reflux 10 years after Belsey fundoplication and Heller myotomy [23], increased reflux and dysphagia caused by poor emptying 10 years after surgery [24], and increased reflux 17 years after Heller myotomy without fundoplication [25], support the need for an antireflux procedure. Most authors routinely perform an antireflux procedure when a laparoscopic myotomy is required.

13.2.5
Partial versus 360° Fundoplication

There is little data available to guide the choice of fundoplication. Both partial and complete fundoplications offer effective therapy for reflux esophagitis in GERD [26]. However, abnormal esophageal motility is usually considered a relative contraindication to Nissen fundoplication, because of the purported risk of postoperative dysphagia. Early good results are usually obtained following Heller myotomy and Nissen fundoplication but, even if uncommon, overly competent Nissen fundoplication can occur [27]. Topart et al. [27] reported deterioration with recurrence of symptoms and retention. In their series, 29% of the patients had to be reoperated for dysphagia, because of overly competent distal esophageal wraps. On the other hand, Heider et al. [28] showed that Nissen fundoplication was not associated with increased dysphagia in patients with manometric criteria for abnormal esophageal motility. Most authors, however, prefer to perform partial fundoplication to reduce the incidence of postoperative dysphagia.

When partial fundoplication is considered, both anterior and posterior wraps likely provide adequate antireflux protection with minimal outflow resistance. Anterior (Dor) fundoplication has the advantage of protecting against microperforation, as the stomach covers the exposed esophageal mucosa, and not requiring disruption of the normal posterior gastroesophageal attachments (a theoretical advantage in preventing postoperative reflux). Partial fundoplications (Dor or Toupet) could have a lower incidence of immediate dysphagia but may be associated with increased postoperative esophageal acid exposure. However, long-term results are not well characterized. These data lead most authors to perform partial fundoplication, with a slight predilection for anterior fundoplication.

13.2.6
Management of Patients with Markedly Dilated Esophagus

It has been conventionally advised that myotomy will not reduce dysphagia in patients with markedly dilated or sigmoid shaped esophagus, and esophagectomy has been recommended in these patients [29]. Patti et al. [30] reported their results in a series of patients with varying degrees of esophageal dilatation. They concluded that laparoscopic Heller myotomy and Dor fundoplication was no more difficult in patients with dilated and tortuous esophagus, was associated with no more postoperative complications, and gave just as good relief of dysphagia. They proposed that myotomy should be considered as initial treatment of achalasia with dilated esophagus, and that esophagectomy be reserved for patients with persistent dysphagia who are not amenable to second myotomy. It should be noted, however, that there is only one such report to date.

13.3
Summary

- Reports are now available, showing that laparoscopic treatment outperforms balloon dilatation or botulinum toxin injection. With the high success rate of laparoscopic myotomy for achalasia, a shift in practice should occur: surgery should be the preferred treatment for achalasia.
- The extent of myotomy remains an unresolved question. Most authors perform a 4- to 6-cm proximal myotomy with 1- to 2-cm gastric myotomy. When this technique is used, the addition of an antireflux procedure is recommended.

— Although the need for an antireflux procedure in conjunction with Heller myotomy is controversial, there is a growing consensus that it is necessary when a laparoscopic approach is used.

— The choice of fundoplication could be trivial. However, partial wraps may avoid the risk of making an overly competent wrap. Anterior fundoplication has the interest to cover the myotomy and prevent microperforations, especially in redo cases.

— In conclusion, laparoscopic Heller cardiomyotomy extending 4–6 cm above the gastroesophageal junction and 1–2 cm onto the stomach, plus partial anterior (Dor) fundoplication, could be one of the optimal surgical treatment for patients with achalasia.

References

1. Brücher BL. Achalasia and esophageal cancer: incidence, prevalence and prognosis. World J Surg 2001;25:745–9.
2. Feldman M. Sleisenger and Fortran's gastrointestinal and liver disease, 7th edition; 2002. Philadelphia: WB Saunders. p. 577–84.
3. Heller E. Extramukose Cardioplastik beim Chronischen Cardiospasmus mit Dilatation des Oesophagus. Mitt Grenzgeb Med Chir 1913;27:141–9.
4. Patti MG, Feo CV, Arcerito M, De Pinto M, Tamburini A, Diener U, Gantert W, Way LW. Effects of previous treatment on results of laparoscopic Heller myotomy for achalasia. Dig Dis Sci 1999;44:2270–6.
5. Mikaeli J, Fazel A, Montazeri G, Yaghoobi M, Malekzadeh R. Randomized controlled trial comparing botulinum toxin injection to pneumatic dilatation for the treatment of achalasia. Aliment Pharmacol Ther 2001;15:1389–96.
6. Annese V, Bassotti G, Coccia G, Dinelli M, D'Onofrio V, Gatto G, Leandro G, Repici A, Testoni PA, Andriulli A; GISMAD Achalasia Study Group. A multicenter randomized study of intrasphincteric botulinum toxin inpatients with oesophageal achalasia. Gut 2000;46:597–600.
7. Felix VN, Cecconello I, Zilberstein B, Moraes-Filho JP, Pinotti HW, Carvalho E. Achalasia: a prospective study comparing the results of dilatation and myotomy. Hepatogastroenterology 1998;45:97–108.
8. Csendes A, Braghetto I, Henriquez A, Cortes C. Late results of a prospective randomized study comparing forceful dilatation and oesophagomyotomy in patients with achalasia. Gut 1989;30:199–304.
9. Spiess AE, Kahrilas PJ. Treating achalasia: from whalebone to laparoscope. JAMA 1998;19:638–42.
10. West RL, Hirsch DP, Bartelsman JF, et al. Long term results of pneumatic dilatation in achalasia followed for more than 5 years. Am J Gastroenterol 2002;97:1346–51.
11. Ellis FH Jr. Oesophagomyotomy for achalasia: 22-year experience. Br J Surg 1993;80:882–5.
12. Hunter JG. Laparoscopic Heller myotomy and fundoplication for achalasia. Ann Surg 1997;225:655–64.

13. Sabharwal T. Balloon dilatation for achalasia of the cardia: experience in 76 patients. Radiology 2002;224:719–24.

14. Luketich JD, Fernando HC, Christie NA, Buenaventura PO, Keenan RJ, Ikramuddin S, Schauer PR. Outcomes after minimally invasive esophagomyotomy. Ann Thorac Surg 2001;72:1909–12.

15. Sharp KW, Khaitan L, Scholz S, Holzman MD, Richards WO. 100 consecutive minimally invasive Heller myotomies: lessons learned. Ann Surg 2002;235:631–8.

16. Patti MG, Pellegrini CA, Horgan S, Arcerito M, Omelanczuk P, Tamburini A, Diener U, Euanks TR, Way LW. Minimally Invasive surgery for achalasia: an 8-year experience with 168 patients. Ann Surg 1999;130:587–93.

17. Patti MG, Arcerito M, De Pinto M, Feo CV, Tong J, Gantert W, Way LW. Comparison of thoracoscopic and laparoscopic Heller myotomy for achalasia. J Gastrointest Surg 1998;2:561–6.

18. Ramacciato G, Mercantini P, Amodio PM, Corigliano N, Barreca M, Stipa F, Ziparo V. The laparoscopic approach with antireflux surgery is superior to the thoracoscopic approach for the treatment of esophageal achalasia. Experience of a single surgical unit. Surg Endosc 2002;16:1431–7.

19. Cade R. Heller's myotomy: thoracoscopic or laparoscopic? Dis Esophagus 2000;13:279–81.

20. Ellis FH Jr. Surgical management of esophageal motility disturbances. Am J Surg 1980;139:752–759.

21. Jordan P. Longterm results of esophageal myotomy for achalasia. J Am Coll Surg 2001;193:137–45.

22. Andrello NA, Carlam RJ. Heller's myotomy for achalasia: is an added anti-reflux procedure necessary? Br J Surg 1987:74:765–8.

23. Malthauer RA, Todd TR, Miller L, Pearson FG. Long-term results in surgical managed esophageal achalasia. Ann Thorac Surg 1994;58:1343–7.

24. Ellis FH, Watkins E, Gibbs SP, Heatley GJ. Ten to 20 year clinical results after short esophagomyotomy without an anti-reflux procedure (modified Heller operation) for esophageal achalasia. Eur J Cardiothorac Surg 1992;6:86–90.

25. Jara FM, Toledo-Pereyra H, Lewis JW, Magilligan DJ Jr. Long-term results of esophagomyotomy for achalasia of esophagus. Arch Surg 1979;114:935–6.

26. Laws HL, Clements RH, Swillie CM. A randomized, prospective comparison of the Nissen fundoplication versus the Toupet fundoplication for gastroesophageal reflux disease. Ann Surg 1997;225:647–53.

27. Toppart P, Deschamps C, Taillefer R, Durancean A. Long-term effect of total fundoplication on myotomized esophagus. Ann Thorac Surg 1992;54:1046–52.

28. Heider TR, Farrell TM, Kircher AP, et al. Complete fundoplication is not associated with increased dysphagia in patients with abnormal esophageal motility. J Gastrointest Surg 2001;5:36–41.

29. Peters JH, Kauer WK, Crookes PF, Ireland AP, Bremner CG, DeMeester TR. Esophageal resection with colon interposition for end-stage achalasia. Arch Surg 1995;130:632–6.

30. Patti MG, Feo CV, Diener U, Tamburini A, Arcerito M, Safadi B, Way LW. Laparoscopic Heller myotomy relieves dysphagia in achalasia when the esophagus is dilated. Surg Endosc 1999;13:843–7.

Commentary

GARY R. GECELTER

This is an excellent summary of the major controversies facing surgical palliation of achalasia of the esophagus. Our own experience, involving 62 laparoscopic esophagomyotomies, has largely mirrored the same issues and conclusions of the authors. The two areas that I would like to enlarge upon are our technical considerations and experience with the "end-stage esophagus".

There are two aspects of the lapararoscopic operation that we have employed to assist us in optimizing the length and safety of the myotomy. Firstly, we have used intraoperative esophagoscopy routinely. In this way we have identified the rosette of mucosa that represents the proximal commencement of the high-pressure zone. We have often been surprised by the proximal location of the esophageal caliber change and always ensure that the myotomy extends above the rosette, which is easily seen by transillumination of the mucosa as viewed from the esophagoscope. The added benefit of flexible esophagoscopy is the air insufflation, which helps confirm the absence of mucosal perforation. The second technical facilitation has been in the use of a flexible laparoscope. This device allows us to advance our proximal extent as far as necessary while maintaining an *en face* view of the anterior esophagus high into the posterior mediastinum. These two evolutions have aided us in improving our clinical outcomes significantly since we first began recording our data in 1996.

To wrap or not to wrap? I have always felt that wrapping an esophagus after an operation to treat dysphagia is counter-intuitive, especially if it will only benefit 50% of patients at most. I believe that reflux is minimized by maintaining an intra-abdominal esophagus and, as a result, we have used a modification of the Watson "physiologic" repair in which we suture the angle of His and medial fundus to the left lateral esophagus, including bites through the crus. This tends to elongate the intra-abdominal esophagus while pulling the lateral myotomized muscle bundle open [1].

A further observation of ours has been the positive symptomatic results that we have been able to achieve in patients with end-stage mega-esophagi (>6 cm). In our series, we have performed laparoscopic Heller myotomies on 12 patients who had previously undergone forceful pneumatic dilatation or repeated botulinum toxin injection and were now symptomatic enough to be considered for esophagectomy but were unwilling to undertake a major procedure. At 1 year, 7 of 12 patients were significantly less symptomatic and regarded themselves as "cured", three patients improved initially but by 1 year were back to pre-procedural dysphagia, and two patients had no change in their condition and went on to esophagectomy. Of the latter five patients, all were considered to have a sigmoid esophagus with elongation and tortuosity. A curious finding on lateral esophagram in three patients was that the posterior esophagus extended to the posterior costophrenic recess inferiorly and actually ascended to the hiatus, thereby creating a dependent trough from which contents had to ascend to exit the esophagus. We therefore differentiate between mega-esophagus and sigmoid esophagus and will only offer the prior a laparoscopic mytomy. The authors are to be commended on their insightful and detailed review.

Reference

1. Gecelter G, Gellman L, Geiss A, Alexander K, Meslin K, Simms H. Heller Myotomy with angle of his repair – a four-year comparative follow-up study. Surg Endosc 2002;16: S280.

Minimally Invasive Esophagectomy

Alberto de Hoyos, James D. Luketich

> **Key Controversies**
> A. Extent of resection of the primary tumor and extent of lymphadenectomy
> B. Choice of endoscopic technique
> C. Site and technique of construction of the anastomosis
> D. Need for pyloric drainage

14.1
Introduction

Esophagectomy for carcinoma of the esophagus should include several objectives: (1) complete resection of all disease, (2) lymph node sampling or complete dissection of regional lymph nodes, and (3) replacement of the esophagus with a gastric or intestinal conduit with anastomosis in the upper chest or in the neck. Regardless of the surgical procedure used, avoidance of local recurrence, minimizing complications and rapid return to preoperative performance status are obvious goals.

Conventional open esophagectomy is associated with significant morbidity and mortality. A recent report from a single institution for a 10-year period revealed a complication rate of 50% and a mortality rate of 10% [1]. This is consistent with a more comprehensive review of the morbidity and mortality across centers in the United States, which showed the mortality rates of esophagectomy range from 8% in high volume centers to an alarming 22% in centers with low volumes of these complex cases [2]. With the development of minimally invasive techniques, surgeons have accomplished reductions in the morbidity of many foregut procedures and, in some cases, made them technically easier to perform while maintaining sound surgical principles. In an effort to decrease the morbidity associated with esophagectomy, these minimally invasive techniques have been applied to resection of the esophagus. In our own experience, minimally invasive esophagectomy (MIE) appears to achieve the goals of complete resection, good functional outcomes and less morbidity. In this chapter we will review the results of our own experience with MIE and review other recent series, and discuss some of the controversies of this approach. It is important to note that many of the controversies associated with standard open esophagectomy have not been overcome, such as operative approach, radicality of the resection, conduit of choice and use of neoadjuvant therapies. These controversies continue to challenge us in the era of less invasive techniques.

14.2
Discussion

14.2.1
Extent of Resection of the Primary Tumor and Extent of Lymphadenectomy

One of the most controversial aspects of treating esophageal and esophagogastric cancers is the appropriate extent of resection to achieve the best outcome [3]. Some surgeons believe that surgery for esophageal cancer is mainly palliative and cure is attained only in those with very early tumors. Transhiatal esophagectomy (THE) is, in part, based on this reasoning [4]. THE requires a laparotomy and blunt mediastinal dissection without inclusion of the adjacent intrathoracic lymph nodes. Conventional transthoracic esophagectomy (TTE) requires a thoracotomy and allows a standard thoracic lymphadenectomy. In addition, a laparotomy is also required for mobilization of the gastric or intestinal conduit (Ivor Lewis procedure) [5]. More aggressive surgeons perform extended radical resection of the primary tumor as well as lymphadenectomy of the neck, chest and abdomen (three-field lymphadenectomy) [6, 7]. All of these approaches require a laparotomy, thoracotomy, or both and are associated with significant morbidity and mortality [8]. One recent randomized trial showed no statistically significant survival advantage of a more radical resection versus a transhiatal esophagectomy but did suggest some advantages of better local control with the extended resection group [9]. In the absence of consistent data to show a benefit for a more radical operation, the choice of surgical approach remains debatable and the only definitive information is that the surgeon or group of surgeons in any given center should have significant experience and maintain a high volume of cases to minimize the morbidity and mortality of the operation [2, 10].

14.2.2
Choice of Minimally Invasive Approach

In an effort to decrease the morbidity associated with esophagectomy, surgeons have begun to apply minimally invasive techniques to resection of the esophagus (Tables 14.1, 14.2). Initial reports focused on thoracoscopic mobilization of the esophagus in combination with a standard open laparotomy to complete the esophagectomy [11]. Subsequently, several authors demonstrated the feasibility and safety of minimally invasive total laparoscopic approach with transhiatal esophagectomy in combination with a cervical anastomosis [12]. While this technique avoided a thoracotomy, it had the same disadvantage of the traditional THE, namely the inability to perform a standard lymphadenectomy. Total laparoscopic approaches also suffer from limited visibility and technical difficulties of operating through the hiatus well up into the mediastinum. These early reports demonstrated feasibility but did not demonstrate an advantage over conventional open approaches. This was not surprising because most of these cases included an access thoracotomy or laparotomy which was similar in size to standard incisions.

Total laparoscopic esophagectomy has been reported by our group and others [13, 14]. However, concerns with the technical aspects of the completeness of the esophageal mobilization and lymph node dissection prompted us and others to utilize a combined thoracoscopic and laparoscopic approach to MIE [15, 16]. This technique has allowed us to achieve a full esophageal mobilization and a complete lymphadenectomy under direct endoscopic visualization similar to the one achieved with standard open techniques and is currently our preferred approach to esophagectomy.

Other approaches to the local treatment of Barrett's esophagus with high-grade dysplasia and small, mucosal cancers include endoscopic mucosal resection (EMR) and photodynamic therapy (PDT). Photodynamic therapy using Photofrin has been recently approved by the FDA for the endoscopic ablation of high-grade dysplasia and small mucosal cancers. Overholt and colleagues have published the largest series with impressive short-term results [17]. In his study of 103 patients with Barrett's esophagus, they claimed a 94% complete ablation of the areas of high-grade dysplasia (60 of 65 patients). They did note some local recurrences and the requirement of both YAG-laser and PDT to achieve these results. In addition, repeated endoscopic treatments and surveillance endoscopies were required in the majority of the patients. Overall the stricture rate was 30% and was dependent on the number of interventions performed. In our own experience, we have treated 20 patients with high-grade dysplasia or T1 tumors who were medically unfit for surgery or who refused MIE. At a median follow-up of 20 months, 50% of patients remained free of recurrence, 30% required additional treatments or had some

Table 14.1. Endoscopic esophagectomy (LOS length of hospital stay, NA not available)

Study [ref.]	No. of patients	Approach	No. of nodes	Conversion (%)	Operative time (min)	LOS (days)	Compli- cations (%)	Leak (%)	Mortality at 30 days
Akaishi et al. [11]	39	thoracoscopy laparotomy	19±11 12±9	0	448	NA	21/39	5	0
Swanstrom and Hansen [13]	9	laparoscopy, thoracoscopy	NA	0	390	6.4		0	0
Nguyen et al. [16]	18	thoracoscopy, laparoscopy	12±9	0	364	11	50	11	0
Osugi et al. [33]	75	thoracoscopy, thoracotomy, laparotomy	34±13	0	226	NA	33	NA	0
Law et al. [34]	22	thoracoscopy, laparotomy	7	18	240	NA	?	0	4
Smithers et al. [35]	153	thoracoscopy, laparotomy	11	7	299	14	35	4	3.3
Kawahara et al. [36]	23	thoracoscopy, laparotomy	29			26	39	4	0
Luketich et al. [15]	222	thoracoscopy, laparoscopy	16	5	450	7	55	15[a]	1.4

Leak rate dependent on diameter of gastric tube used

Table 14.2. Endoscopic Approaches to Esophagectomy

Approach	Advantage	Disadvantage
Thoracoscopic and laparotomy	Esophageal mobilization Standard lymphadenectomy Reduced pulmonary morbidity	Requires laparotomy Position change Double lumen tube
Laparoscopic	Avoids laparotomy Avoids thoracotomy Reduces pulmonary morbidity Avoids double lumen tube Single position	No standard lymphadenectomy Risk of mediastinal hemorrhage Poor visualization of thoracic dissection
Combined Thoracoscopic/ Laparoscopic	Avoids thoracotomy Avoids laparotomy Reduces pulmonary morbidity Excellent view of esophageal mobilization Allows standard lymphadenectomy	Increased operative time Learning curve Double lumen intubation Position change

degree of residual high-grade dysplasia, and 20% had recurrence and died of their disease [18]. Our current practice is to reserve PDT for patients who are not surgical candidates for whom this less invasive therapy offers a very reasonable option but requires intensive endoscopic follow-up.

Endoscopic mucosal resection has been recently utilized as a therapeutic option for treatment of small mucosal esophageal carcinomas [19–24]. It is known that mucosal cancers in which invasion depth is limited to the lamina propria have only a 4% incidence of lymph node involvement. As opposed to this, cancers showing submucosal invasion have a 35% rate of lymph node metastases. Therefore, only mucosal cancers (m1, representing superficial mucosal carcinoma *in situ*, or m2, representing deep mucosal carcinoma into lamina propria but not reaching muscularis mucosa) are considered appropriate candidates for mucosal resection in attempts to permanently cure the disease. In addition, the superficial spread of carcinoma should be limited to less than half the circumference of the esophageal lumen.

On the other hand, proponents of a more radical approach to high grade dysplasia or early carcinoma argue that esophagectomy can be accomplished with a low mortality rate and that a large number of patients have invasive carcinoma in the resected specimen despite a preoperative diagnosis of only high grade dysplasia [25, 26]. In addition, the 5-year survival is excellent even if invasive cancer is present, and these patients are liberated from rigorous surveillance for the rest of their lives. Therefore, they reserve EMR for high-grade dysplasia to patients who are poor operative risks.

14.2.3
Site and Technique to Construct the Anastomosis

Another area of controversy entails the site and technique to construct the esophagogastric anastomosis. Muller et al. reviewed all published reports of surgical therapy of esophageal carcinoma from 1980 to 1988 (59 published reports) [27]. In most reports the risk of anastomotic leak from a cervical anastomosis is higher than that reported for an intrathoracic anastomosis. In patients experiencing leaks, however, morbidity and mortality related to the leak itself were lower if the anastomosis is located in the neck rather than in the chest, but this is not always true [28]. The anastomotic leak rate in Muller and colleagues' review was 11% for intrathoracic anastomosis compared with 19% for cervical anastomosis. However, the mortality rate for an intrathoracic anastomotic leak was three times higher than that for cervical anastomotic leak (69% versus 20%, respectively). More recent experience in centers with a high volume of esophageal surgery report anastomotic leak rates to be less than 3% for cervical anastomosis and less than 2% for intrathoracic anastomosis [29, 30].

Beitler and Urschel's review of four randomized and seven nonrandomized comparative studies showed that stapled anastomosis and hand-sewn anastomosis have equivalent leak rates, but strictures are more common in stapled anastomosis [31]. Orringer et al. have recently published their experience with a stapled anastomosis and have demonstrated significantly lower leak rates of (3%) and less stricture problems utilizing a linear stapler (Autosuture Endo-GIA II stapler) [29].

14.2.4
Need for Pyloric Drainage

In another meta-analysis of nine randomized trials, Urschel and colleagues showed that if surgeons did not perform a pyloric drainage procedure, the incidence of gastric outlet obstruction was significantly increased [32]. However, delayed gastric emptying is not solely due to pyloric obstruction. Other reasons for delayed gastric emptying are obstruction at the level of the diaphragmatic spiraling of the gastric conduit, or redundant intrathoracic stomach lying in the posterior costophrenic gutter. This results in a J-shaped configuration of the stomach before passage through the hiatus. These problems are best avoided by an adequate drainage procedure at the time of the operation, enlargement of the hiatus, not pulling the stomach too tightly into the chest and avoiding excess stomach in the chest. Routine pyloric drainage procedures, however, are not done at all centers with experience in esophageal surgery. Experience has shown that keeping the gastric tube narrow (3–4 cm) and enlarging the hiatus improve its rate of emptying, and may avoid the need for a pyloric drainage procedure. We have found, however, that by constructing a narrow gastric conduit, the blood supply to the tip of the fundus may be jeopardized, resulting in an increased rate of anastomotic leak [16]. We currently advocate performing a pyloroplasty in all patients.

14.2.4.1
University of Pittsburgh Results of MIE

Recently, we published our results of MIE in 222 patients [15]. We encountered many of the controversies discussed above and as our experience increased, our technique evolved to some degree. Initially, we approached the operation totally laparoscopically but were dissatisfied with the visualization and ability to perform an adequate lymph node dissection. We therefore added thoracoscopy to fully mobilize the intrathoracic esophagus and perform a complete lymphadenectomy. Other modifications included an attempt to create a very narrow gastric tube of 3 cm in an effort to avoid the need for pyloric drainage. We encountered an increased leak rate with a tendency for some of these leaks to drain along the narrow conduit and into the right chest creating a more difficult technical approach to management. This led us to modify our approach and to construct a slightly larger diameter gastric tube of 5–6 cm, with creation of a very high cervical anastomosis. In addition, we now preserve the mediastinal pleura above the level of the azygos vein. All of these modifications were done in an attempt to minimize ischemia to the gastric tube tip, lower the leak rate, and improve the likelihood that if a cervical leak occurs it would be associated with minimal necrosis of the gastric tip, and would more likely drain out of the neck making management easier.

Our 222 patients included 186 (83.6%) men and 36 (16.2%) women. Median age was 66.5 years (range 39–89). Preoperative indications for esophagectomy included carcinoma in 175 (78.8%) and high-grade dysplasia in 46 (21.2%). Neoadjuvant therapy was used in 78 (35.1%) patients and radiation in 36 (16.2%) patients. The 30-day operative mortality was 1.4% ($n=3$). One patient died of pneumonia and necrosis of the gastric conduit. One patient died of a postoperative myocardial infarction and one patient died of pericardial tamponade on the third postoperative day. The anastomotic leak rate was affected by the size of the gastric tube. In patients with the standard diameter of 6 cm, leak occurred in 10 our of 164 patients (6.1%). In those patients where a narrow gastric tube was used (3–4 cm) the leak rate was 26.6% (15 of 58 patients).

Follow-up dysphagia scores were excellent with a mean score of 1.4 (1 indicating no dysphagia; 5 indicating severe dysphagia). The mean health-related quality of life (HRQOL) score was 4.6, which represents a normal score. Only 4% of the patients complained of significant reflux symptoms (HRQOL >15). Our results demonstrate that MIE is feasible and can produce therapeutic outcomes comparable to those reported in most series.

14.3
Summary

— MIE is a technically demanding operation requiring advanced laparoscopic and thoracoscopic skills. The addition of thoracoscopy has allowed us to perform a totally endoscopic and an oncologically sound esophagectomy.
— Proper patient selection, adequate preparation of the patient, attention to technical detail and diligent postoperative care allow this procedure to be performed safely and with a mortality rate of 1.4% in our first 222 patients.
— We continue to perform a drainage procedure routinely to avoid postoperative gastric outlet obstruction.
— Our preferred method for construction of the esophagogastric anastomosis is by utilizing an end-to-end stapled anastomosis. Our reported morbidity and mortality is superior to many published series utilizing open approaches but we acknowledge this is a single institution series and is not randomized. As experience is gained with this procedure, results are expected to improve.
— Prospective trials with longer follow-up will be required to confirm any advantages of MIE over conventional approaches. Recently, we have opened a multicenter study to further assess results (Eastern Cooperative Group Trial ECOG-2202). Open surgical approaches should remain the standard operation for esophagectomy in most institutions.
— We continue to advocate MIE in good surgical candidates with high-grade dysplasia and early mucosal carcinomas. We reserve endoscopic based interventions to patients who are at high surgical risk.

References

1. Bailey SH, Bull DA, Harpole DH, et al. Outcomes after esophagectomy: a ten-year prospective cohort. Ann Thorac Surg 2003;75:217–22.
2. Birkmeyer JD, Stukel TA, Siewers AE, et al. Surgeon volume and operative mortality in the United States. N Engl J Med 2003;349:2117–27.

3. Hulscher JB, Tijssen JG, Obertop H, et al. Transthoracic versus transhiatal resection for carcinoma of the esophagus: a meta-analysis. Ann Thorac Surg 2001;72:306–13.
4. Orringer MB, Marshall B, Iannetoni MD. Transhiatal esophagectomy: clinical experience and refinements. Ann Surg 1999;230:392–400.
5. King RM, Pairolero PC, Trastek VF, et al. Ivor Lewis esophagogastrectomy for carcinoma of the esophagus: early and late functional results. Ann Thorac Surg 1987;44:119–25.
6. Altorki NK, Lerut T. Three field lymph node dissection for cancer of the esophagus. In: Pearson FG, Cooper JD, Deslauries J, eds. Esophageal surgery. New York: Churchill Livingstone; 2002. pp. 866–70.
7. Tachibana M, Kinugasa S, Yoshimura H, et al. Extended esophagectomy with 3-field lymph node dissection for esophageal cancer. Arch Surg 2003;138:1383–9.
8. Shahian DM, Neptune WB, Ellis FH, et al. Transthoracic versus extrathoracic esophagectomy: mortality, morbidity, and long-term survival. Ann Thorac Surg 1986;41:237–41.
9. Hulschler JB, van Sandick JW, de Boer AG, et al. Extended transthoracic resection compared with limited transhiatal resection for adenocarcionma of the esophagus. N Engl J Med 2002;347:1662–9.
10. Patti MG, Corvera C, Glasgow RE, et al. A hospital's annual rate of esophagectomy influences the operative mortality rate. J Gastrointest Surg 1998;2:186–92.
11. Akaishi T, Kaneda I, Higuchi N, et al. Thoracoscopic en bloc total esophagectomy with radical mediastinal lymphadenectomy. J Thorac Cardiovasc Surg 1996;112:1533–41.
12. DePaula AL, Hashiba K, Ferreira EA, et al. Transhiatal approach for esophagectomy. In: Tooli J, Gossot D, Hunter JG, eds. Endosurgery. New York: Churchill Livingstone; 1996. pp. 293–9.
13. Swanstrom LL, Hansen P. Laparoscopic total esophagectomy. Arch Surg 1997;132:943–9.
14. Luketich JD, Nguyen N, Schauer P. Laparoscopic transhiatal esophagectomy for Barrett's esophagus with high-grade dysplasia. J Soc Laparoendosc Surg 1988;2:75–7.
15. Luketich JD, Alvelo-Rivera M, Buenaventura PO, et al. Minimally invasive esophagectomy: outcomes in 222 patients. Ann Surg 2003;238:486–95.
16. Nguyen NT, Roberts P, Follette DM, et al. Thoracoscopic and laparoscopic esophagectomy for benign and malignant disease: lessons learned from 46 consecutive procedures. J Am Coll Surg 2003;197:902–13.
17. Overholt BF, Panjehpour M, Halbert DL. Photodynamic therapy for Barrett's esophagus with dysplasia and or early stage carcinoma: long-term results. Gastrointest Endosc 2003;58:183–8.
18. Luketich JD, Christie NA, Lovas KE, Weigel TL. Photodynamic therapy: results of curative intent for esophageal cancer and Barrett's with high grade dysplasia in high risk patients. In: Abstracts of International Biomedical Optics Symposium, San Jose, CA, 23–28 January 2000.
19. Inoue H, Fukami N, Yoshida T, et al. Endoscopic mucosal resection for esophageal and gastric cancers. J Gastroenterol Hepatol 2002;17:382–8.
20. Noguchi H, Naomoto Y, Kondo H, et al. Evaluation of endoscopic mucosal resection for superficial esophageal carcinoma. Surg Laparosc Endosc Percutan Tech 2000;10:343–50.

21. Nijhawan PK, Wang KK. Endoscopic mucosal resection for lesions with endoscopic features suggestive of malignancy and high-grade dysplasia with Barrett's esophagus. Gastrointest Endosc 2000;52:328–32.

22. Takeo Y, Yoshida T, Shigemitu T, et al. Endoscopic mucosa resection for early esophageal cancer and esophageal dysplasia. Hepatogastroenterology 2001;48:453–7.

23. Soetikno RM, Gotoda T, Nakanishi Y, et al. Endoscopic mucosal resection. Gastrointest Endosc 2003;57:567–79.

24. Pech O, May A, Gossner L, et al. Barrett's esophagus: endoscopic resection. Gastrointest Endosc Clin North Am 2003;13:505–12.

25. Korst RJ, Altorki NK. High grade dysplasia: surveillance, mucosal ablation or resection? World J Surg 2003;27:1030–4.

26. Fujita H, Sueyoshi S, Yamana H, et al. Optimum treatment strategy for superficial esophageal cancer: endoscopic mucosal resection versus radical esophagectomy. World J Surg 2001;25:424–31.

27. Muller JM, Erasmi H, Stelzner, et al. Surgical therapy of oesophageal carcinoma. Br J Surg 1990;77:845–57.

28. Walther B, Johansson J, Johnson F, et al. Cervical or thoracic anastomosis after esophageal resection and gastric tube reconstruction: a prospective randomized trial comparing sutured neck anastomosis with stapled intrathoracic anastomosis. Ann Surg 2003;238:803–14.

29. Orringer MB, Marshall B, Iannettoni MD. Eliminating the cervical esophagogastric anastomotic leak with a side-to-side stapled anastomosis. J Thorac Cardiovasc Surg 2000;119:277–88.

30. Mathisen DJ, Grillo HC, Wilkins EW, et al. Transthoracic esophagectomy: a safe approach to carcinoma of the esophagus. Ann Thorac Surg 1988;45:137–42.

31. Beitler AL, Urschel JD. Comparison of stapled and hand-sewn esophagogastric anastomoses. Am J Surg 1998;175:337–40.

32. Urschel JD, Blewett CJ, Young JE, et al. Pyloric drainage (pyloroplasty) or no drainage in gastric reconstruction after esophagectomy: a meta-analysis of randomized controlled trials. Dig Surg 2002;19:160–4.

33. Osugi H, Takemura M, Higashino M, Takada N, et al. Video-assisted thoracoscopic esophagectomy and radical lymph node dissection for esophageal cancer. A series of 75 cases. Surg Endosc 2002;16:1588–93.

34. Law S, Fok M, Chu KM, Wong J. Thorascopic esophagectomy for esophageal cancer. Surgery 1997;122:8–14.

35. Smithers BM, Gotley DC, McEwan D, et al. Thoracoscopic mobilization of the esophagus. A 6 year experience. Surg Endosc 2001;15:176–82.

36. Kawahara K, Maekawa T, Okabayashi K, Hideshima T, et al. Video-assisted thoracoscopic esophagectomy for esophageal cancer. Surg Endosc 1999;13:218–23.

Commentary

Mark B. Orringer

The described combined thorascopic/laparoscopic approach to esophageal resection and reconstruction represents an extraordinary technologic achievement by Dr. Luketich and his associates. In this balanced presentation of their results, the authors point out that this procedure requires advanced laparoscopic and thorascopic skills. Even in their hands, the average reported operative time (Table 14.1) is 7.5 h, 55% of their patients experience postoperative complications, and the anastomotic leak rate is 15%. These are far from acceptable results for modern esophageal surgery.

While our experience at the University of Michigan with nearly 1,800 "open" transhiatal esophagectomies (THEs) and cervical esophagogastric anastomoses (CEGAs) has been refined over a 25-year period and no longer represents our "learning curve" with the operation, our comparative date are quite different than that of the University of Pittsburgh group. The operative "flow" of a THE and CEGA in our hands is now sufficiently orchestrated that the procedure is often completed in 3–4 h. With the current onslaught of patients with esophageal carcinoma and Barrett's esophagus with high-grade dysplasia we now see, we frequently perform one THE in the morning and one in the afternoon. We absolutely could not do this with average operative times 7+ hours for the operations.

A growing number of our patients with esophageal complications of gastroesophageal reflux disease (Barrett's mucosa with high-grade dysplasia and adenocarcinoma) are severely obese (body mass index of 35 or more). Routine use in these patients of deep table-mounted self-retaining retractors (e.g., the Buchwalter), extra-long right, angle clamps and electrocautery extensions, greatly facilitates THE. I question the applicability of MIE in this population. Of our THE patients, 80% have an uneventful, uncomplicated postoperative course [1], and our CEGA leak rate is approximately 3% using the side-to-side stapled anastomotic technique we have described [2].

There is no question that the mortality and *acute* morbidity of a CEGA leak is substantially less than that associated with an intrathoracic esophageal anastomotic leak. Unfortunately, the story does not stop there. Approximately 50% of patients who experience a CEGA leak develop a CEGA stricture as the cervical wound heals (and scars) by secondary intent. And an operation performed with the expressed intent of relieving dysphagia but resulting in the need for lifelong esophageal anastomotic dilatations to maintain comfortable swallowing represents a poor functional result.

Over the years that I have been performing THE and a CEGA, I have learned that gentle handling of the stomach during its mobilization and subsequent positioning through the posterior mediastinum and into the neck is of para-mount importance. The rule that we use is a "pink stomach in the abdomen and a pink stomach in the neck ensure a successful anastomosis". The tip of the gastric fundus to which the cervical esophagus will be anastomosed is relatively ischemic after division of the left gastric and left gastroepiploic ves-sels, and while the gastric submucosal collateral circulation is extraordinarily rich, gastric trauma must be minimized. Once the cervical esophagus is di-vided and the intrathoracic esophagus delivered downward into the abdomen and along with the stomach placed on the anterior chest wall, the stomach is divided approximately 5–6 cm distal to the esophagogastric junction when-ever possible, preserving as much gastric submucosal collateral circulation as possible.

There is *no* advantage to creating a narrow gastric tube, which as these authors have verified, is more vulnerable to an anastomotic leak. In preparing the gastric conduit, the GIA stapler is applied several times beginning along the lesser curvature of the stomach, gently and progressively "straightening" the stomach as the stapler is fired, an average of three times. The staple suture line is carefully oversewn with a running 4-0 monofilament polypropylene suture. I avoid suturing traction drains to the tip of the stomach to help pull it to the posterior mediastinum. Before placing the stomach in the posterior mediastinum, the surgeon's hand and forearm passed upward through the hi-atus ensure a wide mediastinal "tunnel", free of unrecognized fibrous bands. The stomach is gently manipulated through the posterior mediastinum by the surgeon's hand until the fundus can be palpated through the cervical wound. A Babcock clamp (not ratcheted closed) is used to grasp the tip of the stomach and help guide it into the neck wound until it can be grasped by the finger-tips. In order to minimize a traction injury, the stomach is pushed upward through the posterior mediastinum from below, not dragged upward from above. Approximation of a healthy, well-vascularized stomach to a healthy divided cervical esophagus is the goal. I question the ability of the surgeon using the "no-hands-on" minimally invasive technique of gastric mobiliza-tion to perform as gentle and atraumatic creation of the longest gastric "tube" possible, a generous Kocher maneuver to maximize pyloroduodenal mobility, or manipulation of the stomach through the widened hiatus.

I have always performed a gastric drainage procedure with a THE and CEGA. The incidence of gastric outlet obstruction without a drainage pro-cedure may be low, but one has only to experience an uncontrolled massive CEGA leak or postoperative aspiration pneumonia due to gastric outlet ob-struction in such a patient to convince himself that it is better to do a drainage procedure at the time of the initial esophagectomy than to "come back" to do it after a disaster has occurred. My preference is a pyloromyotomy, since this avoids the pyloroplasty suture line of the authors' technique at a right angle to the upward pull of the stomach.

The debate regarding the "oncologic superiority" of a direct mediastinal lymphadenectomy in the patient undergoing an esophagectomy for cancer continues. An open THE does *not* preclude removal of paraesophageal, subcarinal, and upper abdominal lymph nodes, though I concede that the dissection is not en bloc or as thorough as that possible under direct vision with a thoracoscope. The question is whether removal of involved mediastinal lymph nodes significantly improves survival in these patients. In my practice, preoperative chemotherapy and radiation therapy are used routinely in operative patients with esophageal cancer who are under the age of 75 years. If this therapy is successful in eradicating mediastinal lymph node metastases, the effort to remove every mediastinal lymph node at the time of esophagectomy is not worthwhile. If tumor persists in mediastinal lymph nodes after chemoradiation, cure is not likely to be achieved whether the nodes are removed or not.

The combined thoracoscopic/laparoscopic esophagectomy and esophageal reconstruction described by Luketich and associated seems to make an already difficult surgical procedure even more challenging. Single lung ventilation must be available, and the operative time is inordinately prolonged, both being factors that may contribute to postoperative pulmonary complications. Less than 2% of our patients undergoing "open" THE experience postoperative atelectasis or pneumonia. The morbidity of an esophagectomy is not in the size of the incision used to perform it, but rather in the physiologic impact of a major abdominal and intrathoracic operation, and adjusting to new eating habits and to postvagotomy "dumping" when it occurs. My patients are well prepared for their esophagectomy – no smoking for 3 weeks before surgery, regular use of an incentive inspirometer, walking 1–3 miles a day to condition themselves for early postoperative ambulation, and maintaining good caloric intake, if necessary, with nasogastric tube feeding supplements. With the use of epidural anesthesia postoperatively, pulmonary complications are rare. My patients go directly from the recovery room to the floor, where early ambulation is begun the next morning. Postoperative mechanical ventilation and an ICU stay are rarely needed. The average hospital stay after open THE and CEGA on my service is 7 days, similar to that of Dr. Luketich's group using MIE.

From my perspective, the standard "open" THE and CEGA performed through upper midline abdominal and cervical incisions is a faster, simpler operation than the minimally invasive technique described in this chapter. I am not certain if the advanced laparoscopic and thorascopic skills needed to perform the Luketich procedure is widely generalizable to the surgical community. And I agree completely that until more experience is gained with the thoracoscopic/laparoscopic approach, the "standard" should be an "open" esophagectomy, and the mini-invasive procedure should be restricted to the few surgeons doing this in large volume.

Having soundly criticized laparoscopic/thoracoscopic esophagectomy and esophageal reconstruction, I am reminded of the harsh criticism I received at the annual meeting of the American Association for Thoracic Surgery when I first presented the concept of esophagectomy without thoracotomy in 1978 [3]. Dr. Alton Oschner, a giant in the field, declared that a "blind" esophagectomy performed without adequate visualization of the esophagus and meticulous hemostasis was a "step backward into the Dark Ages of surgery" – "awkward" – "like trying to make love in a hammock standing up!" A younger, more liberal thoracic surgeon, Dr. Griffith Pearson of Toronto, countered that he had performed several THEs with good results, and "unless you have tried making love in a hammock standing up, don't knock it!" Like those who were most critical of the "blunt" esophagectomy I described but had never performed the operation, I have not personally performed the operation described by Drs. de Hoyos and Luketich. The world of surgery seems to enjoy two surgeons battling for the supremacy of their operative approach to a problem, each being an expert in their own procedure, which they are convinced is superior. With refinements in minimally invasive surgical technology that are occurring so rapidly today, the laparoscopic/thoracoscopic esophagectomy and esophageal reconstruction may someday be the procedure of choice in these patients. I commend the authors for their technical prowess and continuing efforts to improve the results of esophageal resection and reconstruction.

References

1. Orringer MB, Marshall B, Iannettoni MD. Transhiatal esophagectomy (THE) – clinical experience and refinements. Ann Surg, 1999;230:392–400.
2. Orringer MB, Marshall B, Iannettoni MD. Eliminating the cervical esophagogastric anastomotic leak with a side-to-side stapled anastomosis. J Thorac Cardiovasc Surg 2000;119:277–88.
3. Orringer MB, Sloan H. Esophagectomy without thoracotomy. J. Thorac Cardiovasc Surg. 1978;76:643–54.

Gastric Resection
for Advanced Gastric Cancer

Seigo Kitano, Masayuki Ohta, Norio Shiraishi

▶ Key Controversies

A. Reports of laparoscopic gastrectomy for advanced gastric cancer
B. Laparoscopic D2 lymph node dissection
C. Influence of laparoscopic surgery on gastric cancer recurrence

15.1
Introduction

We started to perform laparoscopic gastrectomy for early gastric cancer in December 1991 prior to the initial report of laparoscopic gastrectomy for benign gastric ulcer [1], and have experienced over 110 cases over the last 10 years [2]. Now laparoscopic gastrectomy has been accepted as a treatment of choice for early gastric cancer among laparoscopic surgeons in Japan. Although the operative time for laparoscopic gastrectomy is generally greater than that with conventional open gastrectomy, laparoscopic surgery is superior to open surgery in terms of less blood loss, less pain, a shorter hospital stay and the cosmetic outcome [3–6]. In addition, rapid recovery of gastrointestinal function, less weight loss, and less cost are recognized benefits of laparoscopic gastrectomy [3, 7, 8]. The operative curability, including surgical margins and number of dissected lymph nodes, in laparoscopic gastrectomy is equivalent to that of conventional gastrectomy [3–6]. Postoperative recurrence after laparoscopic gastrectomy for early gastric cancer is very rare, and over the last 10 years we have never experienced such a recurrence [2]. Since there are no recorded long-term results available for a controlled study regarding laparoscopic gastrectomy, we are now doing a randomized controlled trial for laparoscopic distal gastrectomy [9]. However, we believe that laparoscopic gastrectomy should be a very useful and curative procedure for patients with early gastric cancer. Laparoscopic gastrectomy is probably acceptable for the treatment of early-stage gastric cancer all over the world.

Radical gastrectomy with extended lymph node dissection is usually performed for the treatment of advanced gastric cancer in Eastern countries, especially in Japan. Recently, indications for the use of laparoscopic gastrectomy for gastric cancer have been enlarged to include advanced cancer. Several institutes have started to use laparoscopic gastrectomy in the treatment of advanced gastric cancer [10–16]. However, it is not fully known how laparoscopic surgery including CO_2 pneumoperitoneum may influence tumor growth and promotion, and laparoscopic techniques of extended lymph node dissection for advanced gastric cancer are not standardized. Is laparoscopic radical gastrectomy for advanced gastric cancer less invasive to the patients? Can laparoscopic gastrectomy for advanced cancer be an equivalent treatment to conventional open surgery in terms of the operative curability? Now many questions remain on laparoscopic gastrectomy used in the treatment of advanced cancer. We reviewed the application and associated problems of laparoscopic surgery used to treat patients with advanced gastric cancer.

15.2
Discussion

15.2.1
Reports of Laparoscopic Gastrectomy
for Advanced Gastric Cancer

Results of laparoscopic gastrectomy for advanced gastric cancer in the English literature are shown in Table 15.1. Another two reports probably include advanced gastric cancer but the number of advanced cases are not described [17, 18]. Now most of the operators of laparoscopic radical gastrectomy likely limit the indications of advanced gastric cancer to up to T2 and N1 (Table 15.2). In particular, Japanese laparoscopic surgeons seem to hesitate to operate on more advanced gastric cancer with tumor penetration of serosa (T3) and with extraperigastric lymph node metastasis (N2). This is because it is not known how laparoscopic surgery including CO_2 pneumoperitoneum and laparoscopic handlings may influence tumor recurrence in the more advanced cancer.

Although all reports had a small number of patients, laparoscopic D2 lymph node dissection [19] was mostly undertaken with and without hand-assisted technique (Table 15.1). Since the surgeon's assisting hand is generally useful to perform easier manipulation under the laparoscope, half the operators used the hand-assisted technique in laparoscopic radical gastrectomy. However, the assisting hand often interrupts the operative field and the cosmetic outcome in the hand-assisted laparoscopic surgery is often worse than without the hand-assisted technique. Thus, the use of hand-assisted laparoscopic gastrectomy has generally decreased in Japan.

Table 15.1. Results of laparoscopic gastrectomy for advanced cancer

Authors	No. of cases	Hand-assist	Lymph node dissection	Mortality (%)	Complication rate (%)
Azagra et al. [10]	12	–	D1 or D2	8.3	8.3
Uyama et al. [11, 12]	7	–	D2	0	0
Goh et al. [13]	4	–	D2	0	0
Tanimura et al. [14]	12	+	D2	0	5.0[a]
Ikeda et al. [15]	3	+	D2	0	0
Chau et al. [16]	1	+	D2	0	0

[a]Overall complication rates including early and advanced cases

Table 15.2. Indications of laparoscopic gastrectomy for advanced cancer (*TNM* International Union Against Cancer TNM Classification, *JCGC* Japanese Classification of Gastric Carcinoma),

Authors	Classification			Lymph node dissection
	System	T stage	N stage	
Azagra et al. [10]	TNM	T2	N0	D1
		>T2	>N0	D2
Uyama et al. [11, 12]	JCGC	T2	N0 or N1	D2
Goh et al. [13]	TNM	T2 or T3	N0 or N1	D2
Tanimura et al. [14]	JCGC	T2(MP)[a]	N0	D2
Ikeda et al. [15]	TNM	T2(MP)	N0	D2

[a]*MP* muscularis propria

Low mortality and morbidity were present in the laparoscopic gastrectomy with D2 lymph node dissection (Table 15.1). Azagra et al. experienced one case of complication with intraoperative injury of proper hepatic artery during dissection of the lesser omentum and one case where the patient has died from liver cirrhosis and acute hepatic failure [10]. Tanimura et al. experienced only three postoperative complications in 48 early and 12 advanced cancer patients treated by hand-assisted laparoscopic gastrectomy with D2 lymph node dissection, which included anastomotic leakage, bleeding and stenosis [14]. They also demonstrated that laparoscopic gastrectomy was a superior treatment to open surgery in terms of less blood loss, less pain and a shorter hospital stay, resulting in the same outcome as the studies regarding early gastric cancer [3–6]. Presently, no other report provides a comparison between laparoscopic and open gastrectomy for advanced cancer. Only two reports had data from a follow-up after the operations. The mean follow-ups were 27.5 and 15 months, respectively, and only one patient had tumor recurrence [10, 13]. Therefore, an evaluation indicating that laparoscopic gastrectomy for advanced gastric cancer would be less invasive compared with conventional open surgery is not enough, as there is no result regarding a long-term follow-up after the operations. Besides this, technical difficulty of D2 lymph node dissection and oncological problems remain regarding the laparoscopic treatment of advanced gastric cancer.

15.2.2
Laparoscopic D2 Lymph Node Dissection

In Western countries, recent randomized controlled trials demonstrated that patients treated by D2 lymph node dissection had a higher operative mortality and morbidity than those treated by D1 lymph node dissection [20, 21]. In addition, in the 5-year survival rates in the controlled trials there were no differences between the D1 and D2 lymph node dissections [22, 23]. These results concluded that D2 lymph node dissection should not be used as a standard treatment for Western patients with gastric cancer. However, in Eastern countries, especially in Japan, operative morbidity and mortality after radical gastrectomy are very low even in a non-specialized hospital [24]. It is unknown whether these differences may be due to the physical constitution of the patients and operative techniques for lymph node dissection. In addition, several reports showed that extended lymph node dissection contributed to a better survival rate than the limited dissection [25–27]. Therefore, Japanese guidelines for gastric cancer treatment recommend D2 or D3 lymph node dissection in patients with advanced cancer [28].

Laparoscopic gastrectomy with D2 lymph node dissection was routinely done as the treatment of advanced carcinoma in the actual published papers (Table 15.1). However, some regional lymph nodes containing extraperigastric lymph nodes (group 2 nodes, based on the 13th Japanese edition of Japanese Classification of Gastric Carcinoma) [19] are relatively difficult to dissect using the laparoscopic approach. The lymph nodes along a left gastric artery (no. 7), a common hepatic artery (no. 8a) and a proximal splenic artery (no.

11p) and around a celiac artery (no. 9) can be dissected, relatively easily, and these lymph nodes are often dissected concomitantly with perigastric nodes (group 1 nodes) for the treatment of early gastric cancer [2–9, 29]. It seems to be technically difficult to dissect lymph nodes in hepatoduodenal ligament (along a proper hepatic artery, no. 12a), along a superior mesenteric vein (no. 14v) and a distal splenic artery (no. 11d), and at the splenic hilum (no. 10). It is possible to dissect no. 12a lymph node by means of exposing the proper hepatic artery and taping it with vessel tapes [12]. Regarding no. 14v lymph node dissection, after division of the gastrocolic ligament and exposure of a middle colic vein, the dissection toward the inferior edge of the pancreas head is continued. The lymph node dissection of no. 14v together with no.6 is complete when a superior mesenteric vein, a gastrocolic trunk and a right gastroepiploic vein are all exposed. When laparoscopic splenectomy with gastrectomy is performed, nos. 10 and 11p lymphadenectomy can be performed [11, 15]. However, the hand-assisted technique is probably necessary when the spleen and distal pancreas are mobilized from the retroperitoneum and nos. 10 and 11p lymph nodes are dissected without splenectomy under the laparoscope. We also have experienced several cases treated by laparoscopic D2 lymph node dissection with and without hand-assistance, and it is technically feasible to standardize this procedure. Since D2 lymph node dissection can have a higher operative mortality and morbidity than D1 lymph node dissection even in the conventional open gastrectomy, standard laparoscopic gastrectomy with D2 lymph node dissection, which has a low mortality and morbidity, should be conducted.

15.2.3
Influence of Laparoscopic Surgery on Gastric Cancer Recurrence

Although gastric cancer is declining in incidence in the USA and Western Europe, it is still the second commonest cause of death from cancer in the world. In Britain, about 80% of gastric cancer patients were found to have the advanced and incurable stage IV of the disease, and only 1% were classified in the early stage [30]. Therefore, a staging laparoscopy has been developed to detect peritoneal dissemination and distant metastases before operation in patients with gastric cancer [31, 32]. In regard to the recurrence patterns after curative operation, gastric cancer has a lower incidence in local recurrence than colorectal cancer but a higher incidence in peritoneal dissemination [33]. Detection of microscopic peritoneal dissemination using intraoperative peritoneal lavage is a prognostic factor in patients with gastric cancer after the curative operation (R0) and not in patients with colon cancer [34]. Thus, a scattering of tumor cells should be protected against more carefully for gastric surgery to be a curative treatment of advanced gastric cancer.

The experimental studies demonstrated that pneumoperitoneum induced morphologic peritoneal alterations, which may promote a specific tumor intraperitoneal growth [35, 36]. We showed that the intraperitoneal concentration of hyaluronic acid, which is related to the attachment of cells and extracellular matrix molecules, was increased after CO_2 pneumoperitoneum [37]. In addition, exogenous hyaluronic acid promoted port-site metastases under the pneumoperitoneum [38]. It was also reported that free gastric cancer cells immediately attached to the injured port sites after CO_2 pneumoperitoneum in the experimental study [39]. These phenomena indicated by the experimental studies might all be associated with peritoneal dissemination and port-site metastasis after laparoscopic cancer surgery. Although recent papers in a clinical setting have demonstrated that laparoscopic colectomy in patients with advanced colorectal cancer has an equivalent long-term survival rate compared to open surgery and does not increase port-site metastases [40–42], it is dangerous to apply these results of the colorectal cancer to advanced gastric cancer. There is a risk that the recurrences of peritoneal dissemination and port-site metastasis could be increased after laparoscopic gastrectomy in patients with advanced gastric cancer, especially T3 and T4 cancer, in comparison with conventional open surgery. Actually, most of the operators are limiting the indication up to T2 and N1 (Table 15.2). Randomized controlled trials in patients with advanced gastric cancer are necessary to refute this concern about an increased recurrence after laparoscopic surgery.

15.3
Summary

- Laparoscopic gastrectomy has been accepted as a treatment of choice for early gastric cancer among laparoscopic surgeons in Japan.
- Laparoscopic gastrectomy for advanced gastric cancer is starting to be used.
- Although laparoscopic D2 lymph node dissection for advanced cancer is a relatively difficult procedure, it is technically feasible to standardize this procedure.
- Since gastric cancer has a higher incidence of peritoneal dissemination recurrence than colorectal cancer, it is feared that the recurrence, including peritoneal dissemination and port-site metastasis, could be increased after laparoscopic gastrectomy for advanced gastric cancer.

— Randomized controlled trials are necessary to prove the safety and effectiveness of laparoscopic gastrectomy in patients with advanced gastric cancer.

References

1. Goh P, Tekant Y, Issac J, et al. The technique of laparoscopic Billroth II gastrectomy. Surg Laparosc Endosc 1992;2:258–60.
2. Kitano S, Shiraishi N, Kakisako K, et al. Laparoscopy-assisted Billroth-I Gastrectomy (LADG) for cancer: our 10 year's experience. Surg Laparosc Endosc Percutan Tech 2002;12:204–7.
3. Shimizu S, Uchiyama A, Mizumoto K, et al. Laparoscopically assisted diatal gastrectomy for early gastric cancer. Surg Endosc 2000;14:27–31.
4. Yano H, Monden T, Kinuta M, et al. The usefulness of laparoscopy-assisted distal gastrectomy in comparison with that of open distal gastrectomy for early gastric cancer. Gastric Cancer 2001;4:93–7.
5. Mochiki E, Nakabayashi T, Kamimura H, et al. Gastrointestinal recovery and outcome after laparoscopy-assisted versus conventional open distal gastrectomy for early gastric cancer. World J Surg 2002;26:1145–9.
6. Adachi Y, Shiraishi N, Shiromizu A, et al. Laparoscopy-assisted Billroth I gastrectomy compared with conventional open gastrectomy. Arch Surg 2000;135:806–10.
7. Adachi Y, Suematsu T, Shiraishi N, et al. Quality of life after laparoscopy-assisted Billroth I gastrectomy. Ann Surg 1999;229:80–5.
8. Adachi Y, Shiraishi N, Ikebe K, et al. Evaluation of the cost for laparoscopic-assisted Billroth I gastrectomy. Surg Endosc 2001;15:932–6.
9. Kitano S, Shiraishi N, Fujii K, et al. A randomized controlled trial comparing open vs laparoscopy-assisted distal gastrectomy for the treatment of early gastric cancer: an interim report. Surgery 2002;131:S306–11.
10. Azagra JS, Goergen M, Simone PD, et al. Minimally invasive surgery for gastric cancer. Surg Endosc 1999;13:351–7.
11. Uyama I, Sugioka A, Fujita J, et al. Laparoscopic total gastrectomy with distal pancreatosplenectomy and D2 lymphadenectomy for advanced gastric cancer. Gastric Cancer 1999;2:230–4.
12. Uyama I, Sugioka A, Matsui H, et al. Laparoscopic D2 lymph node dissection for advanced gastric cancer located in the middle or lower third portion of the stomach. Gastric Cancer 2000;3:50–5.
13. Goh PMY, Khan AZ, So JBY, et al. Early experience with laparoscopic radical gastrectomy for advanced gastric cancer. Surg Laparosc Endosc Percutan Tech 2001;11:83–7.
14. Tanimura S, Higashino M, Fukunaga Y, et al. Hand-assisted laparoscopic distal gastrectomy with regional lymph node dissection for gastric cancer. Surg Laparosc Endosc Percutan Tech 2001;11:155–60.
15. Ikeda Y, Sasaki Y, Niimi M, et al. Hand-assisted laparoscopic proximal gastrectomy with jejunal interposition and lymphadenectomy. J Am Coll Surg 2002;195:578–81.
16. Chau C, Siu W, Li MK. Hand-assisted D2 subtotal gastrectomy for carcinoma of stomach. Surg Laparosc Endosc Percutan Tech 2002;12:268–72.

17. Seshadri PA, Mammazza J, Poulin EC, et al. Technique for laparoscopic gastric surgery. Surg Laparosc Endosc Percutan Tech 1999;9:248–52.

18. Reyes CD, Weber KJ, Gagner M, et al. Laparoscopic vs open gastrectomy: a retrospective review. Surg Endosc 2001;15:928–31.

19. Japanese Gastric Cancer Association. Japanese Classification of Gastric Carcinoma, 2nd English edition. Gastric Cancer 1998;1:10–24.

20. Bonenkamp JJ, Songun I, Hermans J, et al. Randomized comparison of morbidity after D1 and D2 dissection for gastric cancer in 996 Dutch patients. Lancet 1995;345:745–8.

21. Cuschieri A, Fayers P, Fielding J, et al. Postoperative morbidity and mortality after D1 and D2 resections for gastric cancer: preliminary results of the MRC randomized controlled surgical trial. Lancet 1996;347:995–9.

22. Bonenkamp JJ, Hermans J, Sasako M, et al. Extended lymph-node dissection for gastric cancer. New Engl J Med 1999; 340:908–14.

23. Cuschieri A, Weeden S, Fielding J, et al. Patient survival after D1 and D2 resections for gastric cancer: long-term results of the MRC randomized surgical trial. Br J Cancer 1999;79:1522–30.

24. Moriwaki Y, Kobayashi S, Kunisaki C, et al. Is D2 lymphadenectomy in gastrectomy safe with regard to the skill of the operator? Dig Surg 2001;18:111–7.

25. Pacelli F, Doglietto GB, Bellantone R, et al. Extensive versus limited lymph node dissection for gastric cancer: a comparative study of 320 patients. Br J Surg 1993; 80:1153–6.

26. Volpe CM, Koo J, Miloro SM, et al. The effect of extended lymphadenectomy on survival in patients with gastric adenocarcinoma. J Am Coll Surg 1995;181:56–64.

27. de Manzoni G, Verlato G, Guglielmi A, et al. Prognostic significance of lymph node dissection in gastric cancer. Br J Surg 1996;83:1604–7.

28. Nakajima T. Gastric cancer treatment guidelines in Japan. Gastric Cancer 2002;5:1–5.

29. Uyama I, Sugioka A, Fujita J, et al. Completely laparoscopic extraperigastric lymph node dissection for gastric malignancies located in the middle or third of the stomach. Gastric Cancer 1999;2:186–90.

30. Allum WH, Powell DJ, McConkey CC, et al. Gastric cancer: a 25 year review. Br J Surg 1989;76:535–40.

31. Burke EC, Karpeh MS, Conlon KC, et al. Laparoscopy in the management of gastric carcinoma. Ann Surg 1997;225:262–7.

32. Shiraishi N, Morimoto A, Sato K, et al. Laparoscopy in the management of scirrhous gastric cancer. Gastric Cancer 1999 2:109–14.

33. Tateishi M, Ichiyoshi Y, Kawano T, et al. Recurrent pattern of digestive tract carcinoma in the Japanese: comparison of gastric cancer to colon cancer. Int Surg 1995;80:41–4.

34. Vogel P, Ruschoff J, Kummel S, et al. Prognostic value of microscopic peritoneal dissemination: comparison between colon and gastric cancer. Dis Colon Rectum 2000;43:92–100.

35. Volz J, Koster S, Spacek Z, et al. The influence of pneumoperitoneum used in laparoscopic surgery on an intraabdominal tumor growth. Cancer 1999;86:770–4.

36. Suematsu T, Hirabayashi Y, Shiraishi N, et al. Morphology of the murine peritoneum after pneumoperitoneum vs laparotomy. Surg Endosc 2001;15:954–8.

37. Yamaguchi K, Hirabayashi Y, Suematsu T, et al. Hyaluronic acid secretion during carbon dioxide pneumoperitoneum and its association with port-site metastasis in a murine model. Surg Endosc 2001;15:59–62.

38. Yamaguchi K, Hirabayashi Y, Shiromizu N, et al. Enhancement of port site metastasis by hyaluronic acid under CO_2 pneumoperitoneum in a murine model. Surg Endosc 2001;15:504–7.
39. Hirabayashi Y, Yamaguchi K, Shiraishi N, et al. Development of port-site metastasis after pneumoperitoneum: a scanning electron microscopy study. Surg Endosc 2002;16:864–8.
40. Franklin ME, Kazantsev GB, Abrego D, et al. Laparoscopic surgery for stage III colon cancer: long-term follow-up. Surg Endosc 2000;14:612–6.
41. Lujan HJ, Plasencia G, Jacobs M, et al. Long-term survival after laparoscopic colon resection for cancer: complete five-year follow-up. Dis Colon Rectum 2002;45:491–501.
42. Lacy AM, Garcia-Valdecasas JC, Delgado S, et al. Laparoscopy-assisted colectomy versus open colectomy for treatment of non-metastatic colon cancer: a randomized trial. Lancet 2002;359:2224–9.

Commentary

David M. Dent

The preceding review comes from one of the major surgical centers in Japan, where Kitano and his colleagues have performed laparoscopic gastrectomies for over a decade. They have extensive, almost unrivalled, experience in the performance of Billroth 1 operations for early gastric cancer, and their views must carry experience and authority.

When commenting on a review of gastrectomy for cancer, it is important to firstly place the goalposts firmly in the ground. One of the past difficulties in assessing results of gastric surgery for cancer, in the West and in Japan, has been with definition, and much misunderstanding has flowed from this. The review concerns "*advanced* gastric cancer", and it is essential at the outset to establish just what this implies. "*Early* gastric cancer" is defined as a cancer confined to the mucosa or submucosa, irrespective of lymph node involvement (and in the majority of cases they are uninvolved). The authors, and others, have defined all stages other than this subset of early gastric cancer as "*advanced* gastric cancer". Given this definition, advanced gastric cancer must comprise the vast majority of cases in both Japan and the West. They cite 99% of cases in Britain [1]. The term advanced gastric cancer must also somewhat paradoxically encompass certain groupings, such as T2N0M0, which are eminently curable.

They have examined the six publications in the English literature which describe laparoscopic gastrectomy (typically accompanied by a D2 dissection) in 39 patients with advanced disease. This is rather odd. Have only 39 of these D2 procedures been reported from the vast reservoir of the majority of cases of the disease? What is the problem?

The first problem would appear to be a technical one. While laparoscopy has become the conventional approach for two categories of gastric operation – antireflux procedures and certain forms of bariatric surgery – this does not seem to be the case with cancer of the stomach. Some endoscopic surgeons make an exception with early gastric cancer, where they believe that a D2 dissection is unnecessary, and a conventional Billroth 1 resection to be appropriate. Kitano and his colleagues share this belief and practice. If, however, the belief is that a D2 dissection is necessary for any more advanced stage of disease (and this is the recommendation in Japan [2]), the technical demands increase greatly. While discounted in randomized trials [3–6], the D2 extragastric lymphadenectomy continues to remain an integral part of gastric surgery in Japan, and in certain other countries, where the randomized trials themselves are discounted as flawed. The technical demands of performing a D2 dissection laparoscopically are great, as has been reported by the most experienced hands: a total gastrectomy with D2 dissection may takes in excess of 10 h [7], or a subtotal proximal procedure with lymphadenectomy in excess of 6 h [8]. The stumbling block would appear to be the D2 lymphadenectomy, which is difficult and time consuming enough with open surgery, and must be more so when performed laparoscopically, if the en bloc principles are to be adhered to. Kitano and colleagues suggest technical difficulty with the nodes in the hepato-duodenal ligament, the superior mesenteric vein and the splenic artery. It would be difficult to associate the established virtues of laparoscopic surgery (less pain, less blood, rapid recovery of gastro-intestinal function, shorter hospital stay) with such lengthy, extensive surgery. Fortunately, four of the six publications report neither morbidity nor mortality from the procedure.

The second problem would appear to be the fear of cancer dissemination by way of the pneumoperitoneum, which may accelerate tumor spread and impair peritoneal defense mechanisms. There has been extensive experimental work to demonstrate this, and Kitano and his colleagues have contributed to it, which they quote. There is also the possibility of port-site seeding, as was reported with laparoscopic colorectal excision. While possibly not a problem with early gastric cancer (with its intact serosa), the spectre of dissemination in more advanced disease haunts the laparoscopic surgeon. Thus the 39 reported cases comprise a subsection, which would appear to be oncologically "safe" from dissemination, and typically not involving the serosa or nodes (T2N0M0), although two reports mention occasional involvement of adjacent perigastric nodes.

The feasibility of laparoscopic subtotal or total gastrectomy, hand assisted or not, is unquestioned, as is the possibility of performing a D2 lymphadenectomy. The problem would appear to be the technical demands of the D2 dissection, and its oncological safety. We are cautioned by two successive Editorials in the dedicated journal *Gastric Cancer*: Aiko suggested that laparoscopic surgery for advanced gastric cancer should be "reserved for selected patients and experienced surgeons" [9]. Hallissey has cautioned that "....it is vital to ensure that the short term gains [reduced post operative discomfort, and hospital stay] do not result in long term losses [of local and distal recurrence]" [10]. Kitano and his colleagues themselves conclude that "randomised controlled trials are necessary...".

In this instance, the art of the possible does not necessarily translate into the science of safe and wise practice.

References

1. Allum WH, Powell DJ, McConkey CC, et al. Gastric cancer: a 25 year review. Br J Surg 1989;76:535–40.
2. Nakajima T. Gastric cancer treatment guidelines in Japan. Gastric Cancer 2002;5:1–5.
3. Dent DM, Madden MV, Price SK. Randomised comparison of R1 and R2 gastrectomy for gastric carcinoma. Br J Surg 1988;75:110–2
4. Robertson CS, Chung SCS, Woods SDS, Griffin SM, Raimes SA, Lau JTF, et al. A prospective randomised trial comparing R1 subtotal gastrectomy with R3 total gastrectomy for antral cancer. Ann Surg 1994;220:176–82.
5. Bonenkamp JJ, Hermans J, Sasako M, Van de Velde CJH; Dutch Gastric cancer group. Extended lymph-node dissection for gastric cancer. N Engl J Med 1999;340:908–14.
6. Cuschieri A, Weeden S, Fielding J, Bancewcz J, Craven J, Joypaul V, et al. Patient survival after D1 and D2 resection for gastric cancer: long term results of the MRC randomised surgical trial. Br J Cancer 1999;79:1522–30
7. Uyama I, Sugioka A, Fujita J, Komoro Y, Matsui H, Hasumi A. Laparoscopic total gastrectomy with distal pancreatico-splenectomy and D2 lymphadenectomy for advanced gastric cancer. Gastric Cancer 1999;2:230–4.
8. Uyama I, Sugioka A, Matsui H, Fujita J, Komori Y, Hatakawa Y, Hasumi A. Laparoscopic side to side esophagogastrostomy using a linear stapler after proximal gastrectomy. Gastric Cancer 2001;4:98–102.
9. Aiko T. Laparoscopic gastrectomy for advanced cancer: a technical challenge [Editorial]. Gastric Cancer 1999;2:199–200.
10. Hallissey MT. Laparoscopically assisted gastric resections: a word of caution [Editorial]. Gastric Cancer 2001;4:53.

Adjustable Gastric Banding (LAGB) for Morbid Obesity

Jacques M. Himpens, Tom P. Vleugels

▶ **Key Controversies**

A. Is the procedure effective?

B. Are the severity and number of complications acceptable?

16.1
Introduction

Adjustable band gastroplasty (ABG), evolved from the nonadjustable gastric banding and characterized by a high stenosis rate [1], was introduced by Kuzmak in the United States in 1986 [2] and at about the same time by Forsell [3] in Sweden. The technique gained widespread acceptance with the advent of laparoscopy. Guy-Bernard Cadière [4, 5] performed the first laparoscopic adjustable gastric band (LAGB) procedure in October 1992, while Belachew [6] was the first to use a device specifically designed for laparoscopic use. Since that time, this procedure has experienced a true explosion in popularity and become the most commonly performed bariatric procedure in Europe [7]; the experience in the USA has been less positive [8]. Considered the final solution in obesity surgery by some, LAGB should be abandoned according to others [8]. In this paper we will look into this controversy.

To our knowledge, there is only one prospective randomized study comparing the US and Swedish bands [9] used in LAGB. Since no differences could be found in outcome or complications, we will discuss the adjustable gastric band procedure without taking the type of band into account.

16.2
Discussion

16.2.1
Is the Procedure Effective?

In order to be effective, a bariatric procedure should create a long-lasting (>5 years) loss of excess weight (EWL) of at least 50% and keep the patient's weight under 30 kg/m^2 body mass index (BMI) [10, 11]. Numerous reports attest to the effectiveness of LAGB but most studies do not reach a high level of evidence. Moreover, very few patients achieve an EWL of 50% or more and/or achieve a BMI of 30 kg/m2 or less [7, 12].

Since the laparoscopic procedure is relatively new, most of the reports cover a rather short follow-up time, and very few papers report a follow-up over 5 years. Doherty et al. [13], in a prospective study on adjustable band gastroplasty by laparotomy, showed a decrease in BMI from 50 to 32.8 kg/m^2 after 3 years but a re-increase to 44.1 kg/m^2 after 8 years and an intra-abdominal reoperation rate of 52.5%. In a Swedish study carried out over 7 years [14], progressive weight regain was documented and 58% of the patients were re-operated on, which resulted into excision of the banding system and conversion to Roux-en-Y gastric bypass (RYGBP) in a majority of cases.

The Swedish inventor of the technique, however, reported great results in laparoscopically treated patients and followed up for at least 4 years [15]. In a Belgian retrospective multicenter study [16] BMI dropped from 42 to 30 kg/m^2 after 4 years but the intra-abdominal reoperation rate was 11%. Zinzindhoue et al. in a prospective non-randomized study on 500 patients [17], reported an EWL of over 50% after 2 and 3 years with the American band. These results were deemed successful, despite an intra-abdominal reoperation rate of 10%. Similar results were achieved in a large multicentric retrospective study in Italy [7], by Vertruyen in Brussels [18] and by Ceelen et al. from Pattyn's team in Ghent, Belgium [19]. Only the Ghent team used a Swedish band. O'Brien and Dixon [20] reported continued good results after up to 6 years. They documented an average EWL of over 50%.

Many authors obtained the best results in patients with lower preoperative BMIs [21, 22]. Favretti's team [23] found a BMI <50 to be a predictor of success (EWL>50%) and found that the success rate was only 30% when BMI was over 45. This is in contradiction with Dixon and O'Brien [24] who reported good results with higher BMIs, be it only after 1 year or more. The same authors also found no difference in outcome between sweet eaters and other obese patients. Interestingly, *non-sweet eating*, especially in male patients, seems to be a predictor of failure (EWL<20%) [23]. This correlates with earlier findings from Sweden [25], but many authors still consider sweet eating a contraindication for LAGB [17, 19]. The unexpected success of a purely restrictive procedure with sweet eaters can only be achieved by thorough screening and by an intensive preoperative psychological intervention [23]. In LAGB, psychological conditioning of the patients before the procedure and a very compulsive psychological follow-up appear to be of the utmost importance [26–28].

LAGB is the only bariatric procedure that requires adjustments. This translates into a number of postoperative office visits required simply for filling up the band. Favretti's team reports an average of 2.7 visits is needed. If one tries to fill up the band more aggressively, clinical results deteriorate [29]. The need for frequent office visits for repeated and sparing band adjustments, along with a strenuous psychological follow-up, makes this procedure very surgeon-demanding.

16.2.2
Severity and Number of Complications

Complications are two-fold: first, general complications, which are specific to any laparoscopic procedure in an obese patient and which we will not discuss here, and second, complications that are either procedure- or device-specific. These latter complications are considered either minor (leaks developing on the band itself, or on the tubing or the port system) or major.

Major complications include: first, dilatation of the proximal part of the stomach, located proximally to the band, and generally referred to as "pouch dilatation"; second, the development of major gastroesophageal reflux and esophageal dilatation; third, erosion of the band through the stomach wall, or "band migration".

16.2.2.1
Pouch Dilatation

The complication of pouch dilatation, the enlargement of the proximal gastric pouch beyond a critical limit, was recognized from the very beginning by Kuzmak and Burak[30]. It is not clear if this complication constitutes a separate entity from band slippage and most often both terms are used to describe the same condition [31]. Band slippage can occur within hours after the procedure and is then considered a technical failure [32]. Treatment consists of immediate repositioning. Late pouch dilation is more insidious. This condition is extremely serious and can be life threatening [33]. It is surprising that some classify this complication as minor [17], whereas others document poor long-term results after pouch dilatation, despite successful repositioning of the band [34]. The most striking symptom is epigastric pain together with complete food intolerance [32]. All series in the literature report a significant number of pouch dilatations varying between 1 and 26% (Table 16.1). Sometimes, simple band deflation deals with this condition. However, if vomiting and/or pain persist, surgical exploration is mandatory. This can be done laparoscopically [35].

The incidence of pouch dilatation seems to depend on the surgical technique. The adjustable band can be placed by three different approaches. The oldest is the perigastric technique where dissection is kept in close vicinity of the gastric wall [5]. A second technique is the so-called pars flaccida ap-

Table 16.1. Incidence of pouch dilatations or band slippage in the literature

Authors [ref.]	No. of patients	Follow-up	No. of pouches	Percentage of pouches
Busetto et al. 2003 [29]	379	3 years	52	13.7
Dargent 2003 [31]	511	4 years	39	6.2
	462	1 year	3	0.6
Ceelen et al. 2003 [19]	625	19.5 months	35	5.6
Ren et al. 2002 [69]	158	9 months	1	0.6
Vertruyen 2002 [18]	543	3 years	24	4.6
Evans et al. 2002 [70]	95	2 years	25	26.3
Suter et al. 2000 [38]	150	17 months	14	9.3
Rubin et al. 2003 [71]	250	3 years	4	1.6
O'Brien et al. 2002 [20]	1120	6 years	153	13.6
Angrisani et al. 2002 [21]	1893	6 years	93	4.9
Victorzon et al. 2002 [56]	110	27 months	3	2.7
Cadière et al. 2002 [72]	652	2 years	25	3.8
Rubenstein 2002 [73]	63	3 years	9	14.2
Szold et al. 2001 [61]	614	2 years	53	8.6
Silecchia et al. 2001 [66]	148	12 months	9	7.5

proach, which was first described by Forsell with the Swedish band [3] and is now routinely used with the American band [36]. With this approach the band is placed around the stomach and perigastric tissues, including vessels and vagus nerves, which supposedly reduces the band's resistance against the gastric contractions [36].

Another technique is the "double-route" or "two-step" approach: dissection through the flaccid part of the lesser omentum is followed by perigastric placement of the prosthesis [37]. It appears that the latter two approaches drastically reduce the number of pouch dilatations [31, 37, 38]. Importantly, the lesser sac should not be entered [38]. Other important factors seem to be: initial pouch size of less than 25 ml or even 15 ml [39–43], thorough fixation, and use of a low pressure band [44]. A less aggressive filling policy (cautious fillings not exceeding a total of 3 ml in the Inamed band) appears to be beneficial as well [45]. There is some question as to the role of the adjustments themselves since reoperations were more frequent with an adjustable than with a non-adjustable band in a prospective randomized study [46].

However, an essential determinant of pouch dilatation is the patient's lack of compliance to the restriction induced by the procedure [34]. Lack of compliance can be anticipated by preoperative screening [47]. Hence the best prevention of pouch dilatation – besides the surgical technique – may very well be patient selection. Scopinaro's team [48] showed that poor compliance is a critical key issue, especially with restrictive procedures for morbid obesity. Patients can indeed become very inventive in bypassing their band gastroplasty [49].

16.2.2.2
Esophageal Dilatation and Gastroesophageal Reflux

Small pouches help to avoid pouch dilatation and bring about good clinical results [50]. The effect of a small pouch is probably dysphagia [51] rather than the induction of early satiety, as was thought earlier [2, 5, 6]. This is not surprising since in "very small pouch gastroplasty", the band is placed around the distal esophagus rather than around the cardia. This placement can have a negative effect on the lower esophageal sphincter (LES) relaxation and on esophageal motility [52]. Hence, esophageal motility problems are more frequent with gastric micropouches than with more conventionally sized pouches [53]. This condition can result in pseudo-achalasia or indeed esophageal dilatation in patients with preoperative LES dysfunction [54]. Esophageal dilatation can explain the poor results in patients with preoperative esophageal dysmotility [55].

Gastroesophagal reflux is associated with abnormal esophageal acid exposure, a common occurrence in morbidly obese patients [56]. Uncomplicated LAGB placement reduces the amount of acid in patients with preoperative abnormal esophageal acid exposure as shown on pH-metry [57, 58]. However, in series where oesogastroscopy was performed systematically postoperatively, objective signs of reflux were found in a high number of patients, even in the ones considered to be a success [14, 56].

Band-induced reflux may be the first step to esophageal dilatation. Aggressive band fillings can trigger this complication [29]. Again, the lack of patient compliance seems to be a determining factor [59]. This underscores once more the importance of patient selection.

16.2.2.3
Band Erosion and Migration

LAGB is confronted with material erosion into the stomach, just like most operative procedures that imply implanting foreign material in the vicinity of a viscus [60]. Almost all series report a number of intragastric band erosions, varying from 1 to 11% (Table 16.2). The time from primary operation to diagnosis of band erosion ranges from a few weeks to several years after implant. Clinical manifestations include weight gain, band system leak, late and/or chronic port site infection, and seldom intraperitoneal abscess [60–62] or even portal vein thrombosis [63]. Treatment consists of laparoscopic [64] or endoscopic removal (in selected centers) [65]. Some advocate delayed rebanding [64] but this approach cannot be recommended [14, 34].

Preventive measures may be: the pars flaccida or the "two-step" approach, the use of low pressure bands [20, 42] and a very cautious dissection at the time of implant since early erosions might be due to gastric wall effraction during the initial operation [32]. The often silent course and delayed appear-

Table 16.2. Incidence of band erosion or band migration in the literature

Authors [ref.]	No. of patients	Follow-up	No. of erosions	Percentage of erosions
Rubin M et al. 2003 [71]	250	3 years	0	0
Abu-Abeid S et al. 2003 [74]	1271	5 years	17	1.3
O'Brien PE et al. 2002 [20]	1120	6 years	34	3
Angrisani L et al. 2002 [21]	1893	6 years	21	1.1
Belachew M et al. 2002 [16]	763	4 years	7	0.9
Victorzon M et al. 2002 [56]	110	27 months	2	1.8
Cadière G et al. 2002 [72]	652	2 years	2	0.3
Rubenstein RB 2002 [73]	63	3 years	1	1.6
Szold A et al. 2001 [61]	614	2 years	3	0.5
Niville E et al. 2001 [64]	301	39 months	5	1.7
Silecchia G et al. 2001 [66]	148	12 months	5	3.4
Westling A et al. 1998 [75]	90	35 months	10	11.1

ance of this complication may warrant systematic and regular upper gastro-intestinal endoscopy in all patients [66]. This obviously will add up to the already demanding follow-up.

16.3
Summary

— Literature implies that the ideal patient for LABG is the occasional female treatment-compliant individual with a BMI below 45 and a normal LES, who may be a sweet eater.
— The band positioning should be around the cardia and not around the distal esophagus, but the pouch should be 15 ml or less and the band should be of the low-pressure type.
— The patient should be committed to a strenuous follow up regimen, which includes psychological support and frequent endoscopies even in an asymptomatic patient. Under these conditions, an excess weight loss of close to 50% can be anticipated.
— The future will tell us if these results will be maintained over a long period of time. If one considers the long-term evolution of a similar [67] procedure, the vertical banded gastroplasty, the future may not be so bright [68].

References

1. Catona A, Gossenberg M, La Manna A, et al. Laparoscopic gastric banding: preliminary series. Obes Surg 1993;3:207–9.
2. Kuzmak LI. A review of seven years' experience with silicone gastric banding. Obes Surg 1991;1:403–8.
3. Forsell P, Hallberg D, Hellers G. Gastric banding for morbid obesity: initial experience with a new adjustable band. Obes Surg 1993;3:369–74.
4. Cadière GB, Favretti F, Bruyns J, et al. Gastroplastie par coelio-vidéoscopie: Technique. J Coeliochir.1994;27:346–9.
5. Cadiere GB, Bruyns J, Himpens J, et al. Laparoscopic gastroplasty for morbid obesity. Br J Surg 1994;81:1524.
6. Belachew M, Legrand MJ, Defechereux T. Laparoscopic Adjustable silicone gastric banding in the treatment of morbid obesity, a preliminary report. Surg Endosc 1994;8:1354–6.
7. Angrisani L, Furbetta F, Doldi B. et al. Lap Band adjustable gastric banding system. Surg Endosc 2003;17:409–12.
8. DeMaria EJ, Sugerman HJ, Meador JG, et al. High failure rate after laparoscopic adjustable silicone gastric banding for treatment of morbid obesity. Ann Surg 2001;233:809–18.

9. Ponson AE, Janssen IM, Klinkenbijl JH. Laparoscopic adjustable gastric banding: a prospective comparison of two commonly used bands. Obes Surg 2002;12:579–82.

10. Brolin RE, Kenler HA, Gorman RC, et al. The dilemma of outcome assessment after operations for morbid obesity. Surgery 1989;105:337–46.

11. Brolin RE. Critical analysis of results: weight loss and quality of data. Am J Clin Nutr 1992;55(2 Suppl):577S–81S.

12. Buchwald H. A bariatric surgical algorithm. Obes Surg 2002;12:733–46.

13. Doherty C, Maher J, Heitshusen D. Late outcome of adjustable gastric banding for surgical treatment of morbid obesity. Obes Surg 2001;11:401–2

14. Gustavsson S, Westling A. Laparoscopic adjustable gastric banding: complications and side effects responsible for the poor long-term outcome. Semin Laparosc Surg 2002;9:115–24.

15. Forsell P, Hellers G. The Swedish adjustable gastric banding (SAGB) for morbid obesity: a 9-year experience and a 4-year follow-up of patients operated with a new adjustable band. Obes Surg 1997;7:345–51.

16. Belachew M, Belva PH, Desaive C. Long-term results of laparoscopic adjustable gastric banding for the treatment of morbid obesity. Obes Surg 2002;12:564–8.

17. Zinzindohoue F, Chevallier JM, Douard R, et al. Laparoscopic gastric banding: a minimally invasive surgical treatment for morbid obesity: a prospective study of 500 consecutive patients. Ann Surg 2003;237:1–9.

18. Vertruyen M. Experience with Lap-band system up to 7 years. Obes Surg 2002;12:569–72.

19. Ceelen W, Walder J, Cardon A, et al. Surgical treatment of severe obesity with a low-pressure adjustable gastric band: experimental data and clinical results in 625 patients. Ann Surg. 2003;237:17–8.

20. O'Brien PE, Dixon JB. Weight loss and early and late complications-the international experience. Am J Surg 2002;184:42–5.

21. Angrisani L, Furbetta F, Doldi SB, et al. Results of the Italian multicenter study on 239 super-obese patients treated by adjustable gastric banding. Obes Surg 2002;12:846–50.

22. Eerten PV, Hunfeld MA, Tuinebreijer WE, Adjustable silicone gastric banding: can we continue the original technique of Kuzmak? Dig Surg. 1999;16:107–10.

23. Busetto L, Segato G, De Marchi F, et al. Outcome predictors in morbidly obese recipients of an adjustable gastric band. Obes Surg 2002;12:83–92.

24. Dixon JB, O'Brien PE. Selecting the optimal patient for LAP-BAND placement. Am J Surg 2002;184:17S–20S.

25. Lindroos AK, Lissner L, Sjoestrom L. Weight change in relation to intake of sugar and sweet foods before and after weight reducing gastric surgery. Int J Obes 1996;20:634–43.

26. Caniato D, Skorjanec B. The role of brief strategic therapy on the outcome of gastric banding. Obes Surg 2002;12:666–71.

27. Sannen I, Himpens J, Leman G. Causes of dissatisfaction in some patients after adjustable gastric banding. Obes Surg 2001;11:605–8.

28. Nicolai A, Ippoliti C, Petrelli MD. Laparoscopic adjustable gastric banding: essential role of psychological support. Obes Surg 2002;12:857–63.

29. Busetto L, Segato G, De Marchi F, et al. Postoperative management of laparoscopic gastric banding. Obes Surg 2003;13:121–7.

30. Kuzmak LI, Burak E. Pouch enlargement: myth or reality? Impressions from serial upper gastrointestinal series in silicone gastric banding patients. Obes Surg 1993;3:57–62.

31. Dargent J. Pouch dilatation and slippage after adjustable gastric banding: is it still an issue? Obes Surg 2003;13:111–5.

32. Chelala E, Cadiere GB, Favretti F, et al. Conversions and complications in 185 laparoscopic adjustable silicone gastric banding cases. Surg Endosc 1997;11:268–71.

33. Kirchmayr W, Ammann K, Aigner F, et al.. Pouch dilatation after gastric banding causing gastric necrosis. Obes Surg 2001;11:770–2.

34. Suter M. Laparoscopic band repositioning for pouch dilatation/slippage after gastric banding: disappointing results. Obes Surg 2001;11:507–12.

35. Niville E, Dams A, Anne T. Laparoscopic repositioning of an adjustable silicone gastric band for pouch dilatation and stoma obstruction. Surg Endosc 1999;13:65–7.

36. Fielding GA, Allen JW. A step-by-step guide to placement of the LAP-BAND adjustable gastric banding system. Am J Surg 2002;184:26S-30S.

37. Rubin M, Benchetrit S, Lustigman H, Laparoscopic gastric banding with Lap-Band for morbid obesity: two-step technique may improve outcome. Obes Surg 2001;11:315–7.

38. Suter M, Bettschart V, Giusti V et al. A 3-year experience with laparoscopic gastric banding for obesity Surg Endosc 2000;14: 532–6

39. Weiner R, Bockhorn H, Rosenthal R, et al. A prospective randomized trial of different laparoscopic gastric banding techniques for morbid obesity. Surg Endosc 2001;15:63–8.

40. Wiesner W, Weber M, Hauser RS, et al. Anterior versus posterior slippage: two different types of eccentric pouch dilatation in patients with adjustable laparoscopic gastric banding. Dig Surg 2001;18:182–6.

41. Belachew M, Zimmermann JM. Evolution of a paradigm for laparoscopic adjustable gastric banding. Am J Surg 2002;184:21S-5S.

42. Spivak H, Favretti F. Avoiding postoperative complications with the LAP-BAND° system. Am J Surg. 2002;184:31S-7S.

43. Favretti F, Cadiere GB, Segato G, et al. Laparoscopic banding: selection and technique in 830 patients. Obes Surg 2002;12:385–90.

44. Zimmermann JM, Blanc M, Mashoyan P. et al. Prevention of slippage. Series of 1410 patients: switching from the 9.5/10.0 band to the new generation 11.0 band. Obes Surg 2001;11:401.

45. Busetto L, Pisent C, Segato G, et al. The influence of a new timing strategy of band adjustment on the vomiting frequency and the food consumption of obese women operated with laparoscopic adjustable silicone gastric banding (Lap-Band). Obes Surg 1997;7:505–12.

46. Fried M, Kasalicky M, Melechovsky D, et al. Current status of non-adjustable gastric banding. Obes Surg 2002;12:395–8.

47. Lang T, Hauser R, Buddeberg C, et al. Impact of gastric banding on eating behavior and weight. Obes Surg 2002;12:100–7.

48. Gandolfo P, Gianetta E, Meneghelli A, et al. Preoperative eating behavior and weight loss after gastric banding for obesity. Minerva Gastroenterol Dietol 1996;42:7–10.

49. Comert M, Ustunda Y, Erdem L. A technique developed by a morbidly obese patient to eat more despite an adjustable gastric band. Obes Surg 2002;12:703–4.

50. Niville E, Vankeirsbilck J, Dams A, et al. Laparoscopic adjustable esophagogastric banding: a preliminary experience. Obes Surg 1998;8:39–43.

51. Capizzi FD, Boschi S, Brulatti M, et al. Laparoscopic adjustable esophagogastric banding: preliminary results. Obes Surg 2002;12:391–4.
52. Weiss HG, Nehoda H, Labeck B, et al. Treatment of morbid obesity with laparoscopic adjustable gastric banding affects esophageal motility. Am J Surg 2000;180:479–82.
53. Weiss H, Nehoda H, Labeck B. Adjustable gastric and esophagogastric banding: a randomized trial. Obes Surg 2002;12:573–8.
54. Wiesner W, Hauser M, Schob O, et al. Pseudo-achalasia following laparoscopically placed adjustable gastric banding. Obes Surg 2001;11:513–8.
55. Greenstein RJ, Nissan A, Jaffin B. Esophageal anatomy and function in laparoscopic gastric restrictive bariatric surgery: implications for patient selection. Obes Surg 1998;8:199–206.
56. Victorzon M, Tolonen P. Intermediate results following laparoscopic adjustable gastric banding for morbid obesity. Dig Surg 2002;19:354–7.
57. Iovino P, Angrisani L, Tremolaterra F, et al. Abnormal esophageal acid exposure is common in morbidly obese patients and improves after a successful Lap-band system implantation Surg Endosc 2002;16:1631–5.
58. Peternac D, Hauser R, Weber M, et al. The effects of laparoscopic adjustable gastric banding on the proximal pouch and the esophagus. Obes Surg 2001;11:76–86.
59. BusettoL, Valente P, Pisent C et al. Eating pattern in the first year following adjustable silicone gastric banding (ASGB) for morbid obesity. Int J Obes 1996;20:539–46.
60. Fobi M, Lee H, Igwe D, Felahy B, et al. Band erosion: incidence, etiology, management and outcome after banded vertical gastric bypass. Obes Surg 2001;11(6):699–707.
61. Szold A, Abu-Abeid S. Laparoscopic adjustable silicone gastric banding for morbid obesity: results and complications in 715 patients. Surg Endosc 2002;16:230–3.
62. Mittermair RP, Weiss H, Nehoda H, et al. Uncommon intragastric migration of the Swedish adjustable gastric band. Obes Surg 2002;12:372–5.
63. Calmes JM, Bettschart V, Raffoul W, et al. Band infection with splenoportal venous thrombosis: an unusual but severe complication of gastric banding. Obes Surg 2002;12:699–702.
64. Niville E, Dams A, Vlasselaers J. Lap-Band erosion: incidence and treatment. Obes Surg 2001;11:744–7.
65. Weiss H, Nehoda H, Labeck B, et al. Gastroscopic band removal after intragastric migration of adjustable gastric band: a new minimal invasive technique. Obes Surg 2000;10:167–70.
66. Silecchia G, Restuccia A, Elmore U, et al. Laparoscopic adjustable silicone gastric banding: prospective evaluation of intragastric migration of the lap-band. Surg Laparosc Endosc Percutan Tech 2001;11:229–34.
67. Ashy AR, Merdad AA.A prospective study comparing vertical banded gastroplasty versus laparoscopic adjustable gastric banding in the treatment of morbid and super-obesity. Int Surg 1998;83:108–10.
68. Balsiger BM, Poggio JL, Mai J, et al. Ten and more years after vertical banded gastroplasty as primary operation for morbid obesity. J Gastrointest Surg 2000;4:598–605.
69. Ren CJ, Horgan S, Ponce J. US experience with the LAP-BAND system. Am J Surg 2002;184:46S–50S.
70. Evans JD, Scott MH, Brown AS, et al. Laparoscopic adjustable gastric banding for the treatment of morbid obesity. Am J Surg 2002;184:97–102.

71. Rubin M, Spivak H. Prospective study of 250 patients undergoing laparoscopic gastric banding using the two-step technique: a technique to prevent postoperative slippage. Surg Endosc 2003;17:857–60.
72. Cadière GB, Himpens J, Hainaux B, et al. Laparoscopic adjustable gastric banding. Semin Laparosc Surg 2002;9:105–14.
73. Rubenstein RB. Laparoscopic adjustable gastric banding at a U.S. center with up to 3 year follow-up. Obes Surg 2002;12:380–4.
74. Abu-Abeid S, Keidar A, Gavert N, et al. The clinical spectrum of band erosion following laparoscopic adjustable silicone gastric banding for morbid obesity. Surg Endosc 2003;17:861–3.
75. Westling A, Bjurling K, Ohrvall M, et al. Silicone-adjustable gastric banding: disappointing results. Obes Surg 1998;8:467–74.

Commentary

WIM P. CEELEN

Morbid obesity increasingly represents a major health care challenge in both industrialized and developing parts of the world. Surgical therapy has been shown to be superior to standard medical care in terms of lasting weight loss, quality of life, and control of comorbidity [1]. Keeping in mind the *primum non nocere* imperative, however, both immediate and long-term side effects should be carefully weighed against any envisaged benefit and this holds especially true for extensive surgery.

Since its introduction in the early 1990s, laparoscopic gastric banding (LGB) has become the most widely performed restrictive bariatric procedure [2, 3]. Contrary to intestinal bypass procedures, LGB does not alter gut anatomy or physiology, as evidenced by the fact that ghrelin concentration is not altered postoperatively [4]. The short-term efficacy and safety of the procedure have been demonstrated in large European and Australian series. Although early results with LGB from the US were disappointing (FDA trial A), recent experience is in keeping with the European and Australian reports [5, 6]. It has by now become clear that the key to success with LGB consists of strict patient selection and education, minimal ("virtual") gastric pouch size and frequent follow-up visits.

However, some questions remain unanswered, the most important of which are long-term results of the procedure and fate of the esophagogastric junction. Medium-term results were recently described by one of the pioneers of the procedure, who demonstrated a mean excess weight loss of 50–60% at 48 months [7]. Mean or median follow-up time is not mentioned, but from the presented data one can deduct that most patients were followed for 4–5 years. Less favorable results were reported by Doherty et al. [8]. In this author's experience, mean BMI increased again (after an initial decrease) starting 1–3 years after gastric banding performed both by open and laparoscopic approach. In interpreting these results, it is important to consider (1) the fact that only 17 of 62 patients (27%) were operated on laparoscopically, (2) the authors employed a rather large (15–25 ml) gastric pouch, and (3) both early and late complication rates are very high, probably related to a learning-curve phenomenon. Nevertheless, long-term (>10 years) results in these predominantly young patients are eagerly awaited to verify whether LGB will stand the test of time.

Another concern with LGB is the effect on the anatomy and physiology of the esphagocardial junction. This concern is justified by a recent increase in acid reflux-associated conditions such as Barrett esophagus and adenocarcinoma of the esophagogastric region. Acid reflux-associated problems in LGB patients usually do not occur in the first 1–3 years postoperatively, unless a pouch dilatation or slippage occurs. In my personal experience, most patients suffering from heartburn preoperatively report substantial amelioration of this symptom after LGB (data not published). Acid reflux-related problems do arise, however, in patients >3 years after LGB who develop a dilatation of the lower esophagus. This "pseudo-achalasia" is usually explained by the fact that these patients use their lower esophagus as a gastric substitute, eventually leading to disturbed function of the esophagogastric junction. The clinical relevance of this development was highlighted recently by Gustavsson and Westling, who reported a 44% prevalence of erosive esophagitis in LGB patients [9]. One has to consider, however, a 58% reoperation rate in this series, which could suggest a suboptimal technique. Based on pre- and postoperative barium radiography and endoscopy, Wiesner et al. identified patients with preoperative insufficiency of the LES to be at risk for esophageal decompensation following LGB [10]. In our experience, despite the fact that we systematically ask for it, patients rarely report heartburn or other reflux-associated complaints unless they develop pouch dilatation or slipping. In order to further investigate this important issue, we are currently performing both pre- and postoperative esophageal manometry and 24-h pH measurement in a group of LGB patients.

In conclusion, the available evidence suggests that laparoscopic gastric banding for severe obesity is safe and effective on short- to medium-term follow-up. Long-term follow-up studies are awaited before any definitive conclusions can be drawn, especially regarding sustained long-term (>10 years) weight loss and development of acid reflux-associated pathology. Finally, it is nothing less than deplorable that despite over 150,000 LGB procedures performed worldwide, hardly any prospective randomized trial (LGB versus gastric bypass, high versus low band placement, etc.) is reported concerning this common surgical indication.

References

1. Colquitt J, Clegg A, Sidhu M, Royle P. Surgery for morbid obesity (Cochrane Review). Cochrane Database Syst Rev 2003;2:CD003641.
2. O'Brien PE, Dixon JB. Laparoscopic adjustable gastric banding in the treatment of morbid obesity. Arch Surg 2003;138:376–82.
3. Ceelen W, Walder J, Cardon A, Van Renterghem K, Hesse U, El Malt M, Pattyn P. Surgical treatment of severe obesity with a low-pressure adjustable gastric band: experimental data and clinical results in 625 patients. Ann Surg 2003;237:10–6.
4. Hanusch-Enserer U, Brabant G, Roden M. Ghrelin concentrations in morbidly obese patients after adjustable gastric banding. N Engl J Med 2003;348:2159–60.
5. DeMaria EJ, Sugerman HJ, Meador JG, Doty JM, Kellum JM, Wolfe L, Szucs RA, Turner MA. High failure rate after laparoscopic adjustable silicone gastric banding for treatment of morbid obesity. Ann Surg 2001;233:809–18.
6. Ren CJ, Horgan S, Ponce J. US experience with the LAP-BAND system. Am J Surg 2002;184:46S-50S.
7. Belachew M, Belva PH, Desaive C. Long-term results of laparoscopic adjustable gastric banding for the treatment of morbid obesity. Obes Surg 2002;12:564–8.
8. Doherty C, Maher JW, Heitshusen DS. Long-term data indicate a progressive loss in efficacy of adjustable silicone gastric banding for the surgical treatment of morbid obesity. Surgery 2002;132:724–7.
9. Gustavsson S, Westling A. Laparoscopic adjustable gastric banding: complications and side effects responsible for the poor long-term outcome. Semin Laparosc Surg 2002;9:115–24.
10. Wiesner W, Hauser M, Schob O, Weber M, Hauser RS. Pseudo-achalasia following laparoscopically placed adjustable gastric banding. Obes Surg 2001;11:513–8.

Vertical Banded Gastroplasty for Morbid Obesity

M. Morino, M. Toppino, G.M. Del Genio

> ▶ **Key Controversy**
>
> A. Long-term results
> B. Quality of life
> C. Why perform a VBG?
> – Why a restrictive procedure?
> – The appropriate candidate?
> – LVBG or LASGB?
> – Which technique for VBG?
> D. Laparoscopic versus open VBG

17.1
Introduction

Since its introduction in 1980, the vertical banded gastroplasty (VBG) gained widespread popularity. This procedure provided a double advantage when compared with other bariatric techniques: lower complication rate compared with that of malabsorptive procedures, minor technical complexity and the possibility of exploring the distal (remnant) stomach, when compared to gastric bypass.

However, since the late 1980s this procedure faced significant criticism with changing trends in favor of laparoscopic adjustable gastric banding in Europe and Australia and gastric bypass and biliopancreatic diversion in the USA.

17.2
Discussion

17.2.1
Long-Term Results

The major reservations with VBG are the frequent weight loss failures and inexorable long-term weight regain. Indeed, reviewing the literature, according to the studies of Mason et al. in 1987, MacLean et al. in 1990, and Deitel and Shahi in 1992, the excess weight loss (EWL) at 5 years seemed to be very satisfactory, at around 60% [1–3]. Even so, after having evaluated the long-term outcome, the data become limited and more unsatisfactory. At 10 years there are only four studies [4–7] available in literature: Fobi (EWL 42%), Sweet (EWL 45%), Toppino et al. (EWL 45%), and Mason. The latter reports in his series a success rate of 78% but considered an EWL >25% to be successful (although this value is judged a failure by the other authors).

With regard to the poor weight loss results, several studies indicated that late disruption of the vertical staple line (rate up to 48%, though not always so important to allow an increase of the caloric intake) was the main cause [8–12]. Therefore, several technical modifications were developed to improve the strength of this staple line, until achieving the modification with complete separation of the pouch from the gastric fundus [12, 13]. In addition, in order to improve the outcome, a precise pouch calibration was suggested [14, 15].

However, these modifications have led to slight improvement, while the reoperation rate increased mainly due to the consequent outlet stenosis and limitation of food intake.

In particular, three randomized studies comparing VBG with gastric by-pass clearly demonstrated a greater weight loss rate with the latter procedure [16–18].

17.2.2
Quality of Life

Several authors criticized the quality of life achieved after VBG and, in particular, the frequent vomiting and the intake intolerance to solid food.

Indeed, in the papers in which the quality of life is evaluated, the outcomes are generally satisfactory. Having once evaluated different parameters, such as improvement of co-morbidities, the health status and well-being, work satisfaction, and personal and social relations, it was possible to recognize a clear improvement after the procedure [19–21].

The criticisms are directed towards the side-effects of the gastroplasty and the alimentary difficulties. Few authors [22, 23] reported that only a few operated patients were able to regain a normal food intake. On the other hand, others expressed a favorable opinion, even while recognizing the trouble. Wyss et al. [24], confirming the clear increase in the quality of life, established the need of patients to have information on postoperative food restrictions. Guisado and colleagues [20] recommend an improvement extended to the compulsive eating behavior and Sabbioni et al. [25] assert that preoperative binge-eating is the most important predictive factor on the quality of life after gastroplasty.

When compared to more complex procedures, VBG resulted in inferior outcomes. In the comparative study by Hell et al. [26], gastric bypass results were superior to those of VBG and laparoscopic adjustable silicone gastric banding (LASGB) with regards to weight loss and quality of life improvement.

17.2.3
Why Perform a VBG?

After reviewing some European series [14, 27, 28], the VBG outcomes appear to be clearly superior to those achieved in the USA. In particular, according to the data of the Italian Registry for Obesity Surgery [28], in the laparoscopic MacLean's vertical banded gastroplasty (1025 cases) EWL was 63% at 5 years. According to the Reinhold classification, 78.1% of the patients at 5 years belonged to the classes „excellent" and „good". The residual excess weight was <50% (in a condition without risk related to obesity). Similarly, the mean residual body mass index (BMI) was 29.3 kg/m^2.

Technical differences do not seem to explain the different results. Possible explanations are the difference in population of morbid obese patients and the selection of these patients.

The mean preoperative BMI in European studies was 44.2 kg/m^2. This means that only a limited number of super-obese patients are included. It is known that this latter category of patients achieves a minor weight loss and represents the main cause of failure of restrictive gastric procedures.

On reviewing the study of MacLean et al. [29], and separating the outcomes of obese and morbid obese from those of super-obese patients, relevant differences can be recognized at 5 years. EWL of 57.1% was found in the first group versus 51% in the super-obese, with residual BMI 30.3 versus 40 kg/m^2, residual excess weight <50% in 80% of cases versus 17%, and residual excess weight >100% in 0% versus 11%, respectively.

17.2.3.1
Why a Restrictive Procedure?

Open gastric bypass and biliopancreatic diversion are feasible, and have been available for many years with an adequate standardization, with the laparoscopic approach. However, these procedures involve unquestionably more complex techniques than VBG, involving longer operating time, greater concentration on the part of the surgeon, along with the consequent rise of costs, as well as increase of long-term complication rate (in particular with the biliopancreatic diversion).

It is true that weight loss outcomes are superior, especially because of the minor risk of failure. Nevertheless, in our opinion, in the European population of morbid obese, VBG can lead to relevant outcomes when applied with correct indications in selected patients; thus, the use of other more complex bariatric techniques should be limited to the cases not receptive to a restrictive gastric procedure.

17.2.3.2
The Appropriate Candidate?

In order to predict an effective outcome after a restrictive gastric procedure, it is necessary to exclude not only super-obese, but also other patients with probable poor compliance to the postoperative eating behavior (especially cases with compulsive eating behavior, as well as binge eating, sweet eating, snacking, nibbling, etc.).

We believe the main cause of failure after restrictive gastric procedures is related to the incorrect selection of patients, due to the enrolment of subjects with eating disorder behavior not diagnosed before the operation. These subjects, as well as all or at least the large majority of super-obese, should be candidates for other types of procedures (more complex, but with higher guaranties of long-term results).

Very important, in our opinion, is the study of Pekkarinen et al. [30], based on the comparison of the results after gastroplasty in „non-binge" and „binge eaters" patients: in the first group EWL was 50%, while in the second it was just 24%.

17.2.3.3
VBG or LASGB?

The explanation of the widespread use of LASGB in Europe is mainly the major technical simplicity and the assumption of achieving a minor complication rate relative to VBG, with comparable results.

One decade after the first LASGB, a lower rate of perioperative complications has been clearly demonstrated compared with that of other bariatric procedures. However, at the beginning of its era, LASGB was accompanied by high and often unacceptable rates of long-term complications. Reoperation rates were high especially for slippage of the distal stomach under the band and the acute dilatation of the gastric pouch (66% in our experience and 40% in Belachew's) [31, 32]. With further technical modifications (virtual pouch, retro-gastric tunnel above the bursa omentalis), this complication dramatically dropped [33, 34], but still continues to be relevant (5–21%, according to the literature). Indeed, the LASGB technique is still under development and the last variant (pars flaccida) aims to give a further reduction, but still awaits a long-term effectiveness demonstration [35].

Nevertheless, a prospective comparative multicenter trial that compares LASGB and laparoscopic vertical banded gastroplasty (LVBG) has demonstrated superior mid-term results of the latter in terms of weight loss and a reduced rate of complications and reoperations [36]. This, however, was at the expense of a slightly higher rate of major perioperative complications and a longer length of stay for LVBG patients.

For this reason our preference among restrictive gastric procedures goes to LVGB, which in our experience, based on more than 450 cases, has lead to completely successful results (EWL 60.2% at 6 years with reoperation rate of 2.2%).

17.2.3.4
Which Technique for VBG?

The creation of a progressively smaller sized gastric pouch, with a shorter vertical staple-line, has led to a reduction in rate of suture disruption. Nevertheless, this complication still occurs in the original Mason's technique and, although it does not represent the only cause of weight loss failure, it can unfavorably affect the outcome.

The variation, which involves the full division between staple-lines, eliminates this risk without presenting a higher incidence of early postoperative leakage. For this reason we prefer to choose the latter procedure, according to our previous experience in open surgery.

In laparoscopy, MacLean's variant is mandatory, because of the unavailability of linear cutting staplers with sufficient length to perform the whole vertical partition with the use of only one cartridge. On the other hand, some authors [15, 27] have, at the beginning, routinely performed a mixed variant (second stapler cartridge with no cutting blade), later abandoned due to the appearance of disruptions in this portion of the staple-line.

17.2.4
Laparoscopic versus Open VBG

Advantages of laparoscopy, especially in the field of morbid obesity, and during the early postoperative period, are well known in terms of lower general and wound morbidity. Even more evident are the subjective advantages of lesser pain, faster recovery, an improved sense of well being and a faster return to normal life activities. Nevertheless, only few studies comparing laparoscopy and laparotomy for morbid obesity are available. In a randomized trial on laparoscopic versus open VBG, Azagra and colleagues [15] found no differences either with early and late complications or results of weight loss. On the other hand, they noted a significant decrease in the incidence of wound infections and later incisional hernias.

The evaluation of operative times of the open and laparoscopic approaches to bariatric surgery shows almost consistently longer times in laparoscopy [15]. This difference is related to the required solid experience in advanced laparoscopy and to the learning curve for the technique of gastroplasty (as well as for the more complex techniques mentioned above). Only in the largest series (in relation to the experience in the field of the specific surgeons) have we found operative times inferior to the open counterpart.

However, we consider that a moderate increase of operative time of the laparoscopic technique is broadly balanced by the advantages mentioned above.

According to the data of the Italian Registry [28], postoperative complications after gastroplasty were 8.2% in the laparoscopic group versus 10% in the open surgery cohorts. It is clear that, when comparing the same technique, there is a decrease in morbidity involving mainly respiratory complications. Interestingly, however, the data have not demonstrated the other known advantages of laparoscopy.

In comparison, the reduction of hospital stay was minimal. Clear differences can be appreciated in the simple techniques, like the LASGB, whereas for all other bariatric procedures, involving multiple sutures, a prudent attitude is reported at least in Europe, which practically eliminates the potential advantages over the open counterpart procedure.

17.3
Summary

— In selected cases (excluding sweet- and binge-eaters), a restrictive procedure is effective.
— VBG is the best restrictive procedure.
— Super-obese patients are not appropriate candidates for VBG.
— A complete staple line division significantly reduces long-term failures.
— Laparoscopic VBG is superior to open VBG.

References

1. Mason EE, Doherty C, Maher JW, Scott DH, Rodriguez EM, Blommers TJ. Super obesity and gastric reduction procedures. Gastroenterol Clin North Am 1987;16:495–502.

2. MacLean LD, Rhode BM, Forse RA. Late results of vertical banded gastroplasty for morbid and super obesity. Surgery 1990;107:20–7.
3. Deitel M, Shahi B. Vertical banded gastroplasty and gastric bypass: long-term results. Obes Surg 1992;2:106–7.
4. Fobi MAL. Vertical banded gastroplasty vs gastric bypass: 10 years follow up. Obesity Surg 1993;3:161–4.
5. Sweet WA. Vertical banded gastroplasty: stable trends in weight control at 10 or more years. Obesity Surg 1994;4:149–52.
6. Toppino M, Morino M, Capuzzi P, Mistrangelo M, Carrera M, Morino F. Outcome of vertical banded gastroplasty. Obes Surg 1999;9:51–4.
7. Mason EE. Gastric surgery for morbid obesity. Surg Clin North Am 1992;72:501–3.
8. Toppino M, Nigra I, Olivieri F, Muratore A, Bosio C, Avagnona S. Staple-line distruptions in vertical banded gastroplasty related to different stapling techniques. Obes Surg 1994;4:256–61.
9. Svenheden KE,Akesson LA, Holmdahl C, Naslund I. Staple disruption in vertical banded gastroplasty. Obes Surg 1997;7:136–8.
10. Camps M, Zervos E, Goode SE, et al. Does inadequate weight loss following bariatric surgery predict staple-line failure? A prospective study. Obes Surg 1996;6:330–5.
11. Melissas J, Christodoulakis M, Schoretsanitis G, Harocopos G, de Bree E, Gramatikakis J, Tsiftsis D. Staple-line disruption following vertical banded gastroplasty. Obes Surg 1998;8:15–20.
12. Baltasar A. Modified vertical banded gastroplasty. Technique with vertical division and serosal patch. Acta Chir Scand 1989;155:107–12.
13. MacLean LD, Rhode BM, Forse RA. A gastroplasty that avoid stapling in continuity. Surgery 1993;113:380–8.
14. Morino M, Toppino M, Bonnet G, et al. Laparoscopic vertical banded gastroplasty for morbid obesity. Assessment of efficacy. Surg Endosc 2002;16:1566–72.
15. Azagra JS, Goergen M, Ansay J, De Simone P, Vanhaverbeek M, Devuyst L, Squelaert J. Laparoscopic gastric reduction surgery. Preliminary results of a randomized prospective trial of laparoscopic vs open vertical banded gastroplasty. Surg Endosc 1999;13:555–8.
16. Howard L, Malone M, Michalek A, Carter J, Alger S, Van Woert J. Gastric Bypass and Vertical Banded Gastroplasty – a prospective randomized comparison and 5-year follow-up. Obes Surg 1995;5:55–60.
17. Surgerman HJ, Starkey JV, Birkenhauer R. A randomized prospective trial of Gastric Bypass versus Vertical Banded Gastroplasty for morbid obesity and their effects on sweet versus non-sweet eaters. Ann Surg 1987;205:613–24.
18. MacLean LD, Rhode BM, Forse RA, Nohr C. Surgery for obesity. An update of a randomized trial. Obes Surg 1995;5:145–53.
19. Isacsson A, Frederiksen SG, Nilsson P, Hedenbro JL. Quality of life after gastroplasty is normal: a controlled study. Eur J Surg 1997;163:181–6.
20. Guisado JA, Vaz FJ, Alarcon J, Lopez-Ibor JJ Jr, Rubio MA, Gaite L. Psychopathological status and interpersonal functioning following weight loss in morbidly obese patients undergoing bariatric surgery. Obes Surg 2002;12:835–40.
21. Papageorgiou GM, Papakonstantinou A, Mamplekou E, Terzis I, Melissas J. Pre- and postoperative psychological characteristics in morbidly obese patients. Obes Surg 2002;12:534–9.

22. Baltasar A, Bou R, Arlandis F, Martinez R, Serra C, Bengochea M, Mirò J. Vertical banded gastroplasty at more than 5 years. Obes Surg 1998;8:29–34.
23. Shai I, Henkin Y, Weitzman S, Levi I. Long-term dietary changes after vertical banded gastroplasty: is the trade-off favorable? Obes Surg 2002;12:805–11.
24. Wyss C, Laurent-Jacard A, Burckhardt P, Jayet A, Gazzola L. Long-term results on quality of life of surgical treatment of obesity with vertical banded gastroplasty. Obes Surg 1995;5:387–92.
25. Sabbioni ME, Dickson MH, Eychmuller S, Franke D, Goez S, Hurny C, Naef M, Balsiger B, de Marco D, Burgi U, Bucheler MW. Intermediate results of health related quality of life after vertical banded gastroplasty. Int J Obes Relat Metab Disord 2002;26:277–80.
26. Hell E, Miller KA, Moorehead MK, Normans S. Evaluation of health status and quality of life after bariatric surgery: comparison of standard Roux-en-Y gastric bypass, vertical banded gastroplasty and laparoscopic adjustable silicone gastric banding. Obes Surg 2000;10:214–9.
27. Alle JL, Poortmam, Chelala E. Five years experience with laparoscopic vertical banded gastroplasty. Obes Surg 1998;8:373–4.
28. Toppino M, Morino F, Morino M. Registry Contributors Italian Registry for bariatric surgery: data up to 6 years. [Abstract]. Obes Surg 2003;4:579.
29. MacLean LD, Rhode BM, Sampalis J, et al. Results of the surgical treatment of obesity. Am J Surg 1993;165:155–60.
30. Pekkarinen T, Koskela K, Hiujuri K et al. Long term results of gastroplasty for morbid obesity: binge eating as a predictor of poor outcome. Obes Surg 1994;4:248–55.
31. Morino M, Toppino M, Garrone C, Disappointing long-term results of laparoscopic adjustable gastric banding. Br J Surg 1997;84:868–9.
32. Belachew M, Legrand M, Vincent V, et al. Laparoscopic adjustable gastric banding. World J Surg 1998;22:955–63.
33. Favretti F, Cadière GB, Segato G, et al. Laparoscopic adjustable silicone gastric banding (Lap-Band): how to avoid complications. Obes Surg 1997;7:352–8.
34. O'Brien PE, Dixon JB, Brown WA, et al.. The laparoscopic adjustable gastric band (Lap-Band) a prospective study of medium-term effect on weight, health and quality of life. Obes Surg 2002;12:652–60.
35. Zimmermann JM, Blanc M, Mashoyan P, Zimmermann E, Grimaldi JM. Lap band, changes in surgical technique: outcome of 1410 surgeries performed from July 1995 through April 2001. Obes Surg 2001;11:379.
36. Basso N, Favretti F, Morino M, Parini U, Silecchia A, Restuccia A, Elmore U, Toppino M. Laparoscopic adjustable silicone gastric banding (LASGB) vs Laparotomic vertical banded gastroplasty (LVBG): intermediate results of a prospective, comparative multicentric trial. Obes Surg 2001;11:392.

Commentary

EDWARD E. MASON

The success or failure of an operation for controlling body weight depends upon one to three known mechanisms: (1) restriction of intake, (2) malabsorption, and (3) changes in the neuro-humoral controls of eating. Only the first of these applies to pure restriction operations, which explains their limitations in weight control. The technical details of VBG are also of major importance in outcome. These were worked out over years of study. The resulting recommendations must be followed. VBG requires a pouch smaller than 20 ml and with an outlet stabilized with a one-layer collar of Marlex mesh 5.0 cm in circumference and 1.5 cm wide.

When gastric bypass was begun in 1966 the pouch was not measured. When pouches were measured, they were decreased in size as patients returned with huge stretched pouches. Decrease in pouch volume continued through the study and abandonment of horizontal gastroplasty and into early use of VBG. The law of Laplace states that the tension in the wall of a pouch is related to the radius. The larger the pouch the more the stretch, and the more problems that develop with emptying and staple-line breakdown.

High rates of breakdown of the staple line, obstruction of the outlet, and migration of the collar into the lumen have resulted from changes that have been made by some surgeons in operative technique, such as use of two layers of mesh and smaller circumference collars [1]. These changes have been made in an effort to increase weight loss. However, obstructing the pouch outlet causes vomiting, aversion to solid and fibrous foods, and complications that require further operative treatment. Uncontrolled vomiting that occurs after any stomach operation for obesity and that continues for 2 months or more may lead to thiamine deficiency and Wernicke-Korsakoff syndrome [2]. This rapidly produces irreversible damage to the central nervous system and death if there is delay in diagnosis and treatment. Obesity surgeons must learn about this syndrome and prevent it by finding and correcting the cause of uncontrolled vomiting, which is not a normal consequence of any of these operations.

The criteria for success or failure of an operation to treat obesity need to include the complications that occur over a lifetime, length of life, and quality of life. We do not have the data needed to decide which operations are best, in large part because of lack of lifelong follow-up. VBG does not cause metabolic bone disease, iron deficiency anemia, stomal ulcers, duodenal ulcers, afferent loop syndrome, acute dilatation of an excluded stomach and other complications that may occur after gastric bypass.

There may be an advantage in an operation that does not divide the stomach and that uses a minimum of foreign material. The operation of Michael Long, as modified by Andrew Jamieson, provides a small pouch, stapled in continuity and with an outlet that is stabilized over a distance of 22 mm by three non-absorbable sutures taken through the staple line and tied over an indwelling 36–38F bougie for calibration [3]. This operation provides a pouch and outlet that is anatomically identical to VBG but avoids the cut and stapled window. It uses less foreign material. The operation has been in use for the same length of time as VBG and Jamieson now has experience with over 4000 patients. The operation needs to be adapted to the laparoscopic approach to make it more acceptable to patients and surgeons. As with any operation it needs evaluation by additional surgeons, who adhere to the current recommendations of the originators. With regard to selection of patients, we need more information about the lifelong weight patterns following properly performed restriction operations for all sizes of patients. We need more studies comparing results between sweet-eaters and non-sweet-eaters [4].

In anticipation of millions of operations for obesity, there may be a total lifelong medical care advantage in starting with a simple restriction operation. For patients with persistent diabetes or inadequate weight control, a malabsorption operation could be added, leaving the restriction operation in place [5]. This needs to be studied in centers where there are investigative review boards and the expertise for clinical investigation of new approaches to treatment. There are promising developments in our understanding of weight control that may lead to medications that will be useful in patients who need more than an operation. Such medications may be effective in certain types of patients without an operation. We need to make greater use of pure restriction operations in anticipation of better selection and new treatment modalities and until we have adequate lifelong data regarding all operations. All of this is discussed in the special issue that is referenced [1].

One of the deficiencies of our present medical system is the limited ability to assure adequate care for these patients over a lifetime. Sjöström recommended a center for each 500,000 population, where the severely obese could be followed. We need to collect data about lifelong treatment and outcome so that we can better inform new patients of the lifelong effects of different operations and combinations of surgical, medical and other treatment modalities [6].

References

1. Mason EE. Development and future of gastroplasties for morbid obesity. Arch Surg 2003;138:361–6.
2. Mason EE. Starvation injury after gastric reduction for obesity. World J Surg 1998;22:1002–7.
3. Jamieson AC. Determinants of weight loss after gastroplasty. In: Mason EE, guest ed.; Nyhus LM, editor-in-chief. Surgical treatment of morbid obesity, vol. 9. Problems in general surgery series. Philadelphia: JB Lippincott; 1992. pp. 290–7.
4. Sjöström L. Surgical intervention as a strategy for treatment of obesity. Endocrine 2000;13:213–30.
5. Kral JG. Overview of surgical techniques for treating obesity. Am J Clin Nutr 1992;55 (2 Suppl):552S–5S.
6. Mason EE, Hesson WW. Informed consent for obesity surgery. Obes Surg 1998;8:419–28.

Gastric Bypass for Morbid Obesity

David S. Tichansky, Adolfo Z. Fernandez, Eric J. DeMaria

▶ **Key Controversies**

A. Gastric bypass is the best procedure for morbid obesity
B. Appropriate length of Roux limb
C. Antecolic versus retrocolic Roux limb placement
D. Type of gastrojejunostomy anastomosis: circular-stapled, linear-stapled, or hand-sewn

---

18.1
Introduction

The integration of laparoscopy into the surgical management of morbid obesity has fueled the tremendous increase in popularity of bariatric surgery in the past few years. By reducing wound infections, incisional hernias, and time to return to normal activity and work [1], surgery by the laparoscopic approach has been accepted more favorably by patients and non-surgical practitioners alike. Most surgeons believe that laparoscopic surgery for obesity is safe and cost-effective with results similar to open gastric bypass [1–5]. The Roux-en-Y gastric bypass (RNYGB) now prevails as the most commonly performed procedure for obesity in the United States, comprising approximately 70% [6, 7]. The RNYGB offers results superior to the restriction-only procedures and fewer complications than the more radical distal malabsorptive procedures. Despite being the most popular procedure, there is considerable variability and controversy in technique. The laparoscopic Roux-en-Y gastric bypass (LapGBP) was first described in the literature in 1994 [8] and is rapidly replacing the open approach.

18.2
Discussion

18.2.1
Gastric Bypass is the Best Procedure for Morbid Obesity

RNYGB combines restriction and altered absorption to cause weight loss. This procedure has proven its superiority to other procedures consistently in many years of open surgery. The improved weight loss compared to the vertical banded gastroplasty (VBG) (50–83% excess weight loss [EWL] versus 25–40%, respectively) has been proven repeatedly in randomized trials [9–15]. Provision of only a restrictive component not only yields less weight loss, but the durability of that result is poor as displayed by long-term data on the VBG. Despite industry and media championing of adjustable gastric banding (AGB), short-term data on this procedure has uniformly shown inferior weight loss results compared with those of the RNYGB in multiple studies [16–18]. No long-term data from the USA exists for AGB. Unfortunately, the AGB has a 30–50% failure rate, either by poor weight loss or device failure [18, 19]. Applying the standard measures of failure due to poor weight loss set forth by Brolin in 1989 [20] (i.e., less than 50% EWL), which have traditionally been used in studies of the RNYGB, the failure rate for AGB is much greater. In defense of the VBG and AGB, the RNYGB adds two gastrointestinal anastomoses, thus significantly increasing the risk of gastrointestinal leak; a potentially fatal postoperative complication. However, VBG and AGB also have significant complications of their own, including outlet obstruction leading to nausea and vomiting, band erosion into the bowel, gastric herniation through the band or band slippage (AGB only), and esophageal dilatation [18]. These complication rates can approach 22% to greater than 50% [16, 18].

RNYGB provides a minimal malabsorptive component for weight loss compared to the more distal bypasses (distal GBP, biliopancreatic diversion, and biliopancreatic diversion with duodenal switch), which yield greater initial weight loss and provide better maintenance of that weight loss with studies reporting 69% to almost 80% EWL with follow-up reported out to 20 years [21, 22]. However, these distal bypasses possess an increased risk of mineral deficiencies and protein-calorie malabsorption.

The procedure described by Wittgrove and colleagues, in 1994 [8], incorporates all of the key elements of the RNYGB. Thus, the procedure done laparoscopically is not changed from the open technique that has been proven superior. Many institutions now perform RNYGB by the laparoscopic approach in a fashion little different from their open techniques [1, 23]. Thus, it is no surprise that incorporation of laparoscopic techniques has not changed the efficacy of the RNYGB in comparison to open techniques. Lastly, the distal procedures are very difficult to perform laparoscopically and have significant perioperative morbidity. Some highly skilled surgeons even advocate performing these distal bypasses as two-stage procedures to reduce morbidity and mortality [24]. Thus, incorporation of laparoscopic techniques has changed the quality of these procedures in comparison to open techniques.

18.2.2
Appropriate Length of Roux Limb

Appropriate length of the Roux limb is widely debated. Theoretically, increased Roux limb length equals increased malabsorption, thus, weight loss should be increased. However, risk of fat-soluble vitamin, mineral, and protein-calorie malnutrition is also increased. The biliopancreatic diversion and biliopancreatic diversion with duodenal switch are the most extreme examples with 50- to 150-cm common channels. Brolin et al. studied the use of a 150 cm Roux limb versus a 50- to 75-cm Roux limb in super obese patients (body mass index, BMI ≥50) and found weight loss in the 150-cm Roux limb group (61% EWL) to be superior to the shorter Roux limb group (56%) [25]. Brolin also studied a third group with a more distal bypass with a 75-cm common channel and found that group to have significantly greater weight loss than the other two groups out to 5 years follow-up. Our experience using a 50-cm Roux limb and a 30-cm biliopancreatic limb has yielded similar weight loss to that reported by Brolin with acceptable resolution of comorbid conditions [23]. Brolin also looked at metabolic complications of the three groups. He found similar metabolic complication rates in the 50–75 cm and 150 cm groups, but increased metabolic complications in the patients with bypasses more distal than 150 cm [25]. A longer Roux limb is also technically more difficult to create as the jejunojejunostomy is in the smaller caliber distal small bowel. Thus, a higher risk of narrowing the efferent common limb exists. Lastly, a Roux limb longer than 100 cm earns the title "long-limb" gastric bypass, which is considered by some to be "experimental". Thus, it inherits many other difficult problems associated with that label. Many surgeons currently use longer Roux limb lengths for patients with BMI ≥50 [1, 11, 23, 25].

18.2.3
Antecolic versus Retrocolic Roux Limb Placement

Antecolic versus retrocolic Roux limb placement is also controversial. Laparoscopic retrocolic placement is a technically more difficult choice, as exposure to create the tunnel and close the mesenteric defect can be difficult. The literature on open procedures is divided on which of these two choices carries a lower risk of postoperative complications including internal hernias [26–29]. However, there is a clear trend toward a greater risk of internal hernia, either through the transverse mesocolon or Petersen's defect, when the retrocolic approach is used in laparoscopic procedures [30, 31]. It should be noted that Petersen's defect is still present when the antecolic approach is used. The clinical significance and hernia risk of this defect with the antecolic approach is also debatable [31]. Despite meticulous closure of the mesenteric defects in the retrocolic approach, hernias still occur in this setting [30] with the potentially disastrous complication of small bowel incarceration and strangulation. Many surgeons do not close the defect in the antecolic approach. An unrelated potential advantage of the retrocolic position is that the excluded portion of the stomach is against the abdominal wall, theoretically facilitating safer percutaneous access should future transgastric procedures be required.

The main problem with the antecolic approach is that excessive tension may be placed on the gastrojejunostomy anastomosis causing an increased leak rate. Schauer et al. directly compared the leak rates for the antecolic and retrocolic techniques and found no significant difference, suggesting this additional tension is not clinically significant [31]. There is also the possibility of obstruction at the transverse colon by the Roux limb itself. Schauer's group did experience one such complication in their antecolic patient group of 231 patients [31]. Thus, this theoretical concern is both valid and clinically significant.

18.2.4
Type of Gastrojejunostomy Anastomosis: Circular-Stapled, Linear-Stapled, or Hand-Sewn

Three basic techniques to create the gastrojejunostomy exist: the circular-stapled anastomosis (CSA), the linear-stapled anastomosis (LSA), and the hand-sewn anastomosis (HSA). Few studies, none randomized, directly compare all three of these anastomoses [32, 33]. The CSA utilizes an end-to-end anastomosis type stapling device. Placement of the anvil into the gastric pouch transorally versus transabdominally is another point of debate. The transoral approach pulls the anvil down the esophagus into the pouch with a pull-wire or tube. Pharyngoesophageal injury with the anvil is reported as high as 10% with this technique [33]. Additionally, wound infections at the abdominal wall where the stapling device is removed from the abdomen occur at a rate up to 9% [11]. The transabdominal method may take more time to perform and leaves little pouch left-over to recover from stapler malfunction. However, proponents of the CSA claim that this approach is faster and a uniform gastrojejunostomy is created every time. The LSA technique utilizes a linear-cutting GIA stapler to create the posterior aspect of the anastomosis.

The stapler opening is closed either by hand-sewing or with a second application of a stapler. This gastrojejunostomy can be created either with or without a hand-sewn outer layer. Supporters of this approach believe that it is faster and cheaper than the CSA, and carries a lower stomal stenosis rate. Problems with this approach are that the anastomosis created may not be uniform from case to case, parallel staple lines created may cause segments of necrosis causing a leak, and small pouch size may be compromised as a larger pouch is required to accept the linear stapler. The HSA technique has the greatest variability of the three techniques. However, many surgeons use hand-sewn techniques during open gastric bypass and prefer to carry this technique into the laparoscopic approach. Gonzalez et al. and Abdel-Galil et al. analyzed these three anastomoses for efficacy and complication rates [32, 33]. The CSA clearly took the longest to perform and the linear-stapled technique was the fastest to perform in both studies [32, 33]. Clinically significant stenosis occurred most commonly in the hand-sewn technique according to Abdel-Galil and most commonly in the CSA according to Gonzalez [32, 33]. In both studies, the LSA had the lowest stomal stenosis rate. The CSA requires two staplers: an EEA stapler for the gastrojejunostomy and a linear stapler to create the gastric pouch. Thus, the cost of this technique is significantly greater than that of the other two techniques [32]. The HSA appears to be the least expensive. In both studies, the LSA had the lowest overall complication rates [32, 33]. This technique is utilized by our group with a 6.6% stomal stenosis rate and 3% leak rate. From these studies, the anastomotic leak rates for the three techniques are not appreciably different [32, 33].

18.3
Summary

— Laparoscopic Roux-en-Y gastric bypass is the most commonly performed procedure for morbid obesity combining superior results to restriction-only procedures and lower morbidity than more radical distal bypasses.

— A Roux limb length between 50 and 100 cm appears to be preferred by most surgeons with similar results. Improved weight loss in super-obese patients without significantly greater morbidity can be obtained utilizing a 150-cm Roux length.

— Antecolic placement of the Roux limb appears equally as safe as the retrocolic position with a lower risk of internal hernia formation. Retrocolic placement may facilitate safer percutaneous access to the excluded stomach should it be needed.

— The LSA can be performed more expeditiously than the HSA or CSA. The LSA has a lower stomal stenosis rate than the other two techniques. All methods appear to have similar leak rates. The CSA is associated with a greater wound infection rate than the other two techniques.

References

1. Nguyen NT, Goldman C, Rosenquist CJ, et al. Laparoscopic versus open gastric bypass: a randomized study of outcomes, quality of life, and costs. Ann Surg 2001;234:279–91.
2. Al-Saif O, Gallagher SF, Banasiak M, et al. Who should be doing laparoscopic bariatric surgery? Obes Surg 2003;13:82–7.
3. Sugerman HJ. Gastric bypass surgery for severe obesity. Semin Laparosc Surg 2002;9:79–85.
4. Gentileschi P, Kini S, Catarci M, Gagner M. Evidence-based medicine: open and laparoscopic bariatric surgery. Surg Endosc 2002;16:736–44.
5. Ali MR, Sugerman HJ, DeMaria EJ. Techniques of laparoscopic Roux-en-Y gastric bypass. Semin Laparosc Surg 2002;9:94–104.
6. American Society for Bariatric Surgery. Membership survey. Gainesville: American Society for Bariatric Surgery; 1999.
7. Fisher BL, Schauer P. Medical and surgical options in the treatment of severe obesity. Am J Surg 2002;184:9S–16S.
8. Wittgrove AC, Clark GW, Tremblay LJ. Laparoscopic gastric bypass, Roux-en-Y: preliminary report of five cases. Obes Surg 1994;4:353–7.
9. Sugerman HJ, Kellum JM, Engle KM, et al. Gastric bypass for treating severe obesity. Am J Clin Nutr 1992;55:560S–6S.
10. Nguyen NT, Ho HS, Palmer LS, et al. A comparison study of laparoscopic versus open gastric bypass for morbid obesity. J Am Coll Surg 2000;191:149–57.
11. Schauer PR, Ikramuddin S, Gourash W, et al. Outcomes after laparoscopic Roux-en-Y gastric bypass for morbid obesity. Ann Surg 2000;232:515–29.
12. Mason EE. Vertical banded gastroplasty for obesity. Arch Surg 1982;117:701–6.
13. Sugerman HJ, Londrey GL, Kellum JM, et al. Weight loss after vertical banded gastroplasty and Roux-en-Y gastric bypass for morbid obesity with selective versus random assignment. Am J Surg 1989;157:93–102.
14. Sugerman HJ, Starkey JV, Birkenhauer R. A randomized prospective trial of gastric bypass versus vertical banded gastroplasty for morbid obesity and their effects on sweets vs. non-sweets eaters. Ann Surg 1987;205:613–24.
15. Brolin RL, Robertson LB, Kenler HA, et al. Weight loss and dietary intake after vertical banded gastroplasty and Roux-en-Y gastric bypass. Ann Surg 1994;220:782–90.
16. Ren CJ, Horgan S, Ponce J. US experience with the LAP-BAND system. Am J Surg 2002;184:46S–50S.
17. Rubenstein RB. Laparoscopic adjustable gastric banding at a US center with up to 3-year follow-up. Obes Surg 2002;12:380–4.
18. DeMaria EJ, Sugerman HJ, Meador JG, et al. High failure rate after laparoscopic adjustable silicone gastric banding for treatment of morbid obesity. Ann Surg 2001;233:809–18.
19. Angrisani L, Furbetta F, Doldi SB, et al. Results of the Italian multicenter study on 239 super-obese patients treated by adjustable gastric banding. Obes Surg 2002;12:846–50.

20. Brolin RE, Kenler HA, Gorman RC, et al. The dilemma of outcome assessment after operations for morbid obesity. Surgery 1989;105:337–46.
21. Buchwald H. A bariatric surgery algorithm. Obes Surg 2002;12:733–46.
22. Scopinaro N, Gianetta E, Adami GF, et al. Biliopancreatic diversion for obesity at eighteen years. Surgery 1996;119:261–68.
23. DeMaria EJ, Sugerman HJ, Kellum JM, et al. Results of 281 consecutive laparoscopic Roux-en-Y gastric bypasses to treat morbid obesity. Ann Surg 2002;235:640–7.
24. Chu CA, Gagner M, Quinn T, et al. Two-stage laparoscopic biliopancreatic diversion with duodenal switch: an alternative approach to super-super morbid obesity. Surg Endosc 2002;16:S187.
25. Brolin RE, LaMarca LB, Kenler, HA, et al. Malabsorptive gastric bypass in patients with superobesity. J Gastrointest Surg 2002;6:195–205.
26. Schweitzer MA, DeMaria EJ, Broderick TJ, et al. Laparoscopic closure of mesenteric defects after Roux-en-Y gastric bypass. J Laparoendosc Adv Surg Tech A 2000;10:173–5.
27. Korenaga D, Yasuda M, Takesue F et al. Factors influencing the development of small intestinal obstruction following total gastrectomy for gastric cancer: the impact of reconstructive route in the Roux-en-Y procedure. Hepatogastroenterology 2001;48:1389–92.
28. Grise K, McFadden D. Anastomotic technique influences outcomes after partial gastrectomy for adenocarcinoma. Am Surg 2001;67:948–50.
29. Renvall S, Niinikoski J. Internal hernias after gastric operations. Eur J Surg 1991;157:575–7.
30. Filip JE, Mattar SG, Bowers SP, et al. Internal hernia formation after laparoscopic Roux-en-Y gastric bypass for morbid obesity. Am Surg 2002;68:640–3.
31. Schauer PR, Ikramuddin S, Hamad G, et al. Antecolic vs. retrocolic laparoscopic Roux-en-Y gastric bypass. Surg Endosc 2003;17:S188.
32. Gonzalez R, Lin E, Venkatesh KR, et al. Gastrojejunostomy during laparoscopic gastric bypass: analysis of 3 techniques. Arch Surg 2003;138:181–4.
33. Abdel-galil E, Sabry AA. Laparoscopic Roux-en-Y gastric bypass-evaluation of three different techniques. Obes Surg 2002;12:639–42.

Commentary

NICOLAS V. CHRISTOU

The authors have tried to clarify the current controversies about laparoscopic gastric bypass using the best data available in the literature. This reviewer concurs with their assessment that there are no prospective randomized trials in the literature to shed light on the controversial issues. Unfortunately, such trials are not planned and they are not easy to do because of the lengthy follow-up required and issues related to funding and ethics. Even more important questions linger, e.g., does surgically induced long term weight loss improve the mortality of obese and severely obese (morbidly obese) patients.

Gastric Bypass is the Best Procedure for Morbid Obesity

The RNYGB is considered the gold standard therapy for severe obesity. The authors list several good randomized trials to support this statement but limit themselves to American studies only. There are several international randomized trials comparing vertical banded gastroplasty to RYNGB that support their viewpoint. Similarly the authors limit their discussion about the efficacy of adjustable gastric banding to USA trials and do not discuss the international trials [1–4] that report sustained weight loss up to 5–6 years after band placement. Certainly, if a bariatric surgeon or patient favors a purely restrictive operation, adjustable gastric banding would be a better option then vertical banded gastroplasty. The only way to settle the controversy is to carry out an adequately powered prospective randomized trial comparing laparoscopic RNYGB to laparoscopic adjustable gastric banding, and to pancreaticobiliary diversion with duodenal switch.

Appropriate Length of Roux Limb

It is usually assumed that longer Roux limbs produce more malabsorption. Data to support this assumption are lacking, although intuitively it makes sense that more small bowel out of circulation should produce more malnutrition. The human gastrointestinal tract has a tremendous capacity to adapt. This is seen clearly with the experience of the jejunoileal bypass patients. The data on Roux limb lengths indicate that significant segments, e.g., at least 100 cm must be bypassed before any effect of excess weight loss is demonstrated. Prospective randomized trials with minimum 5-year follow-up are needed.

Antecolic versus Retrocolic Limb Placement

The data on open gastric resections demonstrate a lower incidence of internal hernias with retrocolic gastrojejunostomies. The opposite has been reported with laparoscopic RNYGB. Antecolic gastrojejunostomies are associated with fewer internal hernias. The lower incidence of adhesion formation with laparoscopic surgery contribute to internal hernia formation. The series where intracorporial suturing is used extensively seem to have a very low incidence of internal hernias through the mesocolic defect or Petersen's defect. Surgeons who are used to hand sewing the gastrojejunostomy and jejunojejunostomy defects may be able to close these mesenteric defects more securely. Antecolic placement of the Roux limb is more difficult in patients with central obesity (usually men) even if the omentum is split or a defect is created through this. In the latter case, the predisposition to internal hernias still exists.

Type of Gastrojejunostomy Anastomosis

The anastomotic technique used in constructing the gastrojejunostomy is not controversial in my mind. We have extensive experience with gastric pouch volume at the McGill University Health Center and have good data to show that very small (<15 ml) pouches produce the best long term results [5]. Since 1991 we have been using small <15 ml vertical gastric pouches, which we feel are responsible for our 10-year excess weight loss of 71%. Since 2002 we have converted our open RNYGB to a laparoscopic technique, which preserves the features of the open technique, i.e., gastric pouches of 5–7 cm long by 1.2 mm diameter (we use a 32-Fr gastric lavage kit tube to size the vertical pouch), which give a calculated volume ($\pi r2l$) of 6.8 ml. Such a small pouch does not permit insertion of anvils or linear staplers without severely compromising its integrity or blood supply. The only way to construct the gastrojejunostomy is a hand-sewn technique. As the authors state this is also quicker and less costly than stapled anastomosis. Also, in experienced hands it produces the lowest incidence of leaks [6]. Having said this, I must defer to the previous discussion that the controversy as to the optimum technique for the gastrojejunostomy will only be settled with an adequately powered prospective randomized trial.

References

1. Zinzindohoue F, Chevallier JM, Douard R, Elian N, Ferraz JM, Blanche JP, Berta JL, Altman JJ, Safran D, Cugnenc PH. Laparoscopic gastric banding: a minimally invasive surgical treatment for morbid obesity: prospective study of 500 consecutive patients. Ann Surg 2003;237:1–9.
2. Ceelen W, Walder J, Cardon A, Van Renterghem K, Hesse U, El Malt M, Pattyn P. Surgical treatment of severe obesity with a low-pressure adjustable gastric band: experimental data and clinical results in 625 patients. Ann Surg 2003;237:10–6.
3. O'Brien PE, Dixon JB, Brown W, Schachter LM, Chapman L, Burn AJ, et al. The laparoscopic adjustable gastric band (Lap-Band): a prospective study of medium-term effects on weight, health and quality of life. Obes Surg 2002;12:652–60.
4. O'Brien, PE, Dixon JB. Lap-band: outcomes and results. J Laparoendosc Adv Surg Tech A 2003;13: 265–70.
5. MacLean LD, Rhode BM, Nohr CW. Late outcomes of isolated gastric bypass. Ann Surg 2000;231:524–8.

6. Higa KD, Boone KB, Ho T. Complications of the laparoscopic Roux-en-Y gastric by-pass: 1,040 patients – what have we learned? Obes Surg 2000;10:509–13.

19

Biliopancreatic Diversion for Morbid Obesity

Paul Cirangle, Gregg Jossart

▶ **Key Controversies**

A. Indications and patient selection
   - Which patients are most appropriate to undergo the biliopancreatic diversion procedure
   - Laparoscopic biliopancreatic diversion in the face of previous abdominal surgery
B. Technique
   - Total laparoscopic versus hand-assisted approach
   - Common channel length
   - Gastric pouch volume and logistics of the operation

19.1
Introduction

Obesity has become a primary focus of both medical professionals and the general public. The rate of obesity in the USA has grown to epidemic proportions, currently the number two cause of preventable deaths in the USA [1–4]. Medical management of obesity has been disappointing, with only 3–5% of participants in dietary or exercise programs being successful in the long term [5, 6]. Many surgical procedures have been developed over the course of more than 40 years with varying degrees of success [7, 8]. The interest in weight-loss surgery has increased exponentially over the past 5–10 years due to position statements by the National Institutes of Health [9, 10], and the development of minimally invasive surgical techniques [11, 12]. Currently, there are multiple techniques being utilized by surgeons for the treatment of morbid obesity – the Roux-en-Y gastric bypass (RNY), the adjustable gastric band (AGB), the vertical banded gastroplasty (VBG) and the biliopancreatic diversion with duodenal switch (BPD-DS).

Significant controversy exists as to which procedure provides patients with the best long-term weight loss and the most acceptable complication profile. Few prospective, randomized trials have been completed comparing different techniques (the VBG versus the RNY) [13–16], and these were completed more than 20 years ago when operative techniques were significantly different from those of today. Several recent retrospective reviews, however, have been completed, as well as one randomized review of postoperative complications in laparoscopic versus open RNY procedures [17–23]. From these data, it is clear that minimally invasive bariatric procedures are at least as effective as their open counterparts, and provide real advantages in terms of reduced postoperative disability, reduced pulmonary and wound complications, and shortened hospital stays.

The classic biliopancreatic diversion (BPD) as described by Scopinaro has generally been abandoned by most bariatric surgeons in the USA in favor of the modified BPD-DS as described by Hess and Marceau [17, 24]. The rationale being similar or improved weight loss results and a lower incidence of long-term complications. In a retrospective evaluation of standard BPD versus BPD-DS, Marceau found that his excess body weight loss at 18 months increased from 71 to 84% and the incidence of essentially all complications decreased. This included a decrease in the need for revision of the common channel from 1.7% per year to 0.7% per year (for protein malnutrition or intolerable diarrhea), reduction in the amount of flatulence and malodorous gas by 50%, reduction in the number of daily bowel movements from 4.1 to 2.9, and reducing fatigue, bone pain, and peripheral edema by more than 60%. More recently, minimally invasive surgeons such as Gagner, Jossart, Cirangle, Smith, Baltasar, Sudan and Kim have developed and pioneered laparoscopic techniques to enable the BPD-DS to be performed in a totally laparoscopic manner [20–26, and personal communication]. This chapter will address issues that the authors feel have not been conclusively demonstrated in the medical literature to date.

19.2
Discussion

19.2.1
Indications and Patient Selection

19.2.1.1
Which Patients Are Most Appropriate for the Biliopancreatic Diversion Procedure

There are presently two ways to surgically induce weight loss – restriction and malabsorption. All of the currently accepted surgical weight loss procedures utilize either one or a combination of both. The only way to safely change intestinal absorption (malabsorption) is by diverting the bile and pancreatic secretions distally down the alimentary tract. The RNY and BPD-DS both incorporate differing degrees of malabsorption – the "gold standard" short limb RNY is *mostly restrictive* and the BPD-DS is a *moderately restrictive and moderately malabsorptive* procedure. We know from long-term data (10 years) that after a "short-limb" RNY gastric bypass, the average weight loss is approximately 50%–62% of preoperative excess body weight [27–30]. However, results vary greatly depending on preoperative weight. Patients who are supermorbidly obese (body mass index, BMI >50 kg/m^2) have results that are significantly poorer than those of lighter patients [28]. Brolin and colleagues demonstrated a significant improvement in the long-term weight loss profile by increasing malabsorption with a long Roux limb [31]. Marceau and Hess, who have the largest published series of BPD-DS with long-term follow-up, report a long-term weight loss of 70–77% at 8–14 years, irrespective of BMI [17, 24, 32, 33]. The BPD-DS significantly shortens the absorptive surface of the intestine, selectively decreases the absorption of high-caloric fat, and alters (lowers) the excessive hormonal response of the gut to food intake that seems to be predominant in the supermorbidly obese patient [34]. The BPD-DS is complex and technically difficult to perform and is associated with the increased risk of malnutrition and revision. The RNY is less complex, has a much lower incidence of malnutrition and yields relatively good results in patients with a BMI <50 kg/m^2. Therefore, we believe that the increased complexity and risk of the BPD-DS is best suited for those patients who are considered supermorbidly obese and our most likely to fail a standard RNY. The irony is that those patients with the highest risk require the procedure with the highest risk. In general, our algorithm stratifies patients with BMIs of less than 50 kg/m^2 to the short limb RNY and those above 50 kg/m^{2}to the BPD-DS. Exceptions are often made upon patient request and insurance company policy. This has yielded similar excess weight loss results for patients of all BMIs and minimized the incidence of malnutrition and the revision rate.

19.2.1.2
Laparoscopic Biliopancreatic Diversion in the Face of Previous Abdominal Surgery

When considering whether a laparoscopic BPD-DS will be possible in a patient who has previously undergone abdominal or pelvic surgery, one must consider several variables. First, we feel that the patient who has undergone an open cholecystectomy, open biliary surgery, or an open procedure to address complicated peptic ulcer disease (vagotomy and pyloroplasty, oversew of a bleeding duodenal ulcer, or repair of a perforated duodenal ulcer) is at high risk for a duodenoileal anastomotic complication. A very low threshold should exist to either convert to an open procedure in the face of any intraoperative difficulty, or perhaps more appropriately, to just perform the operation in an open manner from the start in a high risk patient (BMI >60 kg/m², multiple medical comorbidities, age >52 years, male). Any patients with a history of lower extremity cellulitis or venous stasis disease should be have open procedures with the technique of suturing all of the staple lines to make postoperative anticoagulation safer.

Experience and analysis of our data has found that these individuals are at least 20–30% more likely to experience leaks or other serious postoperative complications. Generally, previous open pelvic procedures do not interfere with the performance of a laparoscopic BPD-DS. Laparoscopic surgery in the face of previous *laparoscopic* abdominal or pelvic procedures is routinely not a significant problem. Adhesions are usually minimal and tissue planes are preserved. An exception to this may be a laparoscopic cholecystectomy where stones were spilled into the right upper quadrant or for severe or emphysematous cholecystitis. Again, these individuals are at a significantly higher risk of anastomotic complications at the duodenoileal anastomosis. For any patients who have undergone a prior weight-reduction procedure, we strongly recommend an open procedure. Adhesions and compromised tissues will need to be addressed with additional techniques that may only be available through an open incision.

19.2.2
Technique

19.2.2.1
Total Laparoscopic versus Hand-Assisted Approach

Many surgeons have looked at using hand-assisted techniques to facilitate performing technically challenging operative procedures [35, 36]. Most have concluded that it offers little advantage over an open approach, and increases the economic costs associated with surgery. In our experience, the only advantage over the open approach was a slightly shorter hospital stay and smaller incision size. Wound complications and the incidence of leaks were higher and operative expense was greater. Operative times, and other postoperative complications were similar to a series of BPD-DS procedures performed in an open fashion. Explanations for these findings can be justified by a steep learning curve and the process of standardization of the operative technique. Further modification of this hand-assisted technique to include a hand-sewn duodenoileostomy has significantly reduced our leak rate. The totally laparoscopic approach is now routinely performed in all patients who have a BMI of less than 60 kg/m². Those with higher BMIs are evaluated on a case by case basis (see Section 19.2.1.1). In addition, male patients and nulliparous women can be much more challenging than multiparous women. The totally laparoscopic approach, combined with intracorporeal suturing of the duodeno-ileostomy has yielded an operation that reduces the incidence of pulmonary complications, wound complications, hospital stay, and postoperative pain in comparison with those patients undergoing open procedures.

19.2.2.2
Common Channel Length

Scopinaro has meticulously documented in numerous papers his methods and results in systematically determining the appropriate length of the alimentary limb (AL) and common channel (CC) for the BPD procedure [37–41]. His long-term reported revision rate (elongation of the CC or AL, or restoration of intestinal continuity) to address nutritional deficiencies (protein malnutrition) and intolerable diarrhea is 7.2–10.5%, depending on the anatomical changes that were made. Most other surgeons' rates have been even higher (15%) especially with reoperative BPD procedures [33, 42–49]. Marceau and Hess felt that gastrointestinal side effects of the BPD could be minimized by lengthening the CC, and eliminating the postgastrectomy effects of a distal gastric resection. They employed a technique originally developed by DeMeester for the treatment of alkaline gastritis [50]. They theorized that lengthening the CC to 100 cm and keeping the AL 250 cm in combination with preservation of the antrum and pylorus should minimize the problem of protein malnutrition as well as peptic ulcer disease and the dumping syndrome, which was seen in approximately 8%–12% of standard BPD patients postoperatively. In addition, they felt that preservation of a more functional stomach (by employing a sleeve gastrectomy rather than a distal partial gastrectomy) would help with protein digestion and maintain the stomach's role in satiety. They figured that these benefits were worth the decrease in long-term weight loss that may occur. Unexpectedly, not only did complications decrease (incidence of diarrhea, protein malnutrition, bloating, vomiting, etc.) but excess weight loss increased from 71% to 84% at 18 months [51, 52]. The initial mild "short-gut syndrome" that is produced by the anatomic changes following surgery is sufficient to significantly impair absorption of fat but only mildly impair absorption of protein. In time, the intestine compensates by elongating, dilating, and developing hyperplastic villi and enlarged valvulae conniventes [53, 54].

At this point, the patient has a "fixed" intestinal absorption capacity for fat and starch, which will prevent late regain of lost weight. This was demonstrated nicely by overfeeding studies in post-BPD patients by Scopinaro [41]. We believe that in order to minimize the incidence of protein malnutrition and the need for future revision of the BPD-DS, a CC length of 100 cm and AL length of 250 cm should always be used. This should be measured by lightly stretching the bowel midway between the mesenteric and antimesenteric surface. This allows for the most reproducible measurements and results. Reducing the length of these limbs in patients with higher BMIs to maximize weight loss is reasonable but they must be counseled on the increased incidence of serious long-term complications.

19.2.2.3
Gastric Pouch Volume and Logistics of the Operation

The standard BPD gastric pouch volume as described by Scopinaro is 250–500 cc (65% distal gastrectomy) [55]. The modification described by Marceau requires a sleeve or vertical gastrectomy leaving intact the distal antrum and approximately 250 cc gastric volume [17, 32]. Marceau believes that a larger stomach aids in protein digestion and Scopinaro believes that the larger stomach slows the transit time of the food bolus increasing absorption of nutrients.

We believe that the majority of the initial and overall weight loss seen after the BPD-DS is secondary to the restrictive effects of a smaller gastric volume. It is for this reason that we advocate a smaller initial pouch size. This has been supported by our series of patients as well as the series by Feng and Gagner [26], which have undergone a two-stage BPD-DS (initial restrictive vertical gastrectomy followed by completion intestinal bypass and duodenal switch). Patients who are stratified to high surgical risk (cardiac failure, BMI >70, severe pulmonary disease, etc.) and undergo vertical gastrectomy alone, seem to loose weight initially as quickly and in a similar fashion as those who have undergone the single-stage BPD-DS. This strategy also allows us to complete the procedure totally laparoscopically in a minimum of time. More importantly however, the perioperative mortality and morbidity is significantly lower in high risk patients who undergo a staged procedure (mortality >5% vs 0%). These patients generally undergo the second stage of the operation after they have lost 100 to 200 pounds, but before they plateau their weight loss (usually 6–12 months following their restrictive gastrectomy). The intestinal bypass and duodenal switch seems to be critical for the long-term maintenance of the initially lost weight. Over time (8–12 months), the gastric pouch dilates, restoring the stomach capacity to at least twice its original volume.

We tailor the gastric pouch volume based on the preoperative BMI of the patient. Patients with BMIs of less than 50 kg/m^2 will receive gastric pouches of between 150 cc and 200 cc. Patients with BMIs of more than 50 kg/m^2 will have pouches fashioned that are to 60–120 cc. The distal 8 cm of the antrum is preserved as is the proximal 3–4 cm of duodenum. This helps assure appropriate functioning of the gastric pouch.

19.3
Summary

— BPD-DS is very effective for weight loss, especially for those individuals with a higher body mass index.
— It is associated with significant short-term and long-term risks. The laparoscopic approach is technically difficult and should be cautiously applied to those with a BMI greater than 60 kg/m². It is critical to have skilled assistants and keep in mind that the open technique "works well".
— Absolute proof on what size to make the gastric pouch and limb lengths is not available yet but we emphasize that with increasing BMI a smaller pouch should be made and a greater amount of malabsorption should be introduced via a short common limb.

References

1. Allison DB, Fontaine KR, Manson JE, et al. Annual deaths attributable to obesity in the United States. JAMA 1999;282:1530–8.
2. National Center for Health Statistics, Centers for Disease Control and Prevention. http://www.cdc.gov/nchs/products/pubs/pubd/hestats/obese/obse99.htm.
3. Flegal KM, Carroll MD, Kuczmarski RJ, et al. Overweight and obesity in the United States: prevalence and trends 1960–1994. Int J Obes 1998;22:39–47.
4. Kuczmarski RJ, Carrol MD, Flegal KM, Troiano RP. Varying body mass index cutoff points to describe overweight prevalence among US adults: NHANES III (1988–1994). Obes Res 1997;5:542–8.
5. National Institutes of Health; National Task Force on the Prevention and Treatment of Obesity. Very low-calorie diets. JAMA 1993;270:967–74.
6. Snow JT, Harris MB. Maintenance of weight loss after very low calorie diets involving behavioral treatment. Psychol Rep 1995;6:82.
7. DeWind LT, Payne JH. Intestinal bypass surgery for morbid obesity. Long-term results. JAMA 1976;236:2298–301.
8. Livingston EH. Obesity and its surgical management. Am J Surg 2002;184:103–13.
9. National Institutes of Health. Gastrointestinal surgery for severe obesity: National Institutes of Health Consensus Development Conference Statement. Am J Clin Nutr 1992;55 (2 Suppl):615s–19s.
10. National Institutes of Health. Clinical guidelines on the identification, evaluation, and treatment of overweight and obesity in adults. The Evidence Report. NIH Publication No. 98–4083. September 1998.
11. Schauer P, Ikramudin S, Gourash W. Laparoscopic Roux Y gastric bypass: a case report and 1 year follow up. J Laparoendosc Adv Surg Tech 1999;9:101–6.
12. Wittgrove AC, Clark GW, Trembly LJ. Laparoscopic gastric bypass, Roux-en-Y: preliminary report of five cases. Obes Surg 1994;13:353–7.
13. Griffen WO, Young VL, Stevenson CC. A prospective comparison of gastric and jejunoileal bypass procedures for morbid obesity. Ann Surg 1977;186:500–9.

14. Sugerman HJ, Starkey JV, Birkenhauer R. A randomized prospective trial of gastric bypass versus vertical banded gastroplasty for morbid obesity and their effects on sweets versus non-sweets eaters. Ann Surg 1987;205:613–24.
15. Freeman JB, Burchett HJ. A comparison of gastric bypass and gastroplasty for morbid obesity. Surgery 1980;88:433–44.
16. Laws HL, Piantadosi S. Superior gastric reduction procedure for morbid obesity – a prospective, randomized trial. Ann Surg 1981;193:334–40.
17. Marceau P, Hould FS, Simard S, et al. Biliopancreatic diversion with duodenal switch. World J Surg 1998;22:947–54.
18. Higa KD, Boone KB, Ho T. Complications of the laparoscopic Roux-en-Y gastric bypass: 1040 patients– what have we learned? Obes Surg 2000;10:509–13.
19. Schauer PR, Ikramuddin S, Gourash W, Ramanathan R, Luketich J. Outcomes after laparoscopic Roux-en-Y gastric bypass for morbid obesity. Ann Surg 2000;232:515–29.
20. Ren CJ, Patterson E, Gagner M. Early results of laparoscopic biliopancreatic diversion with duodenal switch: a case series of 40 consecutive patients. Obes Surg 2000;10:514–23.
21. O'Brien P, Dixon J. Weight loss and early and late complications– the international experience. Am J Surg 2002;184:42S-45S.
22. Nguyen NT, Lee SL, Goldman C, et al. Comparison of pulmonary function and postoperative pain after laparoscopic versus open gastric bypass a randomized trial. J Am Coll Surg 2001;192:469–76.
23. DeMaria EJ, Sugerman HJ, Kellum JM, Meador JG, Wolfe LG. Results of 281 consecutive total laparoscopic Roux-en-Y gastric bypasses to treat morbid obesity. Ann Surg 2002;235:640–5.
24. Hess DW, Hess DS. Biliopancreatic diversion with a duodenal switch. Obes Surg 1998;8:267–82.
25. de Csepel J, Burpee S, Jossart G, Andrei V, Murakami Y, Benavides S, et al. Laparoscopic biliopancreatic diversion with a duodenal switch for morbid obesity: a feasibility study in pigs. J Laparoendosc Adv Surg Tech 2001;11:79–83.
26. Feng JJ, Gagner M. Laparoscopic biliopancreatic diversion with duodenal switch. Semin Laparosc Surg 2002;9:125–9.
27. Pories WJ, Swanson MS, MacDonald KG, et al. Who would have thought it? An operation proves to be the most effective therapy for adult-onset diabetes mellitus. Ann Surg 1995;222:339.
28. MacLean LD, Rhode B, Norhr CW. Late outcome of isolated gastric bypass. Ann Surg 2000;231:524–528.
29. Sugerman HJ, Kellum JM, Engle KM, Wolfe L, Starkey JV, Birkenhauer R, et al. Gastric bypass for treating severe obesity. Am J Clin Nutr 1992;55:560S-6S.
30. Capella JF, Capella RF. The weight reduction operation of choice. Am J Surg 1996;171:74–9.
31. Brolin RE, Kenler HA, Gorman JH, Cody RP. Long-limb gastric bypass in the super-obese. A prospective randomized study. Ann Surg 1992;215:387–95.
32. Marceau P, Hould FS, Lebel S, Marceau S, Biron S. Malabsorptive obesity surgery. Surg Clin North Am 2001;81:1113–27.
33. Marceau S, Biron S, Lagace M, Hould FS, Potvin M, Bourque RA, et al. Biliopancreatic diversion, with distal gastrectomy, 250 cm and 50 cm limbs: Long-term results. Obes Surg 1995;5:302–7.

34. Jones IR, Owens DR, Luzio SD, et al: Obesity is associated with increased post-prandial GIP levels which are not reduced by dietary restriction and weight loss. Diabetes Metab 1989;15:11–22.

35. DeMaria EJ, Schweitzer MA, Kellum JM, Meador J, Wolfe L, Sugerman HJ. Hand-assisted laparoscopic gastric bypass does not improve outcome and increases costs when compared to open gastric bypass for the surgical treatment of obesity. Surg Endosc 2002;16:1452–5.

36. Schweitzer MA, Broderick TJ, Demaria EJ, Sugerman HJ. Laparoscopic-assisted Roux-en-Y gastric bypass. J Laparoendosc Adv Surg Tech A 1999;9:449–53.

37. Scopinaro N, Gianetta E, Civalleri D, et al. Biliopancreatic bypass for obesity: I. An experimental study in dogs. Br J Surg 1979;66:613–17.

38. Scopinaro N, Gianetta E, Civalleri D, et al. Biliopancreatic bypass for obesity: II. Initial experience in man. Br J Surg 1979;66:619–620.

39, Scopinaro N, Gianetta E, Adami GF, Friedman D, Traverso E, Marinari GM, et al. Biliopancreatic diversion for obesity at eighteen years. Surgery 1996;119:261–8.

40. Scopinaro N, Gianetta E, Adami GF, et al. Evolution of biliopancreatic bypass. Clin Nutr 1986;5 (Suppl):137–46.

41. Scopinaro N, Marinari GM, Gianetta E, et al. The respective importance of the alimentary limb (AL) and the common limb (CL) in protein absorption (PA) after BPD. Obes Surg 1997;7:108.

42. Gianetta E, Friedman D, Adami GF, et al. Etiological factors of protein malnutrition after biliopancreatic diversion. Gastroenterol Clin North Am 1987;16:503–4.

43. Wittig J, Wittig VR, Brummer MJ. Effect of common limb length on weight loss, electrolytes, and protein malnourishment in long limb gastric bypass Roux-en-Y. Int J Obes 1987;11:206.

44. Cates JA, Drenick EJ, Abedin MZ, et al. Reoperative surgery for the morbidly obese. Arch Surg 1990;125:1400–4.

45. Fox SR, Fox KM, Oh KH. The gastric bypass for failed bariatric surgical procedures. Obes Surg 1996;6:145–50.

46. Sugerman HJ, Kelum JM, DeMaria DJ. Conversion of proximal to distal gastric bypass for failed gastric bypass for superobesity. J Gastrointest Surg 1997;1:517–26.

47. Holian DK, Clare MW. Biliopancreatic bypass for morbid obesity: late results and complications. Clin Nutr 1986;5 (Suppl):133–6.

48. Clare MW. An analysis of 37 reversals on 504 biliopancreatic surgeries over 12 years. Obes Surg 1993;3:169–73.

49. Lemmens L. Biliopancreatic diversion: 170 patients in a 7-year follow-up. Obes Surg 1993;3:179–80.

50. DeMeester TR, Fuchs KH, Ball CS, et al. Experimental and clinical results with proximal end-to-end duodenojejunostomy for pathologic duodenogastric reflux. Ann Surg 1987;206:414–26.

51. Lagracé M, Marceau P, Marceau S, et al. Biliopancreatic diversion with a new type of gastrectomy: Some previous conclusions revisited. Obes Surg 1995;5:411–8.

52. Biron S, Hould FS, Marceau P. Surgical treatment of obesity. Biliopancreatic diversion: current status. Treatment of obesity and eating disorders. Department of Continuing Medical Education, Harvard Medical School. November 1994.

53. Dowling RH. Small bowel adaptation and its regulation. Scand J Gastroenterol Suppl 1982;74:53–75.

54. Stock-Damge C, Aprahamian M, Raul F, Marescaux J, Scopinaro N. Small intestinal and colonic changes after biliopancreatic bypass for morbid obesity. Scand J Gastroenterol 1986;21:1115–23.
55. Scopinaro N, Gianetta E, et al. Biliopancreatic diversion. In: Griffen WO, Printen KJ, eds. Surgical management of morbid obesity, New York: Marcel Dekker; 1987. pp. 93–162.

Commentary

PICARD MARCEAU

The introduction of the laparoscopic approach has been a major factor for increasing the popularity of bariatric surgery. However, indirectly, it had a negative impact. The search for easier techniques adaptable to laparoscopy has caused a shift away from more fundamental problems that undermine bariatric surgery. The continuous change in technique and the addition of new factors in patient selection will cause further delay for reliable, much needed, long-term results. The new technique, which has attracted new young surgeons without personal experience with the deceptive long-term results of bariatric surgery, has contributed in shifting attention on the short term. Low immediate morbidity was prioritized. Procedures once shown to be inefficient in the long term have returned because of their applicability to laparoscopic surgery. An additional factor in patient selection based on feasibility by laparoscopy is adding another variable that increases confusion. Up to now, there are no reliable data available for selection on the basis of sex, age, or degree of obesity; now another factor is added. All these new elements distract from the fundamental goal, which is a permanent cure with the best quality of life for the rest of these patients' life. The element of immediate easiness is almost irrelevant in regard to the ultimate goal.

Which Patients are Most Appropriate for BPD

To our knowledge, to this day, except for BPD [1–3], 5- or 10-year results that take into account different categories of obesity are not available. Comparison between different surgical techniques is not possible. Global results without stratification for degree of initial obesity and length of follow-up are useless and may even be misleading. At the moment any choice is empiric. For us, BPD has been proven to give good weight-loss maintenance for over 10 years. It is the most efficient procedure to assure maintenance of glycemic and lipidic metabolic improvement [4, 5]. Above all it also preserves normal eating habits and consequently better quality of life. As long as there are no better results available, we see no reason to deprive patients from such an efficient operation that allows them to eat normally. Furthermore, our results with BPD were found to be better for the group of patients with an initial BMI less than 45 kg/m^2. The degree of patients satisfaction was better because the rate of recurrence of morbid obesity (BMI >35 kg/m^2) was lower. Even in this favorable group of patients, recurrence rate was found to be as high as 16% after 10 years [3]. We see no reason to deprive patients with an initial BMI less than 50 kg/m^2 from having an operation that gives good weight maintenance and allows normal eating habits.

Length of the Alimentary Tract

Helpful data for the selection of the alimentary tract length based on sex, age, or type of obesity are not available. The pioneer Scopinaro, seeing no obvious clinical difference between using an alimentary tract representing half the total intestinal length versus a fixed 250 cm, decided for convenience to use 250 cm and reported good results. In the absence of any other data showing the influence of different length, there are no reasons not to use the more convenient 250 cm, which does not require measuring the whole intestinal length. Furthermore, we feel that this alimentary segment need only be less than half the total intestinal length to be on the negative side so as to allow an area for natural recuperation toward patients' need. This process gives the procedure a certain individualization. This segment need be less than half only because it refers to the traditional notion that half the intestine can be removed without much consequence. This was also what initially motivated Scopinaro to use half the intestinal length. Until better data are available the use of 250 cm is simpler.

Length of the Common Tract

There are more data concerning the length of the common channel. Its variation causes rapid direct effects on steatorrhea and clinical consequences. Initially Scopinaro had chosen 50 cm as representing the length giving the maximum fat malabsorption with the minimum side-effects. The experience of others was different and they have found that a 100-cm length improved nutritional status, decreased side-effects, and decreased the need for revision. This was done without compromising weight loss maintenance. Others [6] have suggested varying the length of the common tract according to the total intestinal length. Considering the technical difficulty in measuring adequately the intestine and the great variability from uncontrollable factors, it would seem futile to expect obvious clinical difference from a 20 to 25% range variation. For simplicity we prefer using 100 cm.

Size of the Gastric Remnant

The superiority of sleeve gastrectomy with duodeno-ileostomy over distal gastrectomy with gastrojejunostomy has been rapidly recognized for both its sound physiological basis and clinical evidence [7, 8]. However, the amount of stomach to be preserved is not yet established. There are clinical evidence that smaller gastric remnant increases both weight loss and protein deficiency [9]. A 250-ml remnant size seems to be a landmark [10] under which protein deficiency becomes obvious after distal gastrectomy but there are no data concerning ideal gastric remnant size with sleeve gastrectomy. This was not a major preoccupation for us, our goal being to remove about 65% of stomach to prevent ulcer. Considering Scopinaro's experience, we were more preoccupied with possible malnutrition rather than insufficient weight loss. Our attitude has been to put all emphasis on avoiding other important technical pitfalls. Emphasis was put on constructing a remnant tube 5–6 cm away from the lesser curvature leaving intact the last 8 cm of antrum. Focus was always on preventing an hourglass formation within the tube. Segmental narrowing caused postoperative nausea and vomiting. We grossly estimated the remaining stomach as containing about 250–350 ml. This stomach will eventually increase with time. In a few cases, years later an additional resection has been successful for treating insufficient weight loss by restriction.

Conclusion

To succeed in making a BPD-DS by laparoscopy represents a major contribution and should be encouraged. However its inherent difficulty particularly in its learning period should not be a factor depriving patients from an operation allowing better quality of life. It is worrisome that immediate technical appeal and easiness undermines a more important long-term goal. Laparoscopic technique needs be standardized, stable, used on unselected patients and followed for a long period of observation before being useful for comparison with open technique.

References

1. Scopinaro N, Gianetta E, Adam GF, et al. Biliopancreatic diversion for obesity at eighteen years Surgery 1996;119:261–8.
2. Biron S, Hould FS, Lebel S, Marceau S, Lescelleur O, Marceau P. Twenty years experience with biliopancreatic diversion: assessment need precision. (Poster) In: Abstracts of American Society of Bariatric Surgery (ASBS) Meeting, Boston 17–21 June 2003.
3. Biron S, Hould FS, Lebel S, Marceau S, Lescelleur O, Simard S, Marceau P. Twenty years of biliopancreatic diversion: what is the goal? Obes Surg 2004;14:160–4.
4. Marceau P, Hould F.S., Lebel S, Marceau S, Biron S. Malabsorptive obesity surgery. Surg Clin North Am 2001;81:1113–1127.
5. Brolin R, Bradly LJ, Wilson AC et al. Lipid risk profile and weight stability. Gastrointest Surg 2000;4:464–9.
6. Hess DS. Biliopancreatic diversion with duodenal switch. Obes Surg 1998;8:267–82.
7. Marceau P, Biron S, Bourque RA, Potvin M, Hould FS, Simard S. Biliopancreatic diversion with a new type of gastrectomy. Obes Surg 1993;3:29–35.
8. Marceau P, Hould FS, Simard S, et al. Biliopancreatic diversion with duodenal switch. World J Surg 1998;22:947–54.
9. Marceau P, Biron S, Hould FS, Lebel S, Marceau S. Malabsorption procedure in surgical treatment of morbid obesity. Probl Gen Surg 2000;17:29–39.
10. Gianetta E, Adam GEL, Friedman D. Protein malnutrition after biliopancreatic diversion [Abstract]. Int J Obes 1987;11:50–51.

20

Cholecystectomy

Carol E.H. Scott-Conner

▶ **Key Controversies**

A. Indications
- Acute and gangrenous cholecystitis
- Common duct stones, diagnosis and management
- Cirrhosis
- Pregnancy
- Gallbladder polyps
- Management of incidentally discovered gallbladder cancer
- Cholecystectomy incidental to other laparoscopic operations

B. Technique
- Prophylactic antibiotics
- Gasless laparoscopy
- Fewer ports or smaller ports
- Ultrasonic scalpel, and other gadgets
- Fundus first dissection
- Operative cholangiography and laparoscopic ultrasound
- Outpatient cholecystectomy

20.1
Introduction

Laparoscopic cholecystectomy (LC) was popularized in 1989 and can be credited with introducing a new era of minimal access surgery (MAS). Because LC was the first procedure learned by MAS surgeons, one might suppose that all the issues have been settled and no controversies remain. Indeed, the controversies discussed in this chapter reflect expanding use of the procedure and maturation of the technique.

20.2
Discussion

20.2.1
Indications

20.2.1.1
Acute and Gangrenous Cholecystitis

When LC was initially developed, there was concern that dissection would prove too hazardous if the procedure were attempted for acute and/or gangrenous cholecystitis. Excessive inflammation, increased bleeding, difficulty in identifying crucial structures, and other problems were assumed to produce an increased risk of complications. Spillage of infected bile and gallstones, in the absence of well-developed suction/irrigation methods, was problematic and led to abscess formation in a number of cases. Numerous studies have shown that although the total number of cholecystectomies increased after the introduction of LC, the indications remained relatively similar to those previously accepted for open cholecystectomy [1, 2]. Thus, proportionately more patients with acute cholecystitis underwent LC. Techniques were developed for intra-operative decompression of the swollen gallbladder, better graspers facilitated atraumatic manipulation, and it became evident that LC could be done safely in this setting.

Current opinion favors the use of LC in patients with acute cholecystitis, including those in whom gangrenous cholecystitis is suspected. I feel that surgery should be performed as early as feasible, before the inflammation progresses to scarring and neovascularization. The risk of conversion to an open procedure will be increased-such conversion should not be regarded as a complication, but rather as prudent practice [3–8]. Remember that the enlarged and inflamed gallbladder may be adherent to the common duct (Mirizzi syndrome) or duodenum or both. Dissection in this setting risks injury to these crucial structures. Several maneuvers may help increase the probability of success and minimize the risk of bile duct or duodenal injury. Foremost among these is fundus-down dissection, described in more detail in a subsequent section [9, 10]. Laparoscopic cholecystostomy and subtotal cholecystectomy are two additional bail-out maneuvers that every laparoscopist should be familiar with.

20.2.1.2
Common Duct Stones, Diagnosis and Management

With the increase in number of cholecystectomies performed, there has been a decrease in the number of patients with "silent" common duct stones, presumably because patients undergo surgery earlier in the natural history of their disease. Most patients with common duct stones are now identified preoperatively by clinical presentation, laboratory values, or imaging studies. When common duct stones are suspected, there are several options for management, and the choice will depend upon local expertise. Where available, intraoperative fluorocholangiography with laparoscopic clearance of the common duct is the best choice [11]. It allows the problem to be dealt with in a single procedure. When this expertise is not available, options include pre- or postoperative ERCP (endoscopic retrograde cholangiopancreatography), or an open surgical procedure with open common bile duct exploration [11–14].

20.2.1.3
Cirrhosis

Cholecystectomy is a high-risk procedure in cirrhotics, due to potential collateral vessels, coagulopathy, and decreased hepatic reserve. When cholecystectomy must be done in patients with Childs-Pugh class A or B cirrhosis, LC may be considered. It appears to be neither more nor less safe than open cholecystectomy, although the conversion rate and risk of bleeding are increased when compared with non-cirrhotic patients [15–20]. There is very little data available on the use of LC in Childs-Pugh class C patients and at least one death in this subset has been reported. The possibility that LC might decrease risk of viral contamination to the operating team has been advanced, but there are no real data on this subject.

20.2.1.4
Pregnancy

Twelve percent of all pregnant women harbor gallstones, and a significant number become symptomatic during pregnancy. Medical management fails in more than one-third, and surgery may be required. Early reports, including one that I coauthored, cited an increased risk of fetal demise after laparoscopic cholecystectomy or appendectomy during pregnancy [21]. However, numerous papers have subsequently appeared which document that LC can be safely accomplished in this setting. The second trimester appears to be the optimum window for performing the procedure. Co-management with experienced obstetrical colleagues and an anesthesia team is crucial [22–27].

20.2.1.5
Gallbladder Polyps

Cholecystectomy is indicated for symptomatic gallbladder polyps, polyps that increase in size on ultrasound, or those that measure 1 cm or greater in diameter [28–32]. In one study of 111 polypoid lesions measuring less than 1 cm, 27 patients underwent cholecystectomy (of which 70% proved to be cholesterol polyps); of those followed nonoperatively none developed symptoms of biliary disease, gallstones, or carcinoma and 23.5% of these lesions disappeared [31]. LC is a reasonable approach that has been described as a "reliable, safe, and minimally invasive biopsy procedure" when excision is desired and the risk of malignancy is low [30]. It is not considered appropriate therapy for gallbladder cancer (see Section 20.2.1.6). Risk factors for malignancy included age greater than 60, co-existence of gallstones, and size greater than 1 cm in one study [28].

20.2.1.6
Management of Incidentally Discovered Carcinoma
of the Gallbladder

Carcinoma of the gallbladder is curable only when detected early, usually as an incidental finding during cholecystectomy for other indications. Depth of invasion and positive margins were the most important prognostic factors in one study [33]. Gallbladder perforation, such as may occur during LC, is associated with a significant decrease in survival [34, 35]. Port-site recurrence has been a significant complication of LC (as, indeed, is wound implantation during open cholecystectomy in this disease). The specific mechanism is still being elucidated. For these reasons, LC is definitely not recommended as initial approach to patients suspected of harboring gallbladder cancer [33–38].

If cancer is found on pathologic examination of a gallbladder that has been removed by LC, subsequent management depends upon the stage of the disease and the overall condition of the patient. T1a lesions are, by definition, limited to the mucosa, and may have been adequately treated [33]. T1b and T2 lesions are best treated by radical second operation with excision of port sites, gallbladder bed, and regional lymph nodes [33], if the condition of the patient permits.

20.2.1.7
Cholecystectomy Incidental to Other Laparoscopic Procedures

Because every laparoscopic procedure has an optimum setup, including location of operating ports, there has not been a great deal of enthusiasm for performing incidental procedures. In addition, there is general consensus that asymptomatic gallstones do not require surgery. In the rare patient in whom symptomatic gallstones and other pathology requiring laparoscopy coexist, it is good to know that incidental cholecystectomy may be done safely. The largest such reported series includes 67 LC done during the performance of 1065 laparoscopic antireflux procedures [39]. A handful of LC done during laparoscopic splenectomy for hereditary spherocytosis have been reported [40, 41], as well as an isolated case report documenting the combined management of gallstones and polycystic ovary disease [42]. Incidental cholecystectomy may be combined with laparoscopic bariatric procedures at the expense of significantly increased operative time and postoperative stay [43].

20.2.2
Technique

20.2.2.1
Prophylactic Antibiotics

The use of prophylactic antibiotics is firmly engrained in surgical practice, and many surgeons have continued the practice with the switch to minimal access approaches. It is important to recall that the major demonstrated benefit of prophylactic antibiotics for elective cholecystectomy was in prevention of wound infection. When the "wound" consists only of several trocar sites, where is the benefit? Illig et al. conducted a randomized prospective trial and established that there was no benefit to prophylactic antibiotics in low risk patients [44]. Antibiotics are appropriately used in the management of patients with acute and gangrenous cholecystitis.

20.2.2.2
Gasless Laparoscopy

In a small study of 26 patients randomized to conventional or gasless laparoscopy, there appeared to be hemodynamic advantage to the gasless approach [45]. In a series of 1000 patients, "adjunctive minimal pressure pneumoperitoneum" of 5 mmHg was needed in 46 patients weighing more than 85 kg [46]. Those authors cited advantages in the setting of a developing country, and such advantages might potentially translate to cost savings even in a "developed" nation. Unfortunately, most of the patients in my practice weigh more than 85 kg and with modern anesthesia support there appears to be little benefit to gasless laparoscopy.

20.2.2.3
Fewer Ports or Smaller Ports

LC can be done with three ports, with no degradation in exposure and a slight cosmetic advantage [47]. Unfortunately, postoperative pain was not affected in this study of 159 patients [47]. "Micropuncture" techniques with correspondingly small instruments are quite feasible [47–49] and may decrease pain as well as improving cosmesis. Generally a 10-mm port is still used for the laparoscope, introduced through an umbilical skin crease incision. The laparoscope is then switched to a small scope passed through another trocar and the gallbladder extracted through the larger port-site. Concern over fragility of the instruments has limited widespread adoption of these methods, and the actual benefit over the normal procedure appears to be relatively small.

20.2.2.4
Ultrasonic Scalpel, and Other Gadgets

The original description of LC involved use of laser. It did not take surgeons very long to discover that electrocautery worked very well, was cheaper, and actually had fewer complications. The ultrasonic scalpel has proven of significant benefit in procedures like laparoscopic adrenalectomy, splenectomy, and antireflux procedures. Application to LC shows that it may be used in this setting without increase in bleeding complications but without obvious advantage [50].

The cystic duct is usually secured with nonabsorbable clips during LC. There have been occasional reports of clip migration into the common duct, with subsequent stone formation around this foreign body nidus. There is thus interest in alternative methods; among these, the ultrasonic shears. In one report the ultrasonic shears were used to coapt cystic duct in 461 patients (in half, an additional ligature was added) with very acceptable results [51]. Absorbable clips have also been developed for this purpose, and there is always the option of ligation with an absorbable pre-tied ligature.

20.2.2.5
Fundus-first Dissection

This technique mimics the familiar top-down method used for years during open cholecystectomy. Retraction is achieved with liver retractors. The cystic artery may be identified and clipped at the beginning, or identified as dissection progresses. Generally the cystic duct is not divided until the gallbladder is fully dissected. Kato et al. applied this technique in 81 or 173 patients with success [9]. Mahmud et al felt that selective application of this method allowed them to decrease a potential (estimated) conversion rate of 5.2% to 1.2% [10]. They advocated the use of this method of patients with dense adhesions, Mirizzi syndrome, large stones impacted in Hartmann's pouch, and the short dilated cystic duct.

I use a modification of this technique in most patients [52]. As I create a peritoneal incision across the anticipated region of the cystic duct and cystic artery, I continue these incisions up the lateral peritoneal reflections of the gallbladder for several centimeters. Allowing the gallbladder to remain attached at the top, I develop a window behind the gallbladder in the vicinity of Hartmann's pouch before clipping and dividing cystic artery and cystic duct. I have come to prefer this method in all but the very simplest cases.

20.2.2.6
Operative Cholangiography and Laparoscopic Ultrasound

As mentioned during the discussion of common duct stones, fluorocholangiography and the ability to clear the common duct of stones during LC are important skills for the laparoscopic surgeon to master. Operative cholangiography fulfills two functions during LC: it clarifies ductal anatomy and it allows the diagnosis of previously unsuspected common duct stones [53–57]. The issue of whether operative cholangiography should be used routinely or selectively still rages, and is perhaps one of the most contentious remaining issues in LC. Proponents of routine cholangiography assert that it clarifies anatomy, identifies anomalies, detects previously unsuspected common duct stones, and assures that the surgeon is able to cannulate the cystic duct when needed (a necessary skill for transcystic common duct exploration). On the other side, advocates of a more selective approach cite increased cost and operating time, the relatively low incidence of silent common duct stones, and some studies which show no difference in the rate of common duct injury. While the latter statement is true, it is apparent that the injuries that occur when cholangiography is routinely applied are generally less severe than those noted in its absence. Laparoscopic ultrasound is emerging as an extremely effective method which is complementary to fluorocholangiography and may replace it in most cases [56, 57].

20.2.2.7
Outpatient Cholecystectomy

LC is increasingly being performed as an outpatient procedure in careful selected patients. In a representative series, 269 of 387 patients undergoing LC were successfully managed as outpatients [58]. Predictors of failure were age greater than 50 years, ASA category ≥3, surgery that began after 1 p.m., and duration of surgery [58]. Most surgeons now manage a significant number of their patients as outpatients.

20.3
Summary

- LC is safe and effective for acute and gangrenous cholecystitis. The conversion rate may be higher.
- Common bile duct stones are best managed in the operating room, by laparoscopic clearance. The surgeon who is not facile in this technique has several options, including pre- or postoperative ERCP or open exploration.
- Patients with Childs-Pugh class A and B cirrhosis of the liver may undergo LC with no greater risk than they would open cholecystectomy.
- Pregnant patients may undergo LC safely with careful anesthetic management; optimum time is second trimester.
- Gallbladder polyps that meet criteria for surgery (symptomatic, enlarging, or larger than 1 cm) may be treated by LC.
- Incidental gallbladder cancer found after LC may be managed expectantly (T1a) or by radical reoperation including excision of port sites (T1b). LC should NOT be performed for gallbladder cancer.
- LC may be performed incidental to other indicated laparoscopic procedures.
- Prophylactic antibiotics are not indicated in routine patients who undergo LC.
- Gasless laparoscopy works, but may require adjunctive use of low-pressure pneumoperitoneum.
- LC can be done with smaller and fewer ports; the main advantages are cosmetic.
- LC can be done with the ultrasonic shears; the cystic duct can be coapted closed by this method.
- Fundus-first dissection is an important adjunct in the difficult case.
- There is no consensus on routine intraoperative cholangiography. It should be used liberally when anatomy is in doubt. Laparoscopic ultrasound is an additional adjunct.
- True outpatient management is feasible for a significant number of patients undergoing LC. Older patients, those with ASA classification ≥3, those with long procedures or done late in the day, are less likely to be good candidates for outpatient surgery.

References

1. Safran DB, Sullivan BS, Leveque JE, Williams MD. Cholecystectomy following the introduction of laparoscopy: more, but for the same indications. Am Surg 1997;63:506–11.
2. Steinle EW, VanderMolen RL, Silbergleit A, Cohen MM. Impact of laparoscopic cholecystectomy on indications for surgical treatment of gallstones. Surg Endosc 1997;11:933–5.
3. Kiviluoto T, Siren J, Luukkonen P, Kivilaakso E. Randomised trial of laparoscopic versus open cholecystectomy for acute and gangrenous cholecystitis. Lancet 1998;351:321–5.
4. Merriam LT, Kanaan SA, Dawes LG, Angelos P, Prystowsky JB, Rege RV, Joehl RJ. Gangrenous cholecystitis: analysis of risk factors and experience with laparoscopic cholecystectomy. Surgery 1999;126:680–5.
5. Habib FA, Kolachalam RB, Khilnani R, Preventzq O, Mittal VK. Role of laparoscopic cholecystectomy in the management of gangrenous cholecystitis. Am J Surg 2001;181:71–5.
6. Kanaan SA, Murayama KM, Merriam LT, Dawes LG, Prystowsky JB, Rege RV, Joehl RJ. Risk factors for conversion of laparoscopic to open cholecystectomy. J Surg Res 2002;106:20–4.
7. Ubiali P, Invernizzi R, Prezzati F. Laparoscopic surgery in very acute cholecystitis. J Society Laparoendosc Surg 2002;6:159–62.
8. Bender JS, Duncan MD, Freeswick PD, Harmon JW, Magnuson TH. Increased laparoscopic experience does not lead to improved results with acute cholecystitis. Am J Surg 2002;184:591–4.
9. Kato K, Kasai S, Matsudo M, Onodera K, Kato J, Imai M, Mito M, Saito T. A new technique for laparoscopic cholecystectomy—retrograde laparoscopic cholecystectomy—an analysis of 81 cases. Endoscopy 1996;28:356–9.
10. Mahmud S, Masaud M, Canna K, Nassar AH. Fundus-first laparoscopic cholecystectomy. Surg Endosc 2002;16:581–4.
11. Petelin JB. Laparoscopic common bile duct exploration: Transcystic duct approach. In: Scott-Conner CEH, ed. The SAGES Manual: fundamentals of laparoscopy and GI endoscopy. New York, Berlin, Heidelberg: Springer-Verlag; 1998,.Chap. 14.1. pp. 167–77.
12. Cervantes J, Rojas G. Choledocholithiasis: new approach to an old problem. World J Surg 2001;25:1270–2.
13. Kama NA, Atli M, Dogany M, Kologlu M, Reis E, Dolapci M. Practical recommendations for the prediction and management of common bile duct stones in patients with gallstones. Surg Endosc 2001;15:942–5.
14. Dias MM, Martin CJ, Cox MR. Pattern of management of common duct stones in the laparoscopic era: a New South Wales survey. Aust N Z J Surg 2002;72:181–5.
15. Friel CM, Stack J, Forse A, Babineau TJ. Laparoscopic cholecystectomy in patients with hepatic cirrhosis: a five-year experience. J Gastrointestinal Surg 1999;3:286–91.
16. Poggio JL, Rowland Cm, Gores GJ, Nagorney DM, Donohue JH. A comparison of laparoscopic and open cholecystectomy in patients with compensated cirrhosis and symptomatic gallstone disease. Surgery 2000;127:405–11.

17. Fernandes NF, Schwesinger WH, Hilsenbeck SG, Gross GW, Bay MK, Sirinek KR, Schenker S. Laparoscopic cholecystectomy and cirrhosis: a case-control study of outcomes. Liver Transpl 2000;6:340–4.

18. Morino M, Cavuoti G, Miglietta C, Girando G, Simone P. Laparoscopic cholecystectomy in cirrhosis: contraindication or privileged indication? Surg Laparosc Endosc Percutan Tech 2000;10:360–3.

19. Clark JR, Wills VL, Hunt DR. Cirrhosis and laparoscopic cholecystectomy. Surg Laparosc Endosc Percutan Tech 2001;11:165–9.

20. Leone N, Garino M, DePaolis P, Pellicano R, Fronda GR, Rizzetto M. Laparoscopic cholecystectomy in cirrhotic patients. Dig Surg 2001;18:449–52.

21. Amos JD, Schorr SJ, Norman PF, Poole GV, Thomae KR, Mancino AT, Hall TJ, Scott-Conner CEH. Laparoscopic surgery during pregnancy. Am J Surg 1996;171:435–7.

22. Cosenza CA, Saffari B, Jabbour N, Stain SC, Garry D, Parekh D, Selby RR. Surgical management of biliary gallstone disease during pregnancy. Am J Surg 1999;178:545–8.

23. Barone JE, Bears S, Chen S, Tsai J, Russell JC. Outcome study of cholecystectomy during pregnancy. Am J Surg 1999;177:232–6.

24. Daradkeh S, Sumrein I, Daoud F, Zaidin K, Abu-Khalaf M. Management of gallbladder stones during pregnancy: conservative treatment or laparoscopic cholecystectomy? Hepatogastroenterology 1999;46:3074–6.

25. Sungler P, Heinerman PM, Steiner H, Waclawiczek HW, Holzinger J, Mayer F, Heuberger A. Laparoscopic cholecystectomy and interventional endoscopy for gallstone complications during pregnancy. Surg Endosc 2000;14:267–71.

26. Muench J. Albrink M, Serafini F, Rosemurgy A, Carey L, Murr MM. Delay in treatment of biliary disease during pregnancy increases morbidity and can be avoided by laparoscopic cholecystectomy. Am Surg 2001;67:539–42.

27. Buser KB. Laparoscopic surgery in the pregnant patient—one surgeon's experience in a small rural hospital. J Soc Laparoendosc Surg 2002;6:121–4.

28. Terzi C, Sokmen S, Secklin S, Albayrak L, Ugurlu M. Polypoid lesions of the gallbladder: report of 100 cases with special reference to operative indications. Surgery 2000;127:622–7.

29. Mainprize KS, Gould SW, Gilbert JM, Surgical management of polypoid lesions of the gallbladder. Br J Surg 2000;87:414–7.

30. Huang CS, lien HH, Jeng JY, Huang SH. Role of laparoscopic cholecystectomy in the management of polypoid lesions of the gallbladder. Surg Laparosc Endosc Percutan Tech 2002;11:242–7.

31. Csendes A, Buergos AM, Csendes P, Smok G, Rojas J. Late follow up of polypoid lesions of the gallbladder smaller than 10 mm. Ann Surg 2001;234:657–60.

32. Myers RP, Shaffer EA, Beck PL. Gallbladder polyps: epidemiology, natural history and management. Can J Gastroenterol 2002;16:187–94.

33. Vashney S, Buttirini G, Gupta R. Incidental carcinoma of the gallbladder. Eur J Surg Oncol 2002;28:4–10.

34. Ouchi K, Mikuni J, Kakugawa Y. Organizing Committee, the 30th Annual Congress of the Japanese Society of Biliary Surgery. Laparoscopic cholecystectomy for gallbladder carcinoma: results of a Japanese survey of 498 patients. J Hepatobiliary Pancreat Surg 2002;9:256–60.

35. Wakai T, Shirai Y, Hatakeyama K. Radical second resection provides survival benefit for patients with T2 gallbladder cancer first discovered after laparoscopic cholecystectomy. World J Surg 2002;26:867–71.

36. Box JC, Edge SB. Laparoscopic cholecystectomy and the unsuspected gallbladder cancer. Semin Surg Oncol 1999;16:327–31.

37. Roman F, Fraciosi C, Caprotti R, DeFinas S, Porta G, Visinitini G, Uggeri F. Laparoscopic cholecystectomy and unsuspected gallbladder cancer. Eur J Surg Oncol 2001;27:225–8.

38. Lundberg O, Kristoffersson A. Open versus laparoscopic cholecystectomy for gallbladder cancer. J Hepatobiliary Pancreat Surg 2001;8:525–9.

39. Klaus A, Hinder RA, Swain J, Achem S, Incidental cholecystectomy during laparoscopic antireflux surgery. Am Surg 2002;68:619–23.

40. Patton ML, Moss BE, Haith LR Jr, Shotwell BA, Milliner DH, Simeone MR, Kraut JD, Patton JN. Concomitant laparoscopic cholecystectomy and splenectomy for surgical management of hereditary spherocytosis. Am Surg 1997;63:536–9.

41. Caprotti R, Franciosi C, Romano F, Codescasa G, Musco F, Motto M, Uggeri F. Combined laparoscopic splenectomy and cholecystectomy for the treatment of hereditary spherocytosis: is it safe and effective? Surg Laparosc Endosc Percutan Tech 1999;9:203–6.

42. Ghidirim GHP, Gladun EV, Danch AV, Mishina E. Combined laparoscopic treatment of polycystic ovary disease and gallstones. J Am Assoc Gynecol Laparosc 1996;3:S15.

43. Hamad GG, Ikramuddin S, Gourash WF, Schauer PR. Elective cholecystectomy during laparoscopic Roux-en-Y gastric bypass: is it worth the wait? Obes Surg 2003;13:76–81.

44. Illig KA, Schmidt E, Cavanaugh J, Krusch D, Sax HC. Are prophylactic antibiotics required for elective laparoscopic cholecystectomy? J Am Coll Surg 1997;184:353–6.

45. Koivusalo AM, Kellokumpu I, Scheinin M, Tikkanen I, Makisalo, Lindgren L. A comparison of gasless mechanical and conventional carbon dioxide pneumoperitoneum methods for laparoscopic cholecystectomy. Anesth Analg 1998;86:153–8.

46. Nande AG, Shrikhande SV, Rathod V, Adyanthaya K, Shrikhande V. Modified technique of gasless laparoscopic cholecystectomy in a developing country: a five year experience. Dig Surg 2002;19:366–72.

47. Leggett PL, Brissell CD, Churchman-Winn R, Ahn C. Three-port microlaparoscopic cholecystectomy in 159 patients. Surg Endosc 2001;15:293–6.

48. Uranus S, Peng Z, Kronberger L, Pfeifer J, Salehi B. Laparoscopic cholecystectomy using 2 mm instruments. J Laparoendosc Adv Surg Tech A 1998;8:255–9.

49. Ainslie WG, Catton JA, Davides D, Dexter S, Gibson J, Larvin M, McMahon MJ, Moore M, Smith S, Vezakis A. Micropuncture cholecystectomy versus conventional laparoscopic cholecystectomy. Surg Endosc 2003;17:766–72.

50. Power C, Maguire D, McAnena OJ, Calleary J. Use of the ultrasonic dissecting scalpel in laparoscopic cholecystectomy. Surg Endosc 2000;14:1070–3.

51. Huscher CG, Lirici MM, DiPaola M, Crafa F, Napolitano C, Mereu A, Recher A, Corradi A, Amini M. Laparoscopic cholecystectomy without cystic duct and artery ligation. Surg Endosc 2003;17:442–51.

52. Scott-Conner CEH, Dawson DL. Laparoscopic cholecystectomy, common bile duct exploration, and liver biopsy. In: Scott-Conner CEH, Dawson DL, eds. Operative anatomy, 2nd edn. Philadelphia: Lippincott Williams & Wilkins; 2003. Chap. 57. pp. 378–88.

53. Ludwig K, Bernhardet J, Lorenz D. Value and consequences of routine intraoperative cholangiography during cholecystectomy. Surg Laparosc Endosc Percutan Tech 2002;12:154–9.

54. Ludwig K, Bernhardt J, Steffen H, Lorenz D. Contribution of intraoperative cholangiography to incidence and outcome of common bile duct injuries during laparoscopic cholecystectomy. Surg Endosc 2002;16:1098–104.

55. Birth M, Ehlers KU, Delinikolas K, Weiser HF. Prospective randomized comparison of laparoscopic ultrasonography using a flexible-tip ultrasound probe and intraoperative dynamic laparoscopic cholecystectomy. Surg Endosc 1998;12:30–6.

56. Catheline JM, Turner R, Paries J. Laparoscopic ultrasonography is a complement to cholangiography for detection of choledocholithiasis at laparoscopic cholecystectomy. Br J Surg 2002;89:1235–9.

57. Tranter SE, Thompson MH. A prospective single-blinded controlled study comparing laparoscopic ultrasound of the common bile duct with operative cholangiography. Surg Endosc 2003;17:216–9.

58. Robinson TN, Biffl WL, Moore EE, Heimbach JK, Calkins CM, Burch JM. Predicting failure of outpatient laparoscopic cholecystectomy. Am J Surg 2002;184:515–8.

Commentary

ULRICH SCHÖFFEL

Laparoscopic cholecystectomy (LC) has indeed become the gold standard in the treatment of benign diseases of the gallbladder. Dr. Scott-Connor has provided an excellent overview regarding the key controversies in this field. Almost inevitably, such a project touches on some gray areas, where objective data are sparse or completely lacking, and where subjective judgment must prevail.

Whilst it is certainly not the objective of this commentary to challenge the expert opinion of Dr. Scott-Conner, it is intended to underscore some of her points and to point out where some controversies still require additional evidence before becoming resolved.

During the last decade, a couple of studies dealt with the question of whether LC for acute cholecystitis should be performed early during the acute phase or after a certain "cooling off" period (interval surgery). Expert opinion nowadays seems to favor operating early within the first 3 days, not only because it prevents secondary infection complications. And indeed, it has been shown that LC can be performed relatively safely during the first 3 days when inflammatory edema may even be of help in the dissection of the surrounding planes. Beyond the 3rd day, however, the inflamed tissues become dense and even more hyperemic and conversion rates seem to increase [1–4]. When the acute inflammation has settled down, delayed LC may still be difficult due to dense adhesions and scarring, and conversion and complication rates reported from two small randomized controlled trials range even (insignificantly) higher than those occurring with early surgery [5, 6]. Moreover, throughout those studies, the overall hospital stay was considerably shorter in the group that was operated upon early.

All patients with symptomatic cholecystolithiasis should be assessed for common bile duct stones [7]. When common duct stones have to be suspected preoperatively, the choice between different approaches is, as stated by Dr. Scott-Connor, dictated by local expertise. Up to now, however, there is no hard data available suggesting either preoperative ERCP with endoscopic papillotomy and stone extraction, if necessary, or intraoperative cholangiography with laparoscopic bile duct exploration and clearance as the standard of care [8]. When common duct stones are detected intraoperatively, the latter one-step procedure should be performed.

Concerning gallbladder polyps, it has to be kept in mind that the management of polyps between 5 and 10 mm in diameter remains controversial. Adenocarcinomas have been detected in up to 29% of gallbladder polyps of less than 10 mm [9] and endoscopic ultrasound may be helpful in this differentiation. Single polyps and sessile lesions are additional risk factors, which, if present, may indicate prophylactic LC.

Suggestions as to the optimal management of unexpected gallbladder cancer found incidentally by the pathologist in the (laparoscopically) removed specimen are not unanimous. As Dr. Scott-Connor said, cancer confined to the mucosa (T1a, UICC) does not need further therapy. T1b tumors, however, defined as cancer infiltrating the muscularis propria, have been reported to metastasize at higher rates than originally estimated.

Two points, however, have to be noted. Firstly, many data on metastasizing T1b carcinoma are derived from national surveys using questionnaires [10]. And secondly, it has not been definitively proven that, with negative margins at the primary operation, radical reoperation, including wedge resection of the gallbladder bed or formal resection of liver segments V and IVb, lymphadenectomy in the hepatoduodenal ligament, or excision of port-sites translates into a survival benefit.

Correct identification of the cystic duct is certainly the decisive step during LC. Preparation close to the gallbladder neck allows for visualization of the duct-bladder junction and in most cases also of the cystic artery. Incidental injury of the bile ducts or the right hepatic artery are thus minimized, irrespective of an anterograde (fundus-first) or retrograde dissection technique. This does not relate to the problem of an occasional accessory hepatic duct. Despite many authorities preferring the fundus-first dissection and support from common sense, it has to be stated that in this respect there is no defined standard of care.

It is also true that the issue of routine intraoperative cholangiogaphy is still being hotly debated. Dr. Scott-Connor describes the main arguments. In the absence of hard scientific data supporting the one or the other strategy, it is self-evident that intraoperative visualization of the ductal anatomy should lead to an earlier detection of incidental biliary injury.

Some further controversies, which were not addressed in this chapter, may cross one's mind.

What about the routine use of retrieval bags? Down to what size is it necessary to clear lost stones from the peritoneal cavity? But also here, further evidence is needed before respective recommendations can be given.

References

1. Willsher PC, Sanabria JR, Gallinger S, Rossi L, Strasberg S, Litwin DE. Early laparoscopic cholecystectomy for acute cholecystitis: a safe procedure. J Gastrointest Surg 1999;3:50–3.
2. Eldar S, Eitan A, Bickel A, Sabo E, Cohen A, Abrahamson J, Matter I. The impact of patient delay and physician delay on the outcome of laparoscopic cholecystectomy for acute cholecystitis. Am J Surg 1999;178:303–7.
3. Garber SM, Korman J, Cosgrove JM, Cohen JR. Early laparoscopic cholecystectomy for acute cholecystitis. Surg Endosc 1997;11:347–50.
4. Bittner R, Leibl B, Kraft K, Butters M, Nick G, Ulrich M. Laparoscopic cholecystectomy in therapy of acute cholecystitis: immediate versus interval operation. Chirurgie 1997;68:237–43.
5. Chandler CF, Lane JS, Ferguson P, Thompson JE, Ashley SW. Prospective evaluation of early versus delayed laparoscopic cholecystectomy for treatment of acute cholecystitis. Am Surg 2000;66:896–900.
6. Lo CM, Liu CL, Fan ST, Lai EC, Wong J. Prospective randomized study of early versus delayed laparoscopic cholecystectomy for acute cholecystitis. Ann Surg 1998;227:461–7.
7. Paul A, Millat B, Holhausen U, et al.; Scientific Committee of the European Association for Endoscopic Surgery. Diagnosis and treatment of common bile duct stones. Results of a consensus development conference. Surg Endosc 1998;12:856–864
8. Sarli L, Iusco DR, Roncoroni L. Preoperative endoscopic sphincterotomy and laparoscopic cholecystectomy for the management of cholecystocholedocholithiasis. World J Surg 2003;27:180–8.
9. Choi WB, Lee SK, Kim MW, Seo DW, Kim HJ, Kim DI. A new strategy to predict the neoplastic polyps of the gallbladder based on a scoring system using EUS. Gastrointest Endosc 2000;52:372–9.
10. Ogura Y, Mizumoto R, Isaji S, Kusuda T, Matsuda S, Tabata M. Radical operations for carcinoma of the gallbladder: present status in Japan. World J Surg 1991;15:337–343.

Choledocholithiasis

BIPAN CHAND, JEFFREY PONSKY

> ▶ **Key** Controversies
> A. When should a preoperative ERCP be performed?
> B. What intraoperative techniques can be utilized in stone removal?
> C. What role does ERCP play in stone removal?

21.1
Introduction

The introduction of laparoscopic cholecystectomy a decade ago has now become the gold standard in the treatment of gallbladder disease. Laparoscopic cholecystectomy offers less morbidity, improved cosmesis and has become the platform for other minimally invasive procedures. Skills required to perform laparoscopic cholecystectomy have been adopted by the majority of surgeons trained prior to 1990 and these skills are currently being taught in all general surgery programs. However, the introduction of this new technique in biliary surgery has produced controversy in regard to the management of choledocholithiasis. Prior to laparoscopy, intraoperative cholangiography was routinely performed and common duct stones removed with open duct exploration [1]. Today routine cholangiography is not performed and, if choledocholithiasis is found at the time of laparoscopy, a variety of methods is available for stone removal. Some surgeons believe that routine cholangiography should be performed to master the technique if it is possible that common bile duct exploration is needed [2].

The uses of endoscopic techniques for stone removal have been widely accepted throughout the world, both preoperatively and postoperatively [3–9]. However, advanced laparoscopic surgeons have argued that most stones can be dealt with at the time of cholecystectomy [9–18]. Laparoscopic techniques include transcystic stone removal, laparoscopic choledochotomy with stone removal, and transcystic stenting followed by postoperative ERCP (endoscopic retrograde cholangiopancreatography). Also, a few innovative endoscopists suggested utilizing intraoperative ERCP in combination with laparoscopy [19, 20].

21.2
Discussion

21.2.1
When Should a Preoperative ERCP Be Performed?

After the introduction of laparoscopic cholecystectomy, it was common for all patients with possible choledocholithiasis to undergo preoperative ERCP [4–8]. The rational for this algorithm included the initial lack of laparoscopic skills of the surgeon in managing common duct stones and the greater than 90% success of endoscopic stone removal [4–8]. Patients that had jaundice, elevated cholestatic liver function tests, a history of pancreatitis, or a dilated biliary ductal system on radiographic imaging were all considered candidates for preoperative ERCP. However, it was soon realized that the majority of these patients underwent unnecessary examinations since most of the common bile duct stones had already passed into the duodenum [3–6, 9]. ERCP incurred additional costs and had its own potential for morbidity (10%) and mortality (1%) [4–8, 21, 22]. Current indications for preoperative ERCP include worsening gallstone pancreatitis, cholangitis, and persistent deep jaundice.

21.2.2
What Intraoperative Techniques Should Be Utilized for Stone Removal?

To successfully treat common bile duct stones a good cholangiogram is required. The cholangiogram must show the extra and intrahepatic ductal system, contrast empting into the duodenum, and filling defects. The surgeon must then be able to successfully interpret the cholangiogram. Routine cholangiography is not employed by most surgeons in elective cholecystectomy, but is mandatory if patients have jaundice, elevated liver function tests, a history of gallstone pancreatitis, or dilated dusts on preoperative imaging. It is important to note the characteristics and location of the filling defect once identified within the ductal system. Filling defects can represent air bubbles, stones, or ductal strictures. Stones should be noted for their size, location, and number. Success of stone removal depends not only on stone characteristics but also on the skill of the surgeon as well as the resources available to the surgeon.

21.2.2.1
Laparoscopic Transcystic Removal

Studies have shown a high success rate and low morbidity with transcystic stone extraction [11–13, 15, 16, 18]. After a cholangiogram has been obtained and correctly interpreted, small stones (<4 mm) may be flushed through the duct after the administration of intravenous glucagon to relax the sphincter of Oddi. This should be done under the guidance of fluoroscopy. If this fails to clear the duct and the stone appears small enough to pass through the cystic duct, a wire basket may be used to capture and retrieve the stone. Larger stones may be crushed prior to attempted extraction and smaller cystic ducts can be dilated prior to manipulation. The passage of a 3 mm choledochoscope into the cystic duct allows for direct visualization, capture, and retrieval of stones. Although these methods have been highly effective in the hands of trained surgeons, they are technically demanding and time consuming [8–13].

21.2.2.2
Laparoscopic Choledochotomy

Once the laparoscopic surgeon has acquired the necessary skills to perform intracorporeal suturing, laparoscopic choledochotomy can be completed successfully [14–18]. Stones larger than 15 mm with dilated common bile duct are best managed through this approach [9, 11, 13]. The surgeon must have an adequate cholangiogram prior to making the choledochotomy. The common bile duct is exposed anteriorly by opening the peritoneum parallel to the duct. Bile may then be aspirated from the duct to assure it is identified correctly and two stay sutures can be placed for additional retraction. The duct is then carefully entered in the middle along the vertical axis and an opening created of approximately 1.5 to 2.0 cm. The duct is then irrigated with the use of a 14Fr red rubber catheter passed through a lateral 5 mm trocar. This will typically flush the majority of the common duct stones. A guide wire is then passed into the duodenum under fluoroscopic guidance followed by a balloon catheter. The catheter is then passed up and down the duct to clear any additional stones. Finally a choledochoscope is passed into the duct and duodenum to assure no stones remain. A T-tube is the placed into the choledochotomy and absorbable sutures are placed around the opening to secure the tube and prevent bile leak. A finishing cholangiogram is then obtained through the T-tube to demonstrate no filling defects and no leak from the choledochotomy. The cholecystectomy is then completed and the removed stones as well as the gallbladder are placed in a specimen retrieval bag. This technique is of value when dilated common ducts are encountered and with the increased experience of the laparoscopic surgeon [9, 11, 13–18].

21.2.3
What Role Does ERCP Play in Stone Removal?

21.2.3.1
Intraoperative ERCP

Intraoperative ERCP is an effective method for dealing with common duct stones, particularly stones that are in the common hepatic duct or intrahepatic system [19]). It however does require the transport of endoscopic equipment into the operating room and a skilled endoscopist. The procedure can be best performed by a combination laparoscopic and endoscopic approach. Some authors have suggested the antegrade transcystic passage of a sphincterotome to the ampulla guided by an endoscope positioned in the duodenum [20]. Once the sphincterotome is in proper position, the sphincter is cut and the stones released into the duodenum. Another method involves the laparoscopic passage of a transcystic guide wire into the common bile duct, pass the stone and then into the duodenum. The endoscopist then grasps the wire with a biopsy forceps and pulls the wire out of the working channel. A sphincterotome is then passed over the guide wire through the working channel of the endoscope in its usual manner to the ampulla and a sphincterotomy performed [23]. Stones are then removed endoscopically with the use of baskets or balloon catheters. The use of intraoperative ERCP is plausible and effective but requires additional equipment and additional personnel.

21.2.3.2
Postoperative ERCP

Choledocholithiasis found at laparoscopy can be deferred for postoperative endoscopic management in the majority of patients. The surgeon must determine which stones should be dealt with at the time of surgery and those that can be managed endoscopically. Postoperative ERCP is highly successful in stone removal but still adds additional costs as well as the potential for morbidity and mortality. Large and multiple stones found at laparoscopy may require multiple endoscopic procedures and may be dealt best at the time of initial operation [4–8].

21.2.3.3
Laparoscopic Transcystic Drainage and Postoperative ERCP

Complications that may occur after laparoscopic cholecystectomy with remaining choledocholithiasis include the potential for stone impaction with possible jaundice, cholangitis, and possible cystic duct leak. Also the surgeon is then relying on successful endoscopic treatment for the retained stones. Therefore, an alternative has been suggested that may prevent these complications and bridge the time from surgery to endoscopic therapy. When a stone is discovered at the time of laparoscopy and the surgeon is unable to remove the stone from the common duct a drain may be left transcystically. The tube is placed laparoscopically into the cystic duct with its tip into the common bile duct and the tube secured with a pre-tied ligature. The drain is then brought out through the skin, much as a T-tube would be, and left to gravity drainage. This tube allows for decompression of the biliary system and also future access of the biliary tract. A wire may be passed through this drain into the duodenum to facilitate endoscopic therapy. Once the duct has been swept clear of stones the drain may be capped and subsequently removed after 2–3 weeks, after a secure tract has formed.

21.2.3.4
Transcystic Stenting and Postoperative ERCP

This technique is an extension of the latter method and was first described by Rhodes et al. [24]. It entails the use of a small caliber biliary stent that is passed through the cystic duct into the duodenum. Once a cholangiogram demonstrates a filling defect in the common bile duct, a guide wire is passed transcystically into the duodenum with the use of fluoroscopy. A 7Fr, 5-cm long biliary stent is then passed over the wire and "pushed" into the duodenum with a pusher tube of similar size [23]. The stent is fluoroscopically guided through the cystic duct, common bile duct, and partially into the duodenum. The pusher tube and guide wire are then removed. The cystic duct is then clipped and the cholecystectomy completed. The patient can then be discharged the same day and returns for further endoscopic therapy. The stent has the advantage of allowing for continued internal drainage of the biliary system and therefore preventing potential complications of stone impaction and also aids the endoscopist when ERCP is performed. At the time of endoscopy, the stent can be seen protruding through the ampulla into the duodenal lumen. The endoscopist can then "cut" over the stent and perform an adequate sphincterotomy with subsequent stone removal [23].

21.3
Summary

— Preoperative ERCP should be performed in patients with persistent jaundice, cholangitis, and worsening gallstone pancreatitis.

— Intraoperative cholangiography should be obtained in all patients with a history of jaundice, gallstone pancreatitis, elevated liver function tests, dilated ducts on preoperative imaging, or difficulty discerning the anatomy.

— A variety of laparoscopic techniques can be utilized to remove common duct stones and depends on the experience of the surgeon and the cholangiogram findings.

— Initial laparoscopic techniques include transcystic duct management by flushing the stones or passage of baskets and balloon catheters, followed by laparoscopic choledochotomy in experienced hands.

— Transcystic drains or common bile duct stents can be placed laparoscopically to prevent potential stone impaction and facilitate further clearing of the common bile duct on latter endoscopy.

— ERCP can be utilized intraoperatively if readily available or postoperatively in most situations to successfully remove most stones.

References

1. Way LW, Admirand WH, Dunphy JE. Management of choledocholithiasis. Ann Surg 1972;176:347–59.
2. Berci G. Biliary ductal anatomy and anomalies: the role of intraoperative cholangiography during laparoscopic cholecystectomy. Surg Clin North Am 1992;72:1069–75.
3. Stain SC, Cohen H, Tsuishaysha M, et al. Choledocholithiasis: endoscopic sphincterotomy or common bile duct exploration. Ann Surg 1991;213:627–634.
4. Ponsky, JL. Endoscopic management of common bile duct stones. World J Surg 1992;16,1060–5
5. Delorio AV Jr, Vitale GC, Reynolds M, et al. Acute biliary pancreatitis. The roles of laparoscopic cholecystectomy and endoscopic retrograde cholangiopancreatography. Surg Endosc 1995;9:392–6.
6. Cotton PB. Endoscopic retrograde cholangiopancreatography and laparoscopic cholecystectomy. Am J Surg 1993;1659:474–8.
7. Davis WZ, Cotton PB, Arias R, et al. ERCP and sphincterotomy in the context of laparoscopic cholecystectomy: academic and community practice patterns and results. Am J Gastroenterol 1997;92:597–601.
8. Cotton PB. Endoscopic management of the bile duct stones (apples and oranges). Gut 1984;25:587–91.
9. Cuschieri A, Croce E, Faggioni A, et al. EAES ductal stone study. Preliminary findings of multi-center prospective randomized trial comparing two-stage vs single-stage management. Surg Endosc 1996;10:1130–5.
10. Stoker ME. Common bile duct exploration in the era of laparoscopic surgery. Arch Surg 1995;130:265–9.
11. Petelin JB. Laparoscopic approach to common duct pathology. Am J Surg 1993;165:487–91.

12. Carroll BJ, Phillips EH, Rosenthal R, et al. Update on transcystic exploration of the bile duct. Surg Laparosc Endosc 1996;6:453–8.
13. Hunter JG, Soper NJ. Laparoscopic management of bile duct stones. Surg Clin North Am 1992;72:1077–97.
14. Rhodes M, Nathanson L, O'Rourke N, et al. Laparoscopic exploration of the common bile duct: lessons learned from 129 consecutive cases. Br J Surg 1995;82:664–8.
15. Petelin J. Laparoscopic approach to common duct pathology. Surg Laparosc Endosc 1991;1:33–41.
16. Hunter JG. Laparoscopic transcystic common bile duct exploration. Am J Surg 1992;163:5358.
17. Sackier JM, Berci G, Paz-Partlow M. Laparoscopic transcystic choledochotomy as an adjunct to laparoscopic cholecystectomy. Am Surg 1991;57:323–6.
18. Phillips EH, Carroll BJ, Pearlstein AR, et al. Laparoscopic choledochoscopy and extraction of common bile duct stones. World J Surg 1993;17:22–8.
19. Deslandres E, Gagner M, Pomp A. Intraoperative endoscopic sphincterotomy for common bile duct stones during laparoscopic cholecystectomy. Gastrointest Endosc 1993;39:54–8.
20. Curet MJ, Pitcher DE, Martin DT, Zucker KL. Laparoscopic antegrade sphincterotomy. A new technique for the management of complex choledocholithiasis. Ann Surg 1995;221:149–55.
21. Cotton PB, Lehman G, Vennes J, et al. Endoscopic sphincterotomy complications and their management: an attempt at consensus. Gastrointest Endosc 1991;37:383–93.
22. Frost RA. Prospective multi-center study of British sphincterotomy: initial results and complications. Gut 1984;25:49–55.
23. Ponsky J, Heniford BT, Gersin K. Choledocholithiasis: evolving intraoperative strategies. Am Surg 2000;66:262–8.
24. Rhodes M, Nathanson L, O'Rourke N, Fielding G. Laparoscopic antegrade biliary stenting. Endoscopy 1995;27:676–8.

Commentary

N. Alexakis, J.P. Neoptolemos

Controversy:
When Should a Preoperative ERCP Be Performed?

Endoscopic sphincterotomy (ES) with active stone extraction is the treatment of choice for stone removal from the main bile duct, with initial success rates of 90–95%, and may be supplemented with ancillary techniques such as nasobiliary catheter drainage and an endoscopic stent insertion [1]. ES is associated with an overall complication rate of ~10%, a serious complication rate of ~1.5% and a mortality rate of <0.5%, but these complication rates are increased in high risk elderly patients [1].

There are two situations in which preoperative ERCP is strongly indicated, as follows.

Acute Cholangitis

The evidence strongly favors endoscopic drainage as the initial treatment of choice for acute cholangitis [1–3]. The first important study came from the UK in 1986 that demonstrated a mortality of only 2 (4.7%) out of 43 patient with acute cholangitis treated by ES compared with 6 (21%) deaths out of 28 patients treated by surgical decompression [2].

A subsequent randomized trial from Hong Kong in 1992 confirmed these findings, with 4 (10%) deaths out of 41 patients that had endoscopic decompression compared with 13 (32%) deaths in another 41 patients that had surgical decompression; the morbidity was also significantly reduced (14 patients, 34%, versus 27, 66%, respectively) [3].

Recommendation 1

ERCP ±ES is safer than surgery in acute cholangitis.
[*Recommendation: grade A*]

Acute Pancreatitis Due to Gallstones

The first prospective randomized controlled trial of urgent ES in gallstone-associated acute pancreatitis was performed in the UK [4]. The 121 patients with gallstones were stratified prospectively for the severity of acute pancreatitis prior to randomization [4]. The mortality rate was 1 (2%) in the 59 patients randomized to urgent ERCP±ES compared with 5 (8%) in the 62 patients randomized to conservative treatment, and the complication rates were 10 (17%) and 17 (61%), respectively.

The differences were even more striking when only those with a predicted severe attack were considered; mortality and complications rates were 1 (4%) and 6 (24%), respectively, in the 25 patients predicted severe and treated by ES compared with 5 (18%) and 17 (61%), respectively, in the 28 patients predicted severe in the conservative group [4]. Also the hospital stay was shorter in the predicted severe urgent ES group but the outcome was identical in both groups with predicted mild attacks (morbidity 12%, mortality 0%).

Fan et al. from Hong Kong [5] prospectively randomized 195 patients with acute pancreatitis to either ES within 24 h of presentation or conventional therapy. Overall there was a reduction in biliary sepsis in the urgent ES group compared with that in the conservatively management group (0% vs 12%), with apparently no significant difference in mortality or complications [5]. In fact *only 127 (65%) of the patients actually had gallstones.* Importantly the results in these patients with gallstones were much the same as those from the UK trial: in the 30 patients with severe pancreatitis treated endoscopi-cally there was only 1 (3%) death and 4 (13%) with morbidity compared with 5 (18%) deaths and 15 (54%) with complications in the 28 patients with severe pancreatitis treated conservatively. Moreover ERCP/ES was performed in 18 patients with a severe attack (median 60 h, range 12–288 h). Thus, 64% of the conservative group with severe pancreatitis also had ERCP/ES and mostly within 72 h.

A multicenter study from Germany [6] did not show any benefit, but the study was significantly flawed in a number of ways. It had poor recruitment: 238 patients over 5 years from 22 hospitals. Patients with obstructive jaundice were excluded and underwent emergency ES. The severity was only deter-mined retrospectively and was undefined in some patients. Because ES was performed within 72 h, severity scoring would have been completed after ES in many cases and any apparent positive influence of ES on the course of se-vere disease might have been lost by moving patients to the mild disease cate-gory before completion of the severity scoring. There were 17 (13.5%) patients from the 126 patients in the ES group who developed cholangitis, compared with 13 (11.6%) cases in the 112 patients that had conservative treatment, an observation that indicates an inadequate ES technique. Moreover, there were 10 (38%) related deaths in the 26 patients with severe disease that had an ES compared with 4 (20%) deaths in 20 patients with severe pancreatitis treated conservatively [6]. The high mortality of 38% in the severe patients treated by ES [6] contrasts sharply with mortalities of 4% and 3% in comparable patients in the UK and Hong Kong studies respectively [5, 6]. This observation also suggests an inadequate ES technique in the German study.

Recommendation 2

ERCP ±ES is indicated for all patients with *severe* gallstone-associated acute pancreatitis and significantly improves outcomes.
[*Recommendation: grade A*]

Controversies:
What Intraoperative Techniques Can Be Utilized in Stone Removal? And What Role Does ERCP Play in Stone Removal?

Laparoscopic transcystic stone retrieval and choledocholithotomy are es-tablished as complimentary techniques for laparoscopic bile duct stone clear-ance [1]. It is well established that surgical bile duct exploration is associated with an increased complication rate and mortality in high risk, elderly patients with comorbidity but not for bile duct stone clearance by ES in similar patients

[1]. A multicenter prospective randomized trial from Europe [7] compared two management options in patients with gallstone disease and suspected ductal calculi: 150 patients were randomized to preoperative ERCP with stone extraction followed by laparoscopic cholecystectomy during the same admission, and 150 patients were randomized to a single-stage laparoscopic treatment. The results showed equivalent success rates for stone extraction (82 of 89, 84% vs 92 of 111, 80%, respectively) and patient morbidity (17, 12.8% vs 21, 15.8%, respectively) in the two groups, but a significant shorter hospital stay in the laparoscopic group (median of 9 vs 6 days, respectively).

Another trial from the UK [8], randomized 40 patients to laparoscopic exploration of the main bile duct and 40 patients to postoperative ERCP. The results showed that laparoscopic exploration was as effective as ERCP in clearing the main bile duct (30, 75% vs 37, 93%, respectively) but there was a significant shorter hospital stay for the laparoscopic group (median of 1 day vs 3.5 days, respectively). In both studies laparoscopic transcystic and choledocholithotomy were used according to circumstances. The shorter hospital in the ERCP/ES groups can be ascribed to logistic reasons rather than to treatment-related morbidity.

Recommendation 3

Transcystic and bile duct choledocholithotomy are complementary approaches for laparoscopic bile duct stone clearance.
[*Recommendation grade: B*]

Recommendation 4

Endoscopic therapy is preferable for elderly, high risk patients with main bile duct stones.
[*Recommendation grade: B*]

Recommendation 5

In ASA I/II category patients with main bile duct stones ERCP and ES performed postoperatively is as effective as single-stage laparoscopic treatment.
[*Recommendation grade: A*]

A further randomized trial from the UK [9], compared the results of endoprosthesis insertion over complete initial endoscopic duct clearance in 86 patients with symptomatic main bile duct stones who were at high risk (old age and/or serious comorbidity). The results showed that endoprosthesis insertion was a safe and effective alternative to initial complete duct clearance: the complication rates at 72 h were 7% in the endoprosthesis group and 16% in the duct clearance group. The long term follow-up (median of 20 months) however, showed a higher complication rate in the endoprosthesis group.

Recommendation 6

Endoprosthesis may be used as the initial drainage measure if complete stone clearance is not possible by ES during initial hospitalization.
[*Recommendation grade: A*]

Large series suggest that the performance of routine preoperative cholangiography is associated with a reduced risk (and an earlier diagnosis) of main bile duct injury [1]. A randomized trial from the USA [10] investigated whether intraoperative cholangiography should be performed routinely or on selective basis during laparoscopic cholecystectomy. In this study 56 patients were randomized to routine intraoperative cholangiography and 59 patients allocated to forego cholangiography. The results showed that in patients without indications for cholangiography, the performance of cholangiography markedly increased the operative time and cost of laparoscopic cholecystectomy, whilst it changed the operative management in only four (7.5%) of the patients. There was no mortality or morbidity in the two groups.

Recommendation 7

The routine use of cholangiography may be associated with a reduced risk of main bile duct injury.
[*Recommendation grade: B*]

Recommendation 8

Laparoscopic cholecystectomy without the routine use of cholangiography is associated with an acceptable risk of retained bile duct stones.
[*Recommendation grade: A*]

References

1. Perissat J, Huibregtse K, Keane FBV, Russell RCG, Neoptolemos JP. The management of bile duct stones in the era of laparoscopic cholecystectomy. Br J Surg 1994;81:789–810.
2. Leese T, Neoptolemos JP, Baker AR, Carr-Locke DL. Management of acute cholangitis and impact of endoscopic sphincterotomy. Br J Surg 1986;73:988–92.
3. Lai ECS, Mok FPT, Tan ESY, Lo CM, Fan ST, You KT, et al. Endoscopic biliary drainage for severe acute cholangitis. N Engl J Med 1992;326:1582–6.
4. Neoptolemos JP, London NJ, James D, Carr-Locke DL, Bailey IA, Fossard DP. Controlled trial of urgent endoscopic retrograde cholangiopancreatography and endoscopic sphincterotomy versus conservative treatment for acute pancreatitis due to gallstones. Lancet 1988;2:979–83.
5. Fan ST, Lai CS, Mok FPT, Lo CM, Rheng SS, Wong J. Early treatment of acute biliary pancreatitis by endoscopic papillotomy. N Engl J Med 1993;328:228–32.
6. Fölsch UR, Nitsche R, Ludtke R, Hilgers RA, Creutzfeldt W; the German Study Group of Acute Biliary Pancreatitis. Controlled randomized multi-center trial of urgent endoscopic papillotomy for acute biliary pancreatitis. N Engl J Med 1997;336:237–42.
7. Cuschieri A, Lezoche E, Morino M, Croce E, Lacy A, Toouli J, Faggioni A, Ribeiro VM, Jakimowicz J, Visa J, Hanna GB. EAES multi-center prospective randomized trial comparing two stage vs single stage management of patients with gallstone disease and ductal calculi. Surg Endosc 1999;13:952–7.
8. Rhodes M, Sussman L, Cohen L, Lewis MP. Randomized trial of laparoscopic exploration of common bile duct versus postoperative ERCP for common bile duct stones. Lancet 1998;351:159–61.
9. Chopra KB, Peters RA, O'Toole PA, Williams SG, Gimson AE, Lombard MG, Westaby D. Randomized study of endoscopic biliary endoprosthesis versus duct clearance for bile duct stones in high risk patients. Lancet 1996;348:791–3.
10. Soper NJ, Dunnegan DL. Routine versus selective intra-operative cholangiography during laparoscopic cholecystectomy. World J Surg 1992;16:1133–40.

Cystic Parasitic and Nonparasitic Liver Disease

Selçuk Mercan

> ## Key Controversies
>
> A. Indications
>   - Types and localization of the liver cysts treated by laparoscopic approach
> B. The choice of the laparoscopic technique and its results
>   - Laparoscopic surgery for parasitic cysts of the liver
>   - Laparoscopic surgery for nonparasitic cysts of the liver

22.1
Introduction

Laparoscopic liver surgery has advanced rapidly in the past few years. Recent advances in laparoscopic techniques made possible the laparoscopic treatment of several diseases of liver such as benign cysts and tumors [1, 2], hydatid cysts [3, 4], and even hepatectomies for malignant tumors [5–7]. Laparoscopic fenestration of symptomatic liver cyst was first reported in 1991 [8, 9], followed by the management of polycystic liver disease [10] and hydatid cysts of liver [11]. More than 200 studies have been reported related to this subject but there is still little consensus.

In selected cases laparoscopy can be diagnostic with 87% accuracy [12], can determine the extent of disease and permit application of appropriate therapy. Laparoscopic surgery reduces perioperative morbidity, is less traumatic for the patient, and allows shorter hospital stay and faster recovery [13]. In this chapter I will discuss controversies in the laparoscopic liver cyst surgery, using the available evidence and my personal experience.

22.2
Discussion

22.2.1
Indications

22.2.1.1
Type and Localization of Liver Cysts Treated
by the Laparoscopic Approach

Hepatic cysts are detected incidentally in 2.5–5% of the population [14]). Only about 15–20% of such cysts give rise to symptoms (e.g., pain, gastric outlet obstruction, or jaundice), and require treatment [15]. Asymptomatic peripheral cysts measuring up to 10 cm do not need treatment [16]. Simple solitary and multiple cysts and posttraumatic pseudocysts of the liver and spleen were best treated by laparoscopic approach [8, 17–19]. Patients were selected for the laparoscopic approach according to the ultrasound and/or computed tomography appearance and superficial localization of the cyst [20]. Standard treatment of nonparasitic cyst of liver is fenestration with widest excision of the cyst wall [21].

While some authors named laparoscopic unroofing as the gold standard of the treatment of simple cyst of liver [22–25], others stated that laparoscopic treatment of the true cyst of liver is inadequate unless complete removal of all cyst wall can be assured [26, 27]. Conservative procedures have shown higher recurrence rates and the need for further surgery [28]. The spectrum of treatment options for symptomatic, benign, nonparasitic hepatic cysts ranged from percutaneous aspiration to liver transplantation. Most large series demonstrated that complete resection of the cyst is associated with the lowest rate of recurrence [16, 28, 29]. Laparoscopic complete resection of a large hepatic cyst was successfully performed, using an endoscopic GIA stapling device [30].

Several options are available for the treatment of symptomatic polycystic liver disease (PLD), including liver resection, but surgical morbidity in a benign condition may be unacceptable. Transhepatic fenestration of the liver cyst under laparoscopic guidance carried good outcome and minimal morbidity [31]. Laparoscopic management of PLD should be reserved for patients with large cysts mainly located on the liver surface (type 1), whereas PLD characterized by numerous small cysts all over the liver (type 2) should be considered a contraindication to laparoscopic fenestration [1].

Routine laparoscopic management of patients with echinococcal cysts of liver was not advocated [2]. Recently, however, adequate selection of the patients and meticulous surgical techniques and new instrumentation enables laparoscopic treatment of the hydatid liver cysts, resulting in less morbidity [4, 32–34].

Laparoscopic deroofing allows ample access for surgical treatment of solitary nonparasitic cysts in segments II, III, IVb, V and VIII of the liver; however, the posterior segments VI and VII, and segment IVa are difficult to approach laparoscopically. Endoscopic retroperitoneal approach could be considered to reach the posterior segments of the liver. However, experienced laparoscopic liver surgeons state that all solitary nonparasitic liver cysts, regardless of size and anatomic location, are suitable for laparoscopic management [2].

Selection criteria for laparoscopic pericystectomy for liver hydatid cysts are: solitary cyst located in segment III, IV, V, VI or VIII, diameter less than 7 cm, and no evidence of infection or calcification [35]. There is a reported case of liver hydatid cyst localized in the sixth hepatic segment, which allowed laparoscopic pericystectomy because of its calcified state [36].

22.2.2
The Choice of the Laparoscopic Technique and Its Result

22.2.2.1
Laparoscopic Surgery for Parasitic Cysts of the Liver

The surgical treatment of hepatic hydatid cyst can be discussed in four phases: surgical area isolation, cyst evacuation, treatment of cyst complications (e.g., biliary communications) and treatment of the residual cavity. Hydatid surgery can be "conservative" (marsupialization, cystostomy, simple drainage) or "aggressive" (pericystectomy, partial or subtotal cystectomies, different type of hepatectomies). All these procedures can be achieved by the hands of experienced laparoscopic surgeons, conforming to the standards used in open surgery. Initial attempts at laparoscopic treatment of liver hydatid cysts were reported in 1993 [11, 37] and 1994 [3]. Many studies followed, some of which concluding that hepatic hydatid cysts should be treated conventionally [2, 14], while most advocating laparoscopic approach [4, 32, 38–40] (Table 22.1). There were attempts of developing new instruments [41], for laparoscopic treatment of hepatic hydatid cysts, which may cause disastrous complicatious such as tear of the cyst wall. The best and simple way of puncturing a large hydatid cyst is via an umbrella-shaped locking trochar, which allows safe evacuation of cyst contents [4, 34, 42]. Also, an isolated hypobaric laparoscopic technique is described as an advantagous approach providing a safe and efficacious treatment of almost all types of abdominal hydatid cysts [33].

Packing of the pericystic area with gauze soaked in hypertonic saline may protect from the effects of spillage of cyst content and decrease the risk for anaphylactic shock [43]. After sterilization of the cyst cavity, simple drainage or unroofing and omentoplasty can be done [38]. Infected hydatid liver cysts were also drained using laparoscopic approach without morbidity [44]. Small, partially calcified hydatid cysts favorably located in an anterior hepatic segment can be managed by total pericystectomy [36, 45]. There are many advantages of laparoscopic approach of hydatid cyst of liver, such as lower incidence of infection and it allows through inspection of the cyst cavity to rule out excess germinative membrane and scolocides as well as connection to the biliary tract, both of which are responsible from recurrence or chronical complications.

When this procedure is done with careful selection of patients and proper technique, results are favorable with shorter hospital stay and lower morbidity. The disadvantages are difficulty of reaching posteriorly located cysts and danger of hemorrhage while puncturing the cysts that are located deep in the liver parenchyma. Indiscriminate application of the laparoscopic technique increases the risk of contamination of the abdominal cavity with live scolices. Experienced surgeons can even treat laparoscopically the recurrences hydatid cysts following open surgery [4]. Notably, alveolar echinoccosis is a very rare finding and best treated by chemotherapy [46].

In one study [39], type I and type II hydatid cysts were treated by ultrasound-guided percutaneous drainage plus hypertonic saline and alcohol, type IV and V were treated surgically, and the treatment of type III was by either means, depending on the presence of drainable content; the authors also stated that laparoscopic approach should be limited to uncomplicated cysts. In a large series of 973 cases of hepatic hydatid cyst, the complicated form was 42.3% [47]. An acceptable laparoscopic procedure should enable the treatment of any form of the disease and must conform to standards used in open surgery. Careful examination of the cyst cavity with the laparoscope helps to detect connections to the biliary tree, which are closed by laparoscopic surgery [4]. Postoperative biliary fistulas were treated by endoscopic sphincterotomy [48].

Perioperative albendazole intake may help to prevent the recurrence of echinococal disease in the event of an unrecognized spillage of cyst contents.

22.2.2.2
Laparoscopic Surgery for Nonparasitic Cysts of the Liver

Solitary Cysts. Nonparasitic solitary cysts of the liver become symptomatic when they get large. Complications such as rupture, infection, or intracystic hemorrhage may occur [49]. Different surgical treatments have been proposed for symptomatic hepatic cysts: simple aspiration, enucleation, fenestration, hepatic resection and liver transplantation [1, 50]. In a large series percutaneous aspiration resulted in 100% recurrence within 3 weeks to 9 months, while laparoscopic or open unroofing showed comparable and acceptable recurrence rates (11% for laparoscopy, 13% for open) [51]. Others reported similar results and thus advocated laparoscopic unroofing because of its low morbidity and mortality [29, 33, 52, 53]. Laparoscopic ultrasonography is helpful in obtaining additional information about the structures that cannot be seen by percutaneous ultrasound [54]. Some surgeons found that the recurrence rates of laparoscopic fenestration were higher than expected after long-term follow-up, recommending aggressive techniques such as enucleation or liver resection with lower recurrence rates but higher morbidity and mortality [26, 27, 55]. Laparoscopic unroofing followed by 95% ethanol sclerotherapy can avoid complications of both multisegmental liver resection and extensive fenestration and untoward reactions from a large amount of alcohol [56]. Unroofing in combination with an omental flap, oversewing [14, 22] and ablation of the cyst with an argon beam coagulator [52] were concluded as safe and effective procedures.

Laparoscopic unroofing of solitary liver cysts should be the treatment of choice in carefully selected cases as it is minimally invasive, avoids the morbiditiy of laparotomy, and with shorter hospital stay and faster recovery [57]. Open and "aggressive" operations in nonparasitic cyst of the liver should be rarely needed.

Polycstic Liver Disease. There is much controversy here. The best indication for laparoscopic fenestration seems to be PLD characterized by large cysts mainly located on the liver surface (type l). For PLD characterized by numerous small cysts all over the liver (type2) such a laparoscopic approach is difficult and results in high recurrence rate [l]. (There were some attempts to avoid recurrence problem by adjuvant sclerotherapy with alcohol or tetracycline [56]). After fenestration of multiple cysts the patients are at high risk for recurrence (50–70%) [29]. Open fenestration and partial resection of the liver seem more effective therapeutic alternatives [58]. After open hepatic resection, the morbidity rates (25–50%) and length of hospital stay average (14.3 days to 7 days) twice those of the laparoscopic procedures [29, 59]. Laparoscopic liver resection is feasible today with a morbidity and mortality rate comparable to open surgery [6].

In PLD, adequate fenestration of superficial cysts allows deeper cysts to prolapse and be similarly fenestrated [31]. Additional use of laparoscopic ultrasound enables detection and adequate treatment of deep cystic lesions [54].

There is a wide range of surgical treatment of symptomatic PLD, from laparoscopic fenestration to liver resection and even liver transplation [58]. The best modality of treatment should be decided by further clinical investigations.

22.3
Summary (see Table 22.1)

— Laparoscopic approach should be considered for evaluation and treatment of cystic parasitic and nonparasitic disease of the liver.
— Laparoscopic treatment produces minimal surgical trauma, shorter hospital stay and avoids the morbidity of laparotomy with reduced postoperative adhesions, allowing repeated procedures when necessary.
— Careful selection of the patients and meticulous application of the proper technique makes laparoscopic treatment of this disease feasible, safe and beneficial to the patient.
— Laparoscopic fenestration is the gold standard for the treatment of solitary nonparasitic liver cysts with low morbidity and low recurrence rates.
— Initial treatment of polycystic liver disease should be laparoscopic fenestration with or withhout sclerotherapy in carefully selected patients. In complicated PLD cases open fenestration or liver resection may be a better option.
— Traditional surgical methods should be reserved for cases in which laparoscopic approach is not feasible.

References

1. Morino M, De Ginii M, Festa V, Garrone C. Laparoscopic management of symptomatic non-parasitic cysts of the liver: indications and results. Ann Surg 1994;219:157–64.
2. Katkhouda N, Mavor E. Laparoscopic management of benign liver disease. Surg Clin North Am 2000;80:1203–11.
3. Bickel A, Loberant N. The feasibility of safe laparoscopic treatment of hydatid cysts of the liver. Surg Endosc 1995;9:934–5.
4. Seven R, Berber E, Mercan S, Eminoglu L, Budak D. Laparoscopic treatment of hepatic hydatid cysts. Surgery 2000;128:36–40.
5. Lesurtel M, Cherqui D, Laurent A, Tayar C, Faniez PL. Laparoscopic versus open left lateral lobectomy: a case control study. J Am Coll Surg 2003;196:236–42.
6. Biertho L, Waage A, Gagner M. Laparoscopic hepatectomy. Ann Chir 2002;127:164–70.

Table22.1. Results of laparoscopic management of hydatid cysts of liver

Study [ref.]	Patients/ hydatid cysts	Conversion	Operative time (range, min)	Hospital stay (days)	Morbidity	Mortality	Mean follow-up (months)	Recurrence
Seven et al. 2000 [4]	30/33	7 (23%)	30–120	6±1	1 (4%)	0	17	1 (4%)
Hrubnyk et al. 2001 [40]	39/39	–	40–120	3.6±1.2	8 (20.5%)	0	18	1 (5.9%)
Sinha and Sharma 2001 [39]	42/42	–	–	3.2	7 (16.6%)	0	54	0
Emel'ianov and Khamidov 2000 [32]	37/37	1	–	5.6	4 (4%)	0	–	–
Khoury et al. 2000 [38]	83/108	3%	40–80	3	9 (11%)	0	30	3 (3.6%)

7. Mala T, Edwin B, Gladhaug I, Soride O, Fosse E, Mathisen O, Bergan A. Laparoscopic resection of liver [In Norwegian]. Tidsskr Nor Laegeforen 2002;122:2768–71.

8. Fabiani P, Katkhouda N, Iovine L, Mouiel J. Laparoscopic fenestration of biliary cysts. Surg Laparosc Endosc 1991;1:162–5.

9. Paterson-Brown S, Garden OJ. Laser-assisted laparoscopic excision of liver cyst. Br J Surg 1991;78:1047.

10. Kabbej M, Sauvanet A, Chauveau D, Farges O, Belghiti J. Laparoscopic fenestration in polycystic liver disease. Br J Surg 1996;83:1697–701.

11. Lujan Mompean JA, Parrilla Paricio P, Robles Campos R, Garcia Ayllon J. Laparoscopic treatment of a liver hydatid cyst. Br J Surg 1993;80:907–8.

12. Hersman H, Gardner B, Alfonso A. The value of laparoscopy in general surgery. J Reprod Med 1977;18:235–40.

13. Vogl S, Koperna T, Satzinger U, Schulz F. Nonparasitic liver cysts. Overview of therapy with long-term results [In German]. Langenbecks Arch Chir 1995;380:340–4.

14. Gloor B, Ly Q, Candinas D. Role of laparoscopy in hepatic cyst surgery. Dig Surg 2002;19:494–9.

15. Klotz HP, Schlumpf R, Weder W, Largiader F. Minimal invasive surgery for treatment of enlarged symptomatic liver cyst. Surg Laparoc Endosc 1993;3:351–3.

16. Koperna T, Vogl S, Satzinger U, Schulz F. Nonpurositic cyst of liver results on options of surgical treatment. World J Surg 1997;21:850–4.

17. Targarona EM, Martinez J, Ramos C, Becerra JA, Trias M. Conservative laparoscopic treatment of a posttraumatic splenic cyst. Surg Endosc 1995;91:71–2.

18. Heintz A, Junginger T. Laparoscopic surgery for hepatic, splenic and mesenteric cysts. [In German]. Dtsch Med Wochenschr 1995;120:201–4.

19. Chen BK, Gamagami RA, Kang J, Easter D, Lopez T. Symptomatic post-traumatic cyst of the liver: treatment by laparoscopic surgery. J Laparoendosc Adv Surg Tech A 2001;11:41–2.

20. Zalaba Z, Thianyi TF, Winternitz T, Nehez L, Flautner L. The laparoscopic treatment of non-parasitic liver cyst. Acta Chir Hung 1999;38:221–3.

21. Lange V, Meyer G, Rau H, Schildberg FW. Minimally invasive interventions in solitary liver cyst. Chirurg 1992;63:349–52.

22. Krahenbuhl L, Baer HU, Renzulli P, Z'graggen K, Frei E, Buchler MW. Laparoscopic management of nonparasitic symptom-producing solitary hepatic cysts. J Am Coll Surg 1996;183:493–8.

23. Fabiani P, Mazza D, Toouli J, Bartels AM, Gugenheim J, Mouiel J. Laparoscopic fenestration of symptomatic non-parasitic cyst of the liver, Br J Surg 1997;84:321–2.

24. Klingler PJ, Gadenstatter M, Schmid T, Bodner E, Schwelberger HG. Treatment of hepatic cysts in the era of laparoscopic surgery. Br J Surg 1997;84:838–44.

25. Gigot JF, Metairie S, Etienne J, Horsmans Y, Van Beers BE, Sempoux C, Deprez P, Materne R, Geubel A, Glineur D, Gianello P. The surgical management of congenital liver cyst. Surg Endosc 2001;15:357–63.

26. Ganti AL, Sardi A, Gordon J. Laparoscopic treatment of large true cyst of the liver and spleen is ineffective. Ann Surg 2002;68:1012–7.

27. Gigot JF, Legrand M, Hubens G, de Canniere L, Wibin E, Deweer F, Druart ML, Bertrant C, Devriendt H, Droissart R, Tugilimana M, Hauters P, Vereecken L. Laparoscopic treatment of nonparasitic liver cysts:adequate selection of patients and surgical technique. World J Surg 1996;20:556–61.

28. Tocchi A, Mazzoni G, Costa G, Cassini D, Bettelli E, Agostini N, Miccini M. Symptomatic nonparasitic hepatic cysts: options for and results of surgical management. Arch Surg 2002;137:154–8.

29. Martin IJ, Mc Kinley AJ, Currie EJ, Holmes P, Garden OJ. Tailoring the management of nonparasitic liver cystc. Ann Surg 1998;223:167–72.

30. Libutti SK, Starker PM. Laparoscopic resection of non-parasitic liver cyst. Surg Endosc 1994;8:1005–7.

31. Hodgson WJ, Kuczabski GK, Malhotra K. Laparoscopic management of cystic disease of liver. Surg Endosc 1998;12:46–9.

32. Emel'ianov SI, Khamidov MA. Laparoscopic treatment of hydatid liver cysts [In Russian]. Khirurgiia (Mosk) 2000;11:32–4.

33. Bickel A, Loberant N, Singer-Jordan J, Goldfeld M, Daud G, Eitan A. The laparoscopic approach to abdominal hydatid cysts: a prospective nonselective study using the isolated hypobaric technique. Arch Surg 2001;136:789–95.

34. Kayaalp C. Evacuation of hydatid liver cysts using laparoscopic trocar. World J Surg 2002;26:1324–7.

35. Monterola C, Fernandez O, Munoz S, Vial M, Losada H, Carrasco R, Bello N, Barrosso M. Laparoscopic pericystectomy for liver hydatid cysts. Surg Endosc 2002;16:521–4.

36. Guibert L, Gayral F. Laparoscopic pericystectomy of a liver hydatid cyst. Surg Endosc 1995;9:442–3.

37. Mercan S, Seven R, Ozarmagan S, Bozbora A, Altug K. Laparoscopic treatment of hepatic disorders. In: Proceedings of 1st Asian Pacific Congress of Endoscopic Surgery, 5–8 August 1993, Singapore.

38. Khoury G, Abiad F, Geagea T, Nabbout G, Jabbour S. Laparoscopic treatment of hydatid cyst of liver and spleen. Surg Endosc 2000;14;243–5.

39. Sinha R, Sharma N. Abdominal hydatids: a minimally invasive approach. JSLS 2001;5:237–40

40. Hrubnyk VV, Chetverikov SH, Sabri A Kh. The use of laparoscopic technique in the treatment of hepatic echinococcosis, Klin Khir 2001;7:19–21

41. Saðlam A. Laparoscopic treatment of liver hydatid cysts. Surg Laparosc Endosc 1996;6:16–21.

42. Morris DL. Use of a disposable laparoscopic trocar for the injection and safe evacuation of echinococus cysts of the liver. J Am Coll Surg 1994;179:635–6.

43. Khoury G, Jabbour-Khoury S, Soueidi A, Nabbout G, Baraka A. Anaphylactic shock complicating laparoscopic treatment of hydatid cyst of the liver. Surg Endosc 1998;12:452–4.

44. Sgaurakis G, Gemos K, Dedemadi G, Spetzouris N, Gyftakis H, Salapa P. Laparoscopic drainage of infected hydatid liver cysts. Minerva Chir 2001;56:169–73.

45. Sever M, Skapin S. Laparoscopic pericystectomy of liver hydatid cyst. Surg Endosc 1995;9:1125–26.

46. Liehr H, Richter E. Alveolar echinococcus of the liver. A rare laparoscopic finding. Acta Hepatosplenol 1969;16:46–51.

47. Aliev MA, Seisembaev MA, Ordabekov SO, Aliev RM, Belekov ZhO, Samratow TU. Hepatic echinococcosis and its surgical treatment. [In Russian]. Khirurgiia (Mosk) 1999;3:15–7.

48. Tekant Y, Bilge O, Acarlý K, Alper A, Emre A, Arýoðul O. Endoscopic sphinoterotomy in the treatment of postoperative biliary fistulas of hepatic hydatid disease. Surg Endosc 1996;10:909–11.

49. Sanchez H, Gagner M, Rossi R, et al. Surgical management of nonparasitic cystic liver disease. Am J Surg 1991;161:113.

50. Saini S, Mueller PR, Ferrucci JT, et al. Percutaneous aspiration of hepatic cysts does not provide definitive therapy. AJR Am J Roentgenol 1983;141:559–60.

51. Regev A, Reddy KR, Berho M, Sleeman D, Levi JU, Livingstone AS, Levi D, Ali U, Moliva EG, Schiff ER. Large cystic lesions of the liver in adults: a 15-year experience in a tertiary center. J Am Coll Surg 2001;193:36–45.

52. Kwon AH, Matsui Y, Inui H, Imamura A, Kamiyama Y. Laparoscopic treatment using an argon beam coagulator for non-parasitic liver cyst. Am J Surg 2003;185:273–7.

53. Matevosian VR, Kharnass SS, Lotov AN, Musaev GKh, Safronov VV, Koroleva IM, Kashevarov SB, Avakian VN. Diagnosis and choice of surgery of non-parasitic cyst of the liver. Khirurgiia (Mosk) 2002;7:31–6.

54. Schachter P, Sorin V, Avni Y, Shimonov M, Friedman V, Rosen A, Czerniak A. The role of laparoscopic ultrasound in the minimally invasive management of symptomatic hepatic cyst. Surg Endosc 2001;15:364–7.

55. Schmidbaner S, Hallfeldt KK, Sitzmann G, Kantelhardt T, Trupka A. Experience with ultrasound scissors and blades (Ultracision) in open and laparoscopic liver resection. Ann Surg 2002;235:27–30.

56. Jeng KS, Yang FS, Kao CR, Huang SH. Management of symptomatic polycystic liver disease: laparoscopy adjuvant with alcohol sclero therapy. J Gastroenterol Hepatol 1995;10:359–62.

57. Diez J, Decoud J, Gutierrez L, Suhl A, Merello J. Laparoscopic treatment of symptomatic cysts of the liver. Br J Surg 1998;85:25–7.

58. Ammori BJ, Jenkins BL, Lim PC, Parasad KR, Pollard SG, Lodge JP. Surgical strategy for cystic disease of the liver in a western hepatobiliary center. World J Surg 2002;26:462–9.

59. Petri A, Hohn J, Makula E, Kokai EL, Savanya GI, Boros M, Balogh A. Experience with different methods of treatment of non-parasitic liver cyst. Langenbecks Arch Surg 2002;387:229–33.

Commentary

JEAN EMOND, ADAM GRIESEMER

Dr. Mercan has written a superb review of the laparoscopic treatment of liver cysts. The use of minimally invasive surgery is ideally suited for these conditions, though several key issues are important in implementation. To complement his comprehensive tactical exposition, we propose the following strategic approach, which emphasizes several key issues.

How Do We Evaluate the Patient Referred with a Cyst?

Because the great majority of benign lesions of the liver are discovered incidentally on radiological examination, the hepatobiliary surgeon is faced with a variety of patients referred due to imaging done for unrelated reasons. Although approximately 85% of hepatic cysts are asymptomatic and require no treatment, several conditions – cystadenoma, hydatid cyst, or hepatic solid tumors with a cystic component (exceedingly rare) – require treatment despite the absence of symptoms. Therefore, the central challenge in the asymptomatic patient is to rule out the aforementioned conditions. Ultrasound investigation is the radiological test of choice supplemented by cross-sectional imaging. Simple cysts are anechoic and thin walled. In contrast, cystadenomas typically contain septa. Hydatid cysts have ultrasonographic appearances but the presence of a detached endocyst, of wall calcification, or of septa are typical findings [1]. Antigen and immune complex identification by ELISA (enzyme-linked immunosorbent assay) has 90% sensitivity, while determination of IgE antibody has sensitivity below 95% [2]. When the diagnosis is in doubt, resection is indicated. In a symptomatic patient, investigations should rule out confounding conditions that can cause the vague complaints attributable to liver cysts. Segmental location and depths of the cyst should be noted. In the patient with hydatid cysts, history of jaundice or symptoms consistent with cholangitis may indicate cystobiliary fistulae.

Once It Is Determined that Treatment Is Indicated, What Is the Best Approach?

Single/Dominant Cysts

Simple cysts are currently treated by percutaneous, laparoscopic, and open surgical techniques. Percutaneous aspiration alone has nearly a 100% recurrence rate. Aspiration in combination with chemical sclerosis has been successful in small studies [3]. In our experience, however, sclerotherapy can be extremely painful, often requires multiple treatments, and may result in bacterial contamination. We have also observed contamination of the pleural space, which is often traversed in the right-sided approach. Thus, we remain circumspect about this treatment.

In contrast, laparoscopic fenestration is associated with a low rate of recurrence and minimal morbidity [4]. The combination of fenestration with cyst wall ablation by argon coagulation can result in even lower recurrence rates, but injury to adjacent vascular structures is a potential complication [5]. Cysts located in portions of segments IV, VII and VIII present technical challenges due to difficult exposure. Although fenestration of cysts in these segments is possible, it may be associated with incomplete cyst wall resection, making them prone to recurrence.

Before completion of the operation, pathologic examination should be obtained to rule out the presence of *cystadenoma*. Discovery of a cystadenoma necessitates complete excision, which may require open resection.

Before the advent of laparoscopic surgery, open fenestration was the gold standard for the treatment of simple cysts. Recent studies have shown this approach to have a higher morbidity with recurrence rates equivalent to the laparoscopic approach. However, open surgery is still indicated for some posterior cysts, where there is inability to exclude malignancy, and operator inexperience with advanced laparoscopic techniques. In summary, the great majority of simple cysts are best approached via the laparoscopic approach.

Hydatid Cysts of the Liver

While uncommon in North America, hepatobiliary surgeons in endemic regions have developed remarkable expertise with this challenging disease. For cysts that are fluid filled, with detached endocyst but without daughter cysts, percutaneous aspiration and sterilization has been recommended. This procedure has long been criticized for the risk of spillage and inability to treat daughter cysts [1]. Initial outcomes have been shown to be comparable to open treatment of hydatid cysts [6], but caution must still be advised. Specialized centers report laparoscopic treatment of hydatid cysts with equivalent outcomes to series of open resection. After initiation of albendazole therapy, the standard technique involves aspiration of the cyst contents, instillation of scolicidal solution into the cyst cavity sterilize the cyst, and subsequent unroofing and omentoplasty of the remaining cyst cavity [1]. Development of new instrumentation has facilitated the laparoscopic treatment of these cysts. Inspection of the cyst wall with magnification may allow more accurate identification of cystobiliary communication. However, reports of anaphalyxis resulting from minimally invasive approaches must temper enthusiasm for these early successful results [7]. Open treatment allows easy placement of gauze soaked in hypertonic saline to protect the patient from consequences of spillage. Pericystectomy, in which complete removal of the cyst wall is performed, is most conservative, yet not always possible if vascular or biliary elements comprise part of the wall [8]. Bile staining of cyst contents requires careful inspection and closure of biliary fistulae. We do not perform intraoperative cholangiography, but treat the bile duct separately with endoscopic retrograde cholangiopancreatography (ERCP) in the face of symptoms or abnormal liver function tests. Thus, while in expert hands laparoscopic treatment of these cysts is the treatment of choice, for most practitioners open treatment remains appropriate [9]. In the future, however, refinement of techniques will allow laparoscopy to be employed safely with less morbidity than open resection.

Polycystic Liver Disease

Most patients with polycystic liver disease will not benefit from surgical treatment, and intervention should only be reserved for intractable symptoms of pain, anorexia and malnutrition, or cholestasis and portal hypertension caused by compression of vascular structures. Careful selection should exclude patients with type II PLD, characterized by multiple small cysts distributed throughout the liver. Large peripheral cysts are amenable to surgical therapy, but with a high rate of recurrence [10].

Both percutaneous and laparoscopic treatments are associated with high rates of recurrence. Laparoscopy combined with intraoperative ultrasound allows identification of deep cysts and differentiation of cyst walls from vascular structures. This may allow for more complete treatment at the cost of increased operative time [11]. However, expansion of smaller, untreated cysts or recurrence of fenestrated cysts is to be expected, and the patient should be aware that symptoms are likely to recur. Laparotomy allows for more complete cyst fenestration, but it is also associated with high failure rate. Some authors have combined fenestration with resection of the most involved segments of the liver to reduce the likelihood that small cysts will expand, but this technique has a higher morbidity than fenestration alone [4]. Open surgery also induces adhesion formation, making reoperation for symptomatic recurrence more difficult.

Experience with transplantation for PLD is limited. Transplantation, with or without concomitant renal transplantation, has been performed successfully with comparable morbidity compared with that of other surgical options [12]. The ability to obtain an exception MELD (model for end-stage liver disease) point in the UNOS (United Network for Organ Sharing) system and the application of living related transplantation has allowed these patients to obtain grafts despite the lack of liver failure. It should be emphasized that the use of transplantation is an aggressive approach for a disease entity that rarely develops life-threatening liver failure [13]. We feel that it is appropriate, however, for patients with refractory symptoms who have failed a trial of palliative therapy.

References

1. Sayek I, Onat D. Diagnosis and treatment of uncomplicated hydatid cyst of the liver. World J Surg 2001;25:21–7.
2. Giuliante F, D'Acapito F, Vellone M, Giovannini I, Nuzzo G. Risk for laparoscopic fenestration of liver cysts. Surg Endosc 2003;17:1735–8.
3. Larssen TB, Jensen DK, Viste A, Horn A. Single-session alcohol sclerotherapy in symptomatic benign hepatic cysts. Long-term results. Acta Radiol 1999;40:636–8.
4. Martin IJ, McKinley AJ, Currie EJ, Holmes P, Garden OJ. Tailoring the management of nonparasitic liver cysts. Ann Surg 1998;228:167–72.
5. Kwon AH, Matsui Y, Inui H, Imamura A, Kamiyama Y. Laparoscopic treatment using an argon beam coagulator for nonparasitic liver cysts. Am J Surg 2003;185:273–7.
6. Khuroo MS, Wani NA, Javid G, Khan BA, Yattoo GN, Shah AH, et al. Percutaneous drainage compared with surgery for hepatic hydatid cysts. N Engl J Med 1997;337: 881–7.
7. Khoury G, Jabbour-Khoury S, Soueidi A, Nabbout G, Baraka A. Anaphylactic shock complicating laparoscopic treatment of hydatid cysts of the liver. Surg Endosc 1998;12:452–4.
8. Katkhouda N, Hurwitz M, Gugenheim J, Mavor E, Mason RJ, Waldrep DJ, et al. Laparoscopic management of benign solid and cystic lesions of the liver. Ann Surg 1999;229:460–6.
9. Katkhouda N, Mavor E. Laparoscopic management of benign liver disease. Surg Clin North Am 2000;80:1203–11.
10. Kabbej M, Sauvanet A, Chauveau D, Farges O, Belghiti J. Laparoscopic fenestration in polycystic liver disease. Br J Surg 1996;83:1697–701.
11. Schachter P, Sorin V, Avni Y, Shimonov M, Friedman V, Rosen A, et al. The role of laparoscopic ultrasound in the minimally invasive management of symptomatic hepatic cysts. Surg Endosc 2001;15:364–7.
12. Chen MF. Surgery for adult polycystic liver disease. J Gastroenterol Hepatol 2000;15:1239–42.
13. Pirenne J, Aerts R, Yoong K, Gunson B, Koshiba T, Fourneau I, et al. Liver transplantation for polycystic liver disease. Liver Transpl 2001;7:238–45.

Liver Surgery for Solid Tumors

W.R. Jarnagin, Yuman Fong

▶ **Key Controversies**

A. Technical Considerations, Feasibility and Safety
B. Efficacy
C. Reproducibility

23.1
Introduction

The past two decades have seen dramatic changes in the practice of hepatic resectional surgery. During this time, liver resection has evolved from a high-risk, resource-intensive procedure with limited application to a safe and commonly performed operation with broad indications [1–3]. The improvements in perioperative outcome have been well documented in a number of studies, and have included significant reductions in blood loss, transfusion requirements, hospital stay and mortality. In addition, hepatic resection has been clearly shown to be the most effective therapy for patients with primary and selected secondary hepatic malignancies and the only effective treatment for a wide array of benign conditions [4–10].

The emergence of hepatic resection as a safe and effective treatment option is a relatively recent event, which in part explains the slow incursion of laparoscopic techniques. Progress in this area has also been impeded by a number of other issues, not the least of which are technical factors. These include problems related to mobilization of the liver, adequacy of exposure, achieving vascular control and parenchymal transection. Because of the technical limitations, the safety of laparoscopic hepatectomy remains a concern, primarily as it relates to difficulties controlling hemorrhage and the potential risk of massive gas embolization through openings in the hepatic venous system. In addition, because of the limited access, the question of whether laparoscopic resections have a greater risk of inadequate (i.e., tumor-involved) resection margins has been raised and remains unsettled.

The essence of the controversy is that the basic steps of hepatic resection that one can easily perform at laparotomy have, to this point, proven difficult to reproduce laparoscopically, potentially threatening both the safety and on-cologic adequacy of the procedure. For laparoscopic partial hepatectomy to become a mainstream operative procedure, it must first be shown to be as safe as open hepatic resection, to be equivalent in efficacy, to significantly reduce hospital stay and/or patient discomfort and to be reproducible outside of se-lected centers of expertise [11]. While recent data address some of these issues and suggest that laparoscopic partial hepatectomy is feasible in selected pa-tients, progress has been slow.

23.2
Discussion

23.2.1
Technical Considerations, Feasibility and Safety

Several groups have investigated the feasibility of laparoscopic hepatic re-section, inspired by progress in other areas [12–22]. These efforts have been fostered by a number of technological advances, including the widespread availability of laparoscopic ultrasonography for assessing the extent of liver disease, vascular staplers for controlling major vascular structures, and de-vices that facilitate hepatic parenchymal transection (harmonic scalpel, lap-aroscopic ultrasonic dissectors). The accumulated evidence shows that, for selected patients with benign and malignant hepatic tumors, laparoscopic partial hepatectomy is a technically viable procedure (Table 23.1). However, the evidence also shows that the laparoscopic approach remains quite limited in its application. Indeed, the overwhelming majority of procedures have con-sisted of limited resections (one or two segments) of relatively small tumors at the periphery of the liver (segments 2, 3, 4B, 5 or 6), with very few reported major resections.

This observation underscores a persistent, major barrier to routine lapa-roscopic hepatic resection: adequate mobilization of the liver and safe expo-sure of the vascular pedicles and hepatic veins. The hand-assisted technique using a HandPort or GelPort may be helpful in this regard [12, 22]. Huang et al. recently reported seven hand-assisted resections for tumors in the right posterior sector [12]. The authors suggest that this approach greatly facilitated liver mobilization and, further, provided tactile sense that aided in assessing disease extent and determining the line of parenchymal transection. It should be emphasized, however, that the seven patients comprising this report repre-sented only a third of all patients with similarly located tumors over the study period; the remainder were felt to be inappropriate for laparoscopic resection because of tumor proximity to major hepatic veins. Similarly, Cherqui and

Farges et al. both reported that laparoscopic resection represented a small fraction of the total hepatic resections performed [11, 18].

It has become increasingly apparent that limited hepatic resections performed laparoscopically can be done with a safety profile equivalent to similar resections performed at laparotomy. Operative blood loss, transfusion rates and surgical morbidity are all acceptably low and comparable to the expected results of open resections (Table 23.1); none of the studies listed reported operative mortality. It should be noted that bleeding was a common indication for conversion to an open procedure in these studies, although in general, overwhelming hemorrhage was not encountered [14–16, 19]. Hemodynamically significant gas embolus, a much feared and often discussed potential complication of laparoscopic partial hepatectomy [23], is rarely observed in practice, which may be related to elevated intrahepatic vascular pressures and decreased hepatic tissue blood flow under standard pneumoperitoneum [24]. Nevertheless, given the life-threatening nature of this complication, some investigators advocate the gasless laparoscopic approach [25].

The available data would suggest that, for highly selected patients with small benign or malignant tumors, laparoscopic resection is a safe and feasible alternative to open resection. However, it must be emphasized that proper patient selection is critical. Although major laparoscopic resections have been performed, the number is small, and the safety of such procedures is less clearly established [11, 14, 19, 21, 26].

23.2.2
Efficacy

Whether laparoscopic partial hepatectomy can be done with results similar to those achievable at laparotomy and can offer some improvement in perioperative outcome remains the subject of some controversy. A major concern is the possibility that laparoscopic resections may compromise the resection margins in patients with malignant disease. This is obviously not an issue for patients with benign tumors. On the other hand, it should be pointed out that symptomatic benign tumors are often large and may therefore not be amenable to laparoscopic resection; small benign tumors are less often symptomatic and need not be resected, except for adenomas and cases of diagnostic uncertainty [4].

In the absence of randomized, controlled data, definitive statements regarding the efficacy of laparoscopic hepatectomy are not possible. The best data currently available are from studies that have retrospectively evaluated laparoscopic and comparable open resections [15–18]. These reports provide further evidence of the feasibility and safety of hepatic resection, but because

Table 23.1. Experience with laparoscopic liver resections. (*EBL* estimated blood loss, *LOS* length of stay, *NR* not reported)

Author [ref.]	Year	N	No. of major resections[a]	Benign / malignant	Conversion to open	EBL / transfusions	Hospital LOS (days)	Morbidity / mortality
Linden et al. [13]	2003	5	0	2 / 3	0	41 ml / 0%	2.2	0% / 0%
Laurent et al. [15]	2003	13	0	0 / 13	2	620 ml / 8%	15.3	36% / 0%
Huang et al. [12]	2003	7	0	2 / 5	0	257 ml / 0%	5.3	14% / 0%
Lesurtel et al. [16]	2003	18	0	12 / 6	2	236 ml / 0%	8	11% / 0%
Descottes et al. [14]	2003	87	3	87 / 0	9	NR / 6%	5	5% / 0%
Farges et al. [18]	2002	21	0	21 / 0	0	218 ml / 0%	5.1	10% / 0%
Gigot et al. [19]	2002	37	2	0 / 37	5	NR / 16%	7	22% / 0%
Mala et al. [17]	2002	13	0	0 / 13	0	600 ml / 0%	4	15% / 0%
Descottes et al. [21]	2000	15	1	14 / 2	1	NR / 0%	5.2	7% / 0%
Fong et al. [22]	2000	11	0	1 / 10	6	260 ml / 0%	5	40% / 0%
Ker et al. [20]	2000	9	0	0 / 9	0	NR / 0%	NR	11% / 0%

[a] Lobectomy or greater

of the very small number of patients, conclusions regarding efficacy are limited.

Three studies specifically evaluated oncologic efficacy in patients with malignant disease and found that the resection margins of laparoscopic resections were adequate and comparable with those obtained with open resections [15–17]. Other studies have reported similar results [13, 19], although the report from Gigot et al. did report tumor involved margin in 1 patient and <1 cm margin in six patients [19]. There is little long-term follow-up data available after laparoscopic liver resection for malignancy. However, Laurent et al. suggested a potential survival advantage of laparoscopic resection of hepatocellular carcinoma in cirrhotic patients [15]. The authors observed less postoperative ascites in the laparoscopic group, possibly the result of better preservation of collateral venous channels and reduced intravenous fluid requirements using this approach. While this may be the case, the total number of patients evaluated was small (27) and the observed difference in survival was more likely the result of two postoperative deaths in the open resection group. In this study, as well as in a report from Mala et al. [17], cancer recurrence rates were similar between the open and laparoscopic groups, suggesting that laparoscopic resections do not increase the risk of cancer dissemination. Another consideration is the potential for incomplete laparoscopic disease staging. A number of studies have shown that laparoscopy may not identify some patients with extrahepatic metastatic disease (peritoneal or nodal) [27–29], a finding that in most cases would contraindicate hepatic resection.

The oncologic efficacy of laparoscopic hepatic resection thus appears to be similar to that of open resections, at least with respect to achieving adequate resection margins in the highly selected patients studied to date. On the other hand, a clear-cut improvement in perioperative outcome has not been shown. Operative morbidity and mortality rates are similar between laparoscopic and comparable open resections, and the laparoscopic approach is not associated with obvious reductions in blood loss or transfusion requirements [15–18]. Also, while some studies have shown decreased hospital length of stay [17, 18], others have found no difference [15, 16]. As one would expect, incision-related morbidity is lower with the laparoscopic approach. Farges et al. and Mala et al. both reported significant reductions in duration of postoperative narcotic analgesic usage [17, 18]. By contrast, complications related to the hepatic resection itself, such as bleeding, bile leak/fluid collection, are not necessarily lower after laparoscopic resections.

23.2.3
Reproducibility

In general, liver surgery is technically demanding, requires specific training, and the best results are obtained at high volume referral centers [30].
Major hepatic resections are procedures that most surgeons do not perform
on a regular basis. It is therefore unrealistic to expect that the laparoscopic
approach will easily supplant open resections and become widely applied by
surgeons without a large, parallel practice of open liver surgery. Laparoscopic
liver resections have been largely performed in specialized units, and this
trend is likely to continue for the foreseeable future.

Laparoscopic partial hepatectomy requires considerable expertise in
both open hepatic resectional surgery and advanced laparoscopic surgery,
a relatively unique combination of technical skills. Advanced laparoscopic
training is now quite common, and many surgeons routinely perform large
numbers of complex laparoscopic cases. By contrast, liver surgery is typically
concentrated in high volume, tertiary referral centers. While nearly all surgical trainees now receive considerable exposure to laparoscopic surgery and
many go on to laparoscopic fellowships, adequate exposure to and training in
liver surgery are not widely available. It would therefore be unreasonable for
even a very seasoned laparoscopic surgeon with little exposure to open liver
surgery to undertake laparoscopic liver resections. Similarly, an experienced
liver surgeon with limited laparoscopic ability is not sufficiently trained for
these procedures. Some surgeons have acquired the necessary training and
skills and more are likely to do so with time; however, a collaborative effort
of experienced laparoscopic and liver surgeons would seem to be a rationale
approach [11].

23.3
Summary

— Despite some advances, progress in laparoscopic liver surgery has been
slow. This is not the result of any lack of interest or effort, however. Hepatic resection, unlike other abdominal operations, does not readily lend
itself to laparoscopic approaches, particularly for major procedures. In
addition, although advances in instrumentation have made laparoscopic
resections feasible, a number of technical and other barriers remain.
— The available data would suggest that for selected patients with small, peripheral tumors who require limited resections (one or two segments), the
laparoscopic approach is a safe and effective alternative. In such cases,

there is likely to be a reduction in patient discomfort and hospital length of stay, although this has not been shown definitively.

— In patients with malignant disease, the principles of surgical oncology must be observed, and long-term follow-up data is necessary to fully assess disease-related outcomes.

— While major resections have been performed, the safety, efficacy and potential perioperative benefits are less clearly established. For major resections in particular, given the substantial postoperative physiological changes that require in-hospital observation, it must be established that the minimal access approach offers a significant perioperative benefit over open resections to justify its use.

— Proper patient selection is clearly critical and the availability of laparoscopy should not change the indications for resection, particularly in patients with benign tumors.

References

1. Belghiti J, Hiramatsu K, Benoist S, Massault P, Sauvanet A, Farges O. Seven hundred forty-seven hepatectomies in the 1990s: an update to evaluate the actual risk of liver resection. J Am Coll Surg 2000;191:38–46.
2. Foster JH, Berman MM. Solid liver tumors. Major Probl Clin Surg 1977;22:1–342.
3. Jarnagin WR, Gonen M, Fong Y, DeMatteo RP, Ben-Porat L, Little S, Weber SM, Weber S, Blumgart LH. Improvement in perioperative outcome after hepatic resection: analysis of 1803 consecutive cases over the past decade. Ann Surg 2002;236:397–407.
4. Charny CK, Jarnagin WR, Schwartz LH, Frommeyer HS, DeMatteo RP, Fong Y, Blumgart LH. Management of 155 patients with benign liver tumours. Br J Surg 2001;88:808–13.
5. Fan ST, Lo CM, Liu CL, Lam CM, Yuen WK, Yeung C, Wong J. Hepatectomy for hepatocellular carcinoma: toward zero hospital deaths. Ann Surg 1999;229:322–30.
6. Fong Y, Fortner JG, Sun R, Brennan MF, Blumgart LH. Clinical score for predicting recurrence after hepatic resection for metastatic colorectal cancer: analysis of 1001 consecutive cases. Ann Surg 1999;230:309–21.
7. Gayowski TJ, Iwatsuki S, Madariaga JR, Selby R, Todo S, Irish W, Starzl TE. Experience in hepatic resection for metastatic colorectal cancer: analysis of clinical and pathological risk factors. Surgery 1994;116:703–11.
8. Jarnagin WR, Fong Y, DeMatteo RP, Gonen M, Burke EC, Bodniewicz BJ, Youssef BM, Klimstra D, Blumgart LH. Staging, resectability, and outcome in 225 patients with hilar cholangiocarcinoma. Ann Surg 2001;234:507–17.
9. Nordlinger B, Guiguet M, Vaillant JC, Balladur P, Boudjema K, Bachellier P, Jaeck D; Association Française de Chirurgie. Surgical resection of colorectal carcinoma metastases to the liver. a prognostic scoring system to improve case selection, based on 1568 patients. Cancer 1996;77:1254–62.
10. Scheele J. Liver resection for colorectal metastases. World J Surg 1995;19:59–71.

11. Cherqui D. Laparoscopic liver resection. Br J Surg 2003;90:644–646.

12. Huang MT, Lee WJ, Wang W, et al. Hand-assisted laparoscopic hepatectomy for solid tumor in the posterior portion of the right lobe: initial experience. Ann Surg 2003; 238:674–9.

13. Linden BCH, Humar A, Sielaff TD. Laparoscopic stapled left lateral segment liver resection – technique and results. J Gastrointest Surg 2003;7:777–82.

14. Descottes BG, Glineur D, Lachachi, et al. Laparoscopic liver resection of benign liver tumors. Surg Endosc 2003;17:668.

15. Laurent A, Cherqui D, Lesurtel M, Brunetti F, Tayar C, Fagniez PL. Laparoscopic liver resection for subcapsular hepatocellular carcinoma complicating chronic liver disease. Arch Surg 2003;138:763–9.

16. Lesurtel M, Cherqui D, Laurent A, Tayar C, Fagniez PL. Laparoscopic versus open left lateral hepatic lobectomy: a case-control study. J Am Coll Surg 2003;196:236–42.

17. Mala T, Edwin B, Gladhaug I, Fosse E, Soreide O, Bergan A, Mathisen O. A comparative study of the short-term outcome following open and laparoscopic liver resection of colorectal metastases. Surg Endosc 2002;16:1059–63.

18. Farges O, Jagot P, Kirstetter P, Marty J, Belghiti J. Prospective assessment of the safety and benefit of laparoscopic liver resections. J Hepatobiliary Pancreat Surg 2002;9:242–8.

19. Gigot JF, Glineur D, Santiago AJ, Goergen M, Ceuterick M, Morino M, Etienne J, Marescaux J, Mutter D, van Krunckelsven L, Descottes B, Valleix D, Lachachi F, Bertrand C, Mansvelt B, Hubens G, Saey JP, Schockmel R; Hepatobiliary and Pancreatic Section of the Royal Belgian Society of Surgery and the Belgian Group for Endoscopic Surgery. Laparoscopic liver resection for malignant liver tumors: preliminary results of a multi-center European study. Ann Surg 2002;236:90–7.

20. Ker CG, Chen HY, Juan CC, Chang WS, Tsai CY, Lo HW, Yau MT. Laparoscopic sub-segmentectomy for hepatocellular carcinoma with cirrhosis. Hepatogastroenterology 2000;47:1260–3.

21. Descottes B, Lachachi F, Sodji M, Valleix D, Durand-Fontanier S, Pech DL, Grousseau D. Early experience with laparoscopic approach for solid liver tumors: initial 16 cases. Ann Surg 2000;232:641–5.

22. Fong Y, Jarnagin WR, Conlon KC, DeMatteo RP, Dougherty E, Blumgart LH. Hand-assisted laparoscopic liver resection: lessons from an initial experience. Arch Surg 2000;135:854–9.

23. Schmandra TC, Mierdl S, Bauer H, Gutt C, Hanisch E. Transoesophageal echocardiography shows high risk of gas embolism during laparoscopic hepatic resection under carbon dioxide pneumoperitoneum. Br J Surg 2002;89:870–6.

24. Ricciardi R, Anwaruddin S, Schaffer BK, Quarfordt SH, Donohue SE, Wheeler SM, Gallagher KA, Callery MP, Litwin DE, Meyers WC. Elevated intrahepatic pressures and decreased hepatic tissue blood flow prevent gas embolus during limited laparoscopic liver resections. Surg Endosc 2001;15:729–33.

25. Takagi S. Hepatic and portal vein blood flow during carbon dioxide pneumoperitoneum for laparoscopic hepatectomy. Surg Endosc 1998;12:427–31.

26. Huscher CG, Lirici MM, Chiodini S. Laparoscopic liver resections. Semin Laparosc Surg 1998;5:204–10.

27. Lo CM, Lai EC, Liu CL, Fan ST, Wong J. Laparoscopy and laparoscopic ultrasonography avoid exploratory laparotomy in patients with hepatocellular carcinoma. Ann Surg 1998;227:527–32.
28. Jarnagin WR, Bodniewicz J, Dougherty E, Conlon K, Blumgart LH, Fong Y. A prospective analysis of staging laparoscopy in patients with primary and secondary hepatobiliary malignancies. J Gastrointest Surg 2000;4:34–43.
29. D'Angelica M, Fong Y, Weber S, Gonen M, DeMatteo RP, Conlon K, Blumgart LH, Jarnagin WR. The role of staging laparoscopy in hepatobiliary malignancy: prospective analysis of 401 cases. Ann Surg Oncol 2003;10:183–9.
30. Choti MA, Bowman HM, Pitt HA, Sosa JA, Sitzmann JV, Cameron JL, Gordon TA. Should hepatic resections be performed at high-volume referral centers? J Gastrointest Surg 1998;2:11–20.

Commentary

IBRAHIM DAGHER, DOMINIQUE FRANCO

Will liver resections soon be routinely performed by laparoscopy? In their chapter Jarnagin and Fong are not so optimistic. Their point of view is based on the limited experience published so far. However, a certain number of arguments suggest that liver surgery can safely be done by laparoscopy.

First of all, most procedures that are well validated by laparotomy can be reproduced by laparoscopy. In fact magnification and direct vision often makes them easier and safer. This is true for the approach of portal pedicles of the right and left livers and also of the left lateral lobe. This is even more evident for the approach and control of major hepatic veins. The vision of the terminal part of the left hepatic vein and of its junction with inferior vena cava is much better by laparoscopy, making its dissection and taping easy. The approach of the right hepatic vein is also facilitated by laparoscopy. The position of the optic in the same direction as the inferior vena cava makes easy to lift the posterior aspect of the liver away from the anterior wall of the inferior vena cava upwards and to expose small direct hepatic branches. Division of these branches leads to the inferior border of the right hepatic vein and its left and right walls.

Development of new technologies has helped laparoscopic liver parenchymal transection. The harmonic scalpel on the one hand, and thermofusion on the other, allow one to perform transection without much bleeding. When using these instruments, however, care must be taken not to tear large hepatic branches going across the transection plane particularly in the depth of the right liver. One should learn to use these instruments not uniquely for coagulation of liver tissue but also for gentle blunt dissection. An important point in transecting liver parenchyma is to place the camera right in front of the transection line and to use a cutting instrument on one side and a bipolar coagulation on the other.

Gas embolism was feared in initial experiences and appeared to be infrequent although small gas bubbles are often seen when monitoring the patient by esophageal ultrasonography. Bipolar coagulation is enough to treat most bleeding from the hepatic stump. Only a few clips have to be used on the largest pedicles. New laparoscopic stapling devices allow one to safely divide major portal vessels and hepatic veins. Division of the right hepatic duct requires particular care since there is usually little room for the stapler.

Not all procedures can however be easily reproduced by laparoscopy. For example the exposure of posterior segments of the right liver is difficult. It may require special positioning of the patient on his or her left side, the use of a 30° optic, and/or a hand-assisted technique [1]. Trocars might also be shifted much to the right side. Also, resection of a cube of liver parenchyma away from the anterior border of the liver remains uneasy particularly at the upper part of the right liver.

At the present time, it is not provocative to say that not only laparoscopic left lateral lobectomy [2] is feasible. But also left hepatectomy, right hepatectomy [3] and resection of segments 5 and 6 [4] have become standardized and reproducible in the hands of experienced surgical teams. On the other hand, resection of segments 7 and 8, and posterolateral and anteromedial sectionectomies are not. The will to perform laparoscopy by any means should not lead to modify indications for resection. A small hepatocellular carcinoma in segment 8 should not be treated by a laparoscopic right hepatectomy only because laparoscopic resection of segment 8 is not yet available.

Laparoscopy seems to be oncologically correct. This is a major point since liver resections are now mainly performed for malignant liver tumors. There has been no report of cancer dissemination following surgery. This is quite similar to what is now admitted for other digestive tract cancers [5]. The safety margin around the tumor is similar to what was reported by laparotomy. One should keep in mind that safety margin depends more on the type of resection defined upon preoperative morphological investigations of the liver rather than on the technique of resection itself. Intraoperative ultrasonography remains helpful to confirm that the transection plane remains away from the tumor. Data from small series suggest the recurrence and recurrence-free survival rates are similar to what was observed after conventional liver resections for hepatocellular carcinomas and liver metastases.

Are benefits from laparoscopy worth the burden of training, the increased operative duration and the increased operating room cost? Although this has not yet been studied for liver resection one can bet that it will be much the same as to what has been demonstrated for other types of abdominal surgery concerning postoperative pain, hospital stay, and the rate of postoperative complications. Liver resections by laparotomy usually require a large bisubcostal incision. In cirrhotic patients this exposes particularly to formation of ascites and to incisional leaks. If this were the only benefit of laparoscopy it would be a major step.

It is unfair to write about laparoscopic liver resection without highlighting new issues such as virtual reality and robot-assisted surgery. Computer reconstruction of the liver is now easily achieved [6]. Liver transection can be performed on a screen before doing it in the operating room. This enables to forecast every step of the procedure. Together with the enhanced reality brought up by laparoscopy, it might allow one to perform liver parenchymal transection very safely while remaining at a distance from the tumor and visualizing in advance any vessel or bile duct going across the transection plan. Robots should then be able to achieve parenchymal transection under the surgeon supervision. Laparoscopic liver surgery might be a leading procedure in robot-assisted surgery.

Jarnagin and Fong are quite right when stating that performance of laparoscopic liver resection requires both training and experience in both liver surgery and laparoscopy. Certainly the best way to slow down the development of laparoscopic liver surgery would be to ignore experienced liver surgeons and not encourage them for laparoscopic training. This would leave them with the status quo whereby they are spending long exhausting hours behind the screen to complete a liver resection they would otherwise have completed in only 2 h by laparotomy.

References

1. Huang MT, Lee WJ, Wang W, Wei PL, Chen RJ. Hand-assisted laparoscopic hepatectomy for solid tumor in the posterior portion of the right lobe: initial experience. Ann Surg 2003;238:674–9
2. Lesurtel M, Cherqui D, Laurent A, Tayar C, Fagniez PL. Laparoscopic versus open left lateral hepatic lobectomy: a case-controlled study. J Am Coll Surg 2003;196:236–42
3. O'Rourke N, Fielding G. Laparoscopic right hepatectomy: surgical technique. J Gastointest Surg 2004;8:213–6
4. Morino M, Morra I, Rosso E, Miglietta C, Garrone C. Laparoscopic vs open hepatic resection: a comparative study. Surg Endosc 2003;17:1914–8
5. Ceulemans R, Henri M, Leroy J, Marescaux J. Laparoscopic surgery for cancer: are we ready? Acta Gastroenterol Belg 2003;66:227–30
6. Soler L, Delingette H, Malandain G, Ayache N, Koehl C, Clément JM, Dourthe O, Marescaux J. An automatic virtual patient reconstruction from CT-scans for hepatic surgical planning. Stud Health Technol Inform 2000;70:316–22

Splenectomy

RONALD MATTEOTTI, AHMAD ASSALIA, ALFONS POMP

▶ **Key Controversies**

A. Indications
  – Splenomegaly – massive splenomegaly and the "giant spleen"
B. Persistent splenic tissue
  – The congenital accessory spleen
  – Acquired splenosis
C. Choice of laparoscopic technique
  – Anterior approach
  – Lateral approach

24.1
Introduction

Since the first reported laparoscopic splenectomy in 1991 by Delaitre in Paris this surgery has become the "gold standard" for the removal of benign and normal-sized lesions of the spleen such as those found in idiopathic thrombocytopenic purpura (ITP) [1–15]. In pediatric cases it may also be the procedure of choice as well [16, 17].

Laparoscopic removal of the spleen offers significant advantages when compared to an open approach for the benign, normal sized organ. Laparoscopic surgery that involves mere organ excision obviates the majority of complications associated with incisions without compromising the integrity of the operation. This usually translates into less postoperative pain, faster recovery, decreased morbidity and improved cosmesis [15, 16].

24.2
Discussion

24.2.1
Indications

24.2.1.1
Splenomegaly – Massive Splenomegaly and the "Giant Spleen"

Laparoscopic splenectomy is currently performed also for malignant disorders that may be associated with splenomegaly [18]. There is, however, no standard description of this term in the surgical literature. Computed tomography (CT) scan or ultrasound can be used in order to measure the craniocaudal length or the volume of the spleen. While the weight of the spleen may be measured in open surgery, laparoscopic surgeons almost invariably morcellate and aspirate parts of the spleen during extraction, thus rendering any comparison based on "wet weight" inaccurate. Kercher and colleagues have used a craniocaudal length ≥17 cm or wet weight ≥600 g postoperatively to define splenomegaly, and a craniocaudal length ≥22 cm and a weight ≥1600 g to describe "giant spleens" [18]. Others limit the description of a normal sized spleen to a weight ≤500 g [19]. Many authors use either clinical judgment and determine splenomegaly if the organ is clearly palpable under the left costal margin or observed in this location on CT scan or if the spleen has a final wet weight of >700 g [2].

Laparoscopic splenectomy in cases of massive splenomegaly is clearly associated with greater morbidity and conversion rates, and this occurs not only in inexperienced hands [18, 20]. The laparoscopic exposure of a large organ can be very difficult because of the narrow intra-abdominal working space. This problem can be exacerbated in cases of truncal obesity associated with significant steroid use that is not uncommon in patients who require splenectomy. Furthermore, in cases of splenomegaly, not only is the technical difficulty of the procedure increased, but the retrieval of the specimen from the abdomen may become problematic. It is extremely difficult (and often frustrating) to manipulate a large organ into a large retrieval sac in a small working space. It is thus important to attain a consensus when describing spleen size in order to be able to make the appropriate preoperative decision concerning which surgical technique should be used: open, laparoscopic or a possibly hand-assisted approach. The use of a clinical examination in combination with ultrasound or CT should be sufficient to determine spleen size and a spleen with an estimated weight of >500 g should be considered as splenomegaly, a spleen with a craniocaudal length of greater than 17 cm or 1000 g as massive splenomegaly and a spleen with a craniocaudal length of 22 cm or >1500 g as a giant spleen.

Spleen size in relation to the volume of the patient's abdominal cavity is a major consideration in determining the feasibility of a laparascopic approach to this organ. From a group of 47 patients, in 12 cases it was impossible for the surgeon to complete the operation entirely laparoscopically and the operation had to be converted to a hand-assisted procedure [18]. This is a promising technique because it combines many of the advantages of laparoscopy with the restored tactile function of the surgeons hand, which can be used to guide the vascular staplers and may control inadvertent bleeding as well as facilitate the removal of the specimen. If larger pieces for histological examination are required this can be easily accomplished using a hand-assisted technique, although appropriate tissue for histological examination can usually be obtained when the spleen is morcellated in a durable extraction sac In the small cohort of published series where comparison is possible, hand-assisted laparoscopic splenectomy appears to be superior to a total laparoscopic approach in difficult cases, and does lead to less frequent complications (Tables 24.1, 24.2). The importance of hand-assisted laparoscopic splenectomy in cases of splenomegaly remains to be defined in future larger series.

In our opinion, it seems prudent to propose that only experienced surgeons should attempt a laparoscopic resection of spleens greater than 500 g. Hand-assisted laparoscopy should be considered for cases of massive splenomegaly and giant spleens.

24.2.2
Persistent Splenic Tissue

24.2.2.1
The Congenital Accessory Spleen

An accessory spleen may be defined as splenic tissue other than the normal spleen in its original anatomic site. The most common site for accessory spleens is the hilum, followed by the retroperitoneum, greater omentum and mesentery. The function of an accessory spleen remains controversial primarily because the physiological role in relation to a critical size which will induce a recurrent hematological disease after primary operation is unknown.

There is a wide range in the incidence of accessory spleens in the larger series [7, 10, 12, 21–23] and this has been described as a important shortcoming of the laparoscopic approach in hematologic diseases. It is true that the presence of an accessory spleen can be responsible for relapsing disease in a significant percentage of patients suffering from a hematologic disorder like ITP, but relapsing disease can be present as well without any detectable acces-

Table 24.1. Totally laparoscopic splenectomy in cases of splenomegaly (*NR* not recorded)

Study [ref.]	No. of patients	Age (years)	Spleen weight (g)	Follow-up (months)	Conversion (%)	Operative time (min)	Blood loss (ml)	Length of stay (day)	Complications (%)	Deaths (%)
Kercher et al. [18]	49	54.4	600–4750	14	0	171	114	2.3	0	NR
Terrosu et al. [19]	20	54	500–4800	NR	20	163±56	569±393	5.6±2.5	20	5
Patel et al. [20]	27	57	1000–4750	NR	18.5	170	500–2000	5	55.5	NR
Mahon and Rhodes [36]	39									
Spleen <1 kg	29	NR	360	NR	0	72.5	75	2	6.9	NR
Spleen >1 kg	10	NR	2000	NR	60	94	1150	6	20	NR
Targarona et al. [2]	36	58±13	1425±884	NR	20	177±52	NR	6.3±33	30 mild, 5 severe	0
Ailawadi et al. [37]	19	49.9±14.7	740	NR	36.8	212	550	4.5	32	16
Nicholson et al. [38]	3	80.3	1438.3	NR	0	186.6	203	5	NR	NR
Targarona et al. [39]	19									
Group 1[a]		47±19	638±163	NR	25	184±103	NR	5±2	33	NR
Group 2[b]		55±7	1616±651	NR	25	190±69	NR	6±4	30	NR
Total/Mean	212	–	–	–	30	162	451.5	4.77	17.43	10.5

[a]Spleen 400–1000g, [b]Spleen >1000g

Table 24.2. Hand-assisted laparoscopic splenectomy in cases of splenomegaly (*NR* not recorded)

Study [ref.]	No. of patients	Mean age (years)	Spleen weight (g)	Mean follow-up (months)	Con-version (%)	Mean operative time (min)	Mean blood loss (ml)	Mean length of stay (day)	Compli-cations (%)	Mortality (%)
Kerchet et al. [18]	12 1[a]	54.4 –	600–4750 –	14 –	0 –	146 (7) 295 (5)	137.5 –	2.0 –	0 –	NR –
Targarona et al. [2]	20	58±16	1753±1124	NR	5	135±52	NR	4±1.2	5 mild, 5 severe	0
Ailawadi et al. [37]	22	52±18.3	1394	NR	13.6	161	325	3	18	0
Borazzo et al. [40]	16	56	2008	NR	0	240	425	3.3	6.25	0
Rosen et al. [41]	14	57	1516	–	7.1	177	602	5.4	35.7	0
Total/Mean	82	–	–	–	8.5	193.3	372.4	2.94	13.99	0

[a] One initially attempted laparoscopical

sory spleen [1, 24]. The true functional incidence of the accessory spleen has yet to be defined although there are large studies of laparoscopic surgery for frequent hematological disorder like ITP that show excellent results [11].

There are many modalities available to complement the usual preoperative ultrasound or CT including technetium or indium 111 scanning and intraoperative laparoscopic ultrasound [10, 21, 25]. We suppose, given current data, that a thorough explorative laparoscopy at the beginning of the procedure to search for accessory spleens is sufficient. This, however, may be difficult in the lateral position, especially in an obese patient. There is currently not enough evidence to warrant the routine use of denatured red blood cell scintigraphy (DRBCS) postoperatively to detect residual splenic tissue, as others have suggested [24].

24.2.2.2
Acquired Splenosis

Splenosis may be defined as the autotransplantation of splenic tissue after any injury to the spleen, either after trauma, which is the most frequent cause, or after surgical procedures. The presence of splenic tissue is often asymptomatic but may also lead to pain, recurrent disease or even life-threatening bleeding [26, 27]. Concerns have been raised about tissue dissemination during the morcellation process necessary to remove the specimen that could lead to the recurrence of the original disease. Residual splenic tissue requires enough quantity and adequate architecture to induce a relapse of the initial hematological disorder [25]. A seeding of spilt splenic cells from parenchymal injury might theoretically occur during the high pressure pneumoperitoneum if the integrity of the splenic capsule is breached during manipulation. A recent study by Lee et al. examined port site tumor recurrence rates in a murine model of laparoscopic splenectomy and clearly showed that the rate of port-site "metastasis" is due to the extent of tissue manipulation and the experience of the surgeon rather than the pneumoperitoneum itself [28]. The extraction of the specimen is of utmost importance to reduce the incidence of splenic tissue seeding. Morcellation should be performed in a durable impermeable bag with appropriate precautions to avoid spillage and any method of intraperitonel morcellation should be avoided.

It is troubling that Gigot and colleagues found a 50% rate of residual splenic tissue detected by sequential DRBCS after an early series of laparoscopic splenectomies. In all these cases the specimen was removed using a retrieval bag. Clinical recurrence occurred in five of nine patients. Four had had splenic parenchymal injury during the procedure [24]. The true significance of residual splenic tissue following laparoscopic splenectomy remains unknown and must be addressed in future clinical studies.

24.2.3
Choice of Laparoscopic Technique

There are many different patient positions for laparoscopic splenectomy described in the literature [20, 29–31]. We believe that the lateral approach is the position of choice for laparoscopic splenectomy [32] (Table 24.3).

Table 24.3. Endoscopic approaches in laparoscopic splenectomy

Approach	Advantages	Disadvantages
Anterior	No need for change of position if concomitant procedures are performed	Difficult to expose the dorsal spleen and vessels
	Early vascular control of the splenic artery is possible	Perisplenic adhesions may complicate the procedure
		More trocars needed
		More blood loss?
		Longer operation time
Lateral	Better exposure of the dorsal side of the spleen	Reposition of the patient required if concomitant procedures are performed
	Easier dissection of hilar structures	
	Less trocars needed	
	More suitable in splenomegaly	
	Less blood loss?	
	Shorter operation time	
	Less injuries to the tail of pancreas	

24.2.3.1
Anterior Approach

The anterior approach was the initial laparoscopic technique of choice used to operate on spleens. The exposure and dissection of the more hidden parts of the operative field like the posterior surface of the spleen makes this technique very difficult. This is exacerbated in obese patients where a significant amount of force is needed to overcome the resistance of the trocars to lateral movement in the thick abdominal wall in order to work in the subcostal region. This makes the fine motor control required for dissection arduous. Furthermore, the appropriate retraction of the spleen must be done against gravity, which leads to more capsular tears and increased blood loss as well transfusion rates [33]. This was shown in a study that compared the anterior approach with the lateral approach. Blood transfusion requirements were significantly lower (17%) in the lateral group than in the anterior group (60%) [34]. Advocates of this technique point out that the splenic artery can be approached along the superior border of the pancreas and, therefore, control of the splenic blood supply can be easily accomplished early in the case [15]. The true advantage of this procedure is the ability to perform concomitant procedures like cholecystectomy without the necessity of repositioning the patient. We believe that this approach should only be considered for normal-sized spleens and if additional procedures are planned.

24.2.3.2
Lateral Approach

After its initial description by Gagner and Park [35] this technique has gained almost universal acceptance due to its clear advantages when compared to an anterior approach. The larger the spleen the more obvious the advantage becomes because the spleen can act as an "additional assistant" while hanging in the abdominal cavity. Using the gravity, the dorsal side of the spleen can be easily exposed and the perisplenic ligaments can be dissected without difficulty. Another major concern during laparoscopic splenectomy is the possibility of injuries to the tail of the pancreas because of the close proximity to the hilar structures. Using the lateral approach, and with the spleen elevated, the surgeon has a clear view of the pancreas and can avoid injury to the tail of the pancreas more easily than with the anterior approach [32].

A surgeon can encounter difficulties with any laparoscopic technique. It is always difficult to visualize and access the superior pole attachments in large, barrel-chested males. The short gastric vessels can be problematic to isolate even if dissection and hemostasis is performed with an ultrasonic dissector.

In patients with a history of pancreatitis who have consequently obliterated the lesser sac, the dissection of the spleen can be extremely difficult.

We believe that the lateral approach to laparoscopic splenectomy permits superior exposure of the splenic hilar structures and facilitates the dissection. It is our procedure one of choice especially in cases of splenomegaly because of its clear advantages in this higher risk group. It should be pointed out that, in certain cases of enlarged spleens, modifying the position towards the almost supine, or slight left decubitus, may be advantageous, especially if the heavy and difficult to manipulate spleen obstructs the operative field while performing the medial and inferior dissection.

24.3
Summary

— The spleen should be measured and volume defined preoperatively by means of clinical examination in combination with ultrasound or CT as following:

≥500 g   Splenomegaly
≥1000 g, >17 cm   Massive splenomegaly
≥1500 g, >22 cm   "Giant spleen"

— We suggest that large spleens (≥500 g) should only be removed laparoscopically by experienced surgeons. For massive splenomegaly and giant spleens a hand-assisted approach should be considered to reduce morbidity and mortality.
— A definitive search for congenital or acquired residual splenic tissue should be performed to improve the detection rate and reduce the rate of splenosis following laparoscopic splenectomy:
  – Accessory spleens at the typical anatomic sites should be verified at the beginning of the operation
  – The presence of residual splenic tissue in the abdominal cavity should be verified at the end of the operation
— The spleen should always be removed using an impermeable extraction bag and intraperitoneal morcellation should be avoided to prevent splenosis.
— The lateral approach to the spleen should be considered as the technique of choice

References

1. Pace DE, Chiasson PM, Schlachta CM, Mamazza J, Poulin EC. Laparoscopic splenectomy for idiopathic thrombocytopenic purpura (ITP). Surg Endosc 2003;17:95–8.
2. Targarona EM, Balague C, Cerdan G, Espert JJ, Lacy AM, Visa J, et al. Hand-assisted laparoscopic splenectomy (HALS) in cases of splenomegaly: a comparison analysis with conventional laparoscopic splenectomy. Surg Endosc 2002;16:426–30.
3. Szold A, Kais H, Keidar A, Nadav L, Eldor A, Klausner JM. Chronic idiopathic thrombocytopenic purpura (ITP) is a surgical disease. Surg Endosc 2002;16:155–8.
4. Trias M, Targarona EM, Espert JJ, Cerdan G, Bombuy E, Vidal O, et al. Impact of hematological diagnosis on early and late outcome after laparoscopic splenectomy: an analysis of 111 cases. Surg Endosc 2000;14:556–60.
5. Delaitre B, Blezel E, Samama G, Barrat C, Gossot D, Bresler L, et al. Laparoscopic splenectomy for idiopathic thrombocytopenic purpura. Surg Laparosc Endosc Percutan Tech 2002;12:412–9.
6. Cogliandolo A, Berland-Dai B, Pidoto RR, Marc OS. Results of laparoscopic and open splenectomy for nontraumatic diseases. Surg Laparosc Endosc Percutan Tech 2001;11:256–61.
7. Gigot JF, Legrand M, Cadiere GB, Delvaux G, de Ville de Goyet J, de Neve de Roden A, et al.; Belgian Group for Endoscopic Surgery. Is laparoscopic splenectomy a justified approach in hematologic disorders? Preliminary results of a prospective multicenter study. Int Surg 1995;80:299–303.
8. Yu SC, Yuan RH. Laparoscopic splenectomy: preliminary experience. J Formos Med Assoc 1996;95:635–8.
9. Friedman RL, Fallas MJ, Carroll BJ, Hiatt JR, Phillips EH. Laparoscopic splenectomy for ITP. The gold standard. Surg Endosc 1996;10:991–5.
10. Katkhouda N, Hurwitz MB, Rivera RT, Chandra M, Waldrep DJ, Gugenheim J, et al. Laparoscopic splenectomy: outcome and efficacy in 103 consecutive patients. Ann Surg 1998;228:568–78.
11. Poulin EC, Thibault C, Mamazza J. Laparoscopic splenectomy. Surg Endosc 1995;9:172–6; discussion 176–7.
12. Decker G, Millat B, Guillon F, Atger J, Linon M. Laparoscopic splenectomy for benign and malignant hematologic diseases: 35 consecutive cases. World J Surg 1998;22:62–8.
13. Rege RV, Joehl RJ. A learning curve for laparoscopic splenectomy at an academic institution. J Surg Res 1999;81:27–32.
14. Park A, Marcaccio M, Sternbach M, Witzke D, Fitzgerald P. Laparoscopic vs open splenectomy. Arch Surg 1999;134:1263–9.
15. Park A, Targarona EM, Trias M. Laparoscopic surgery of the spleen: state of the art. Langenbecks Arch Surg 2001;386:230–9.
16. Danielson PD, Shaul DB, Phillips JD, Stein JE, Anderson KD. Technical advances in pediatric laparoscopy have had a beneficial impact on splenectomy. J Pediatr Surg 2000;35:1578–81.
17. Sandoval C, Stringel G, Ozkaynak MF, Tugal O, Jayabose S. Laparoscopic splenectomy in pediatric patients with hematologic diseases. JSLS 2000;4:117–20.
18. Kercher KW, Matthews BD, Walsh RM, Sing RF, Backus CL, Heniford BT. Laparoscopic splenectomy for massive splenomegaly. Am J Surg 2002;183:192–6.

19. Terrosu G, Baccarani U, Bresadola V, Sistu MA, Uzzau A, Bresadola F. The impact of splenic weight on laparoscopic splenectomy for splenomegaly. Surg Endosc 2002;16:103–7.
20. Patel AG, Parker JE, Wallwork B, Kau KB, Donaldson N, Rhodes MR, et al. Massive splenomegaly is associated with significant morbidity after laparoscopic splenectomy. Ann Surg 2003;238:235–40.
21. Torelli P, Cavaliere D, Casaccia M, Panaro F, Grondona P, Rossi E, et al. Laparoscopic splenectomy for hematological diseases. Surg Endosc 2002;16:965–71.
22. Emmermann A, Zornig C, Peiper M, Weh HJ, Broelsch CE. Laparoscopic splenectomy. Technique and results in a series of 27 cases. Surg Endosc 1995;9:924–7.
23. Poulin EC, Thibault C. The anatomical basis for laparoscopic splenectomy. Can J Surg 1993;36:484–8.
24. Gigot JF, Jamar F, Ferrant A, van Beers BE, Lengele B, Pauwels S, et al. Inadequate detection of accessory spleens and splenosis with laparoscopic splenectomy – a shortcoming of the laparoscopic approach in hematologic diseases. Surg Endosc 1998;12:101–6.
25. Targarona EM, Espert JJ, Lomena F, Trias M. Inadequate detection of accessory spleens and splenosis with laparoscopic splenectomy: a shortcoming of the laparoscopic approach in hematological diseases. Surg Endosc 1999;13:196––9.
26. Kumar RJ, Borzi PA. Splenosis in a port site after laparoscopic splenectomy. Surg Endosc 2001;15:413–4.
27. Varkarakis J, Neururer R, Steiner H, Bartsch G, Peschel R. Splenosis mimicking local recurrence after laparoscopic radical nephrectomy. Urology 2003;62:552.
28. Lee SW, Gleason NR, Bessler M, Whelan RL. Port site tumor recurrence rates in a murine model of laparoscopic splenectomy decreased with increased experience. Surg Endosc 2000;14:805–11.
29. Romano F, Caprotti R, Franciosi C, De Fina S, Colombo G, Uggeri F. Laparoscopic splenectomy using Ligasure. Preliminary experience. Surg Endosc 2002;16:1608–11.
30. Hellman P, Arvidsson D, Rastad J. HandPort-assisted laparoscopic splenectomy in massive splenomegaly. Surg Endosc 2000;14:1177–9.
31. Gossot D, Fritsch S, Celerier M. Laparoscopic splenectomy: optimal vascular control using the lateral approach and ultrasonic dissection. Surg Endosc 1999;13:21–5.
32. Park A, Gagner M, Pomp A. The lateral approach to laparoscopic splenectomy. Am J Surg 1997;173:126–30.
33. Tan M, Zheng CX, Wu ZM, Chen GT, Chen LH, Zhao ZX. Laparoscopic splenectomy: the latest technical evaluation. World J Gastroenterol 2003;9:1086–9.
34. Trias M, Targarona EM, Balague C. Laparoscopic splenectomy: an evolving technique – a comparison between anterior and lateral approaches. Surg Endosc Ultrasound Intervent Tech 1996;10:389–392.
35. Gagner MPA, Park A. The lateral approach to laparoscopic splenectomy. Surg Endosc 1994;8:443.
36. Mahon D, Rhodes M. Laparoscopic splenectomy: size matters. Ann R Coll Surg Engl 2003;85:248–51.
37. Ailawadi G, Yahanda A, Dimick JB, Bedi A, Mulholland MW, Colletti L, et al. Hand-assisted laparoscopic splenectomy in patients with splenomegaly or prior upper abdominal operation. Surgery 2002;132:689–94; discussion 694–6.

38. Nicholson IA, Falk GL, Mulligan SC. Laparoscopically assisted massive splenectomy. A preliminary report of the technique of early hilar devascularization. Surg Endosc 1998;12:73–5.
39. Targarona EM, Espert JJ, Balague C, Piulachs J, Artigas V, Trias M. Splenomegaly should not be considered a contraindication for laparoscopic splenectomy. Ann Surg 1998;228:35–9.
40. Borrazzo EC, Daly JM, Morrisey KP, Fischer E, Belmont M, Hogle NJ, et al. Hand-assisted laparoscopic splenectomy for giant spleens. Surg Endosc 2003;17:918–20.
41. Rosen M, Brody F, Walsh RM, Ponsky J. Hand-assisted laparoscopic splenectomy vs conventional laparoscopic splenectomy in cases of splenomegaly. Arch Surg 2002;137:1348–52.

Commentary 1

Seymour I. Schwartz

Splenectomy is indicated for a variety of hematologic disorders. Among the hemolytic anemias, hereditary spherocytosis constitutes the most frequent indication, and is associated with consistent cure of the associated anemia and jaundice. The spleen is usually moderately enlarged and cholelithiasis has been reported in 30 to 60% of cases but is rare in children. The operation should be delayed until the patient reaches the age of 4. Thalassemia, another hereditary anemia with marked splenomegaly, is an indication for splenectomly only if there is a significant transfusion requirement because the postoperative complication rate, particularly infection, is relatively high. Splenectomy can be effficacious in the management of pyruvate kinase (PK) deficiency but is not indicated for glucose-6-phosphate deficiency (G-6-PD).

In patients with idiopathic autoimmune hemolytic anemia, splenectomy is often effective when patients have failed steroid therapy. The patients have a positive Coombs' test and should demonstrate "warm" antibodies. The spleen is palpably enlarged in half the cases and concomitant gall stones have been demonstrated in a quarter of the cases.

ITP is the most common hematologic indication for splenectomy. It may be associated with HIV positivity or AIDS. Splenectomy is rarely required for children with acute onset of thromboctyopenia, and is indicated in adult patients who fail steroid therapy. The spleen is not enlarged. Preoperative platelet transfusions are not indicated. Permanent improvement of the platelet count occurs in about 80% of patients.

Secondary hypersplenism is not an indication for splenectomy in patients with cirrhosis and portal hypertension. In the past, splenectomy was carried out as part of the staging for Hodgkin's disease, but this is no longer done because the assessment of intra-abdominal pathology can be made by CT scan, and most patients are managed with a routine chemotherapeutic regimen. Some patients with chronic lymphocytic leukemia or non-Hodgkin's lymphoma will benefit from splenectomy, which is indicated to improve marked leukopenia in order to allow continuance of chemotherapy.

The largest spleens are encountered in patients with advanced myeloproliferative disorders. Splenectomy might be indicated in these patients with increasing transfusion requirements or symptomatic splenomegaly as manifestations. There is an occasionally associated portal hypertension and esophagogastric varices. Postoperative thrombocytosis and/or thrombosis of the splenic vein extending into the portal vein and superior mesenteric vein has been reported [1]. This can be obviated by preoperative administration of alkylating agents and antiplatelet aggregating drugs and heparinization. Other hematologic disorders that benefit from splenectomy include Felty's syndrome (rheumatoid arthritis, neutropenia, and splenomegaly), sarcoidosis, Gaucher's disease, and systemic mast cell disease. Rarely cysts, abscesses, or tumors, are indications for elective splenectomy.

In most instances, the laparoscopic approach is preferable and particularly in patients with ITP and normal-sized spleens. All patients should receive pneumovax and *Haemophilus influenza* vaccine preoperatively. In all instances, a thorough inspection of the peritoneal cavity should be considered to be an integral part of the procedure. Accessory spleens are reported to be present in 14 to 30% of patients with hematologic disorders [2]. In order of decreasing frequency, they are located in the splenic hilum, along the short gastric vessels, in the splenocolic ligament, greater omentum, presacral region, adnexal region, and mesentery of the small intestine.

In most instances of splenomegaly, laparoscopic removal is possible. The most difficult circumstance relates to patients with myeloproliferative disorders, because the splenomegaly is most marked, there is often a perisplenic peel precluding dissection, and there may be marked venous engorgement due to portal hypertension.

References

1.   Gordon DH, Schaffner D, Bennett JM, Schwartz SI. Postsplenectomy thrombocytosis: its association with mesenteric, portal, and/or renal thrombosis in patients with myeloproliferative disorders. Arch Surg 1978;113:713–5.
2.   Schwartz SI. Role of splenectomy in hematologic disorders. World J Surg 1996;20:1156–9.

Commentary 2

Eduardo M Targarona, Carmen Balagué, Manuel Trias

Laparoscopic splenectomy (LS) has become a definitive alternative to open surgery for removal of the non-enlarged spleen. This is particularly the case in ITP, the most frequent indication for splenectomy in a general hospital. Everyday practice has demonstrated the merits of LS, but the scientific and medical world requires definitive evidence of the advantages of a new procedure obtained through randomized trials, comparing it with open surgery. However, these studies probably never will be performed, as for other infrequently performed surgical procedures such as laparoscopic myotomy or adrenalectomy

The need for a definition and classification of the size of the spleen is obviously of paramount importance in laparoscopic surgery, since the procedure involves the manipulation of a bulky organ. One of the most striking discoveries during the evolution of endoscopic splenic surgery was that even large spleens could be mobilized and dissected inside the abdomen [1, 2]. However, the manipulation and extraction of the organ once it is completely free are cumbersome maneuvers. There are several ways to assess the size of the spleen preoperatively: physical explorative landmarks (spleen border reaching the midline or lower pole palpated in left fossa), measurement of main diameters or CT volume calculation; postoperatively the size may be estimated from the morcellated-specimen weight. This information is of particular importance in the clinical setting for defining the best strategy for operation (anterior, semilateral or lateral approach, pure laparoscopic or hand assisted), and from the academic point of view to allow adequate comparison of these parameters between series. However, there is no reason for rejecting the concepts established in the prelaparoscopic era, when splenomegaly was normally considered over 500 g, massive splenomegaly 1000–1500 g and giant splenomegaly above this figure. Further analysis should be conducted of new parameters (ratio weight or volume of the spleen/body weight), or prediction with three-dimension scans. Undoubtedly, clinical judgment and local factors (lax belly, body habitus, etc.) are helpful to design this operative strategy. There is no reason for rejecting the use of the weight of the morcellated spleen plus the aspirated pulp if this material has been carefully recovered. In the case of splenomegaly, the hand-assisted technique has made it possible to reduce operative time and morbidity, but it is an advanced procedure, which in our experience can be applied only to a very small number of patients (32/260, 12%, of our series); we consider that it should be used in the case of spleens over 700–1000 g and only by experienced surgeons. However, spleens of intermediate enlargement (500–1000 g) can easily be managed with a pure laparoscopic technique.

When treating benign autoimmune hematological diseases it is vital to ensure that all the functional tissue is completely removed. Tissue left in the abdomen may be secondary to missed accessory spleens (AS) or splenosis. Responsibility of accessory spleens for recurrence probably has been over-emphasized. Current data show that, after an intermediate follow-up (up to 5 years), the clinical response after LS for ITP is similar to open surgery, and there is no increase in the incidence of relapsing ITP secondary to missed accessory spleens. In our experience with a systematic follow-up (mean 35 months) of a series of 130 patients with autoimmune cytopenia (ITP, HIV-ITP and Evans syndrome), the overall success rate was 90%, with a partial remission of 10% [3].

Based on this experience, we do not think that there are definitive conceptual or technical reasons for holding that LS is less likely to visualize AS located in the left hypochondria than in the subcostal open approach. However, it is difficult to understand the variations in AS incidence reported by different authors. A number of small AS can be included during stapling of the splenic hilum. The key factor is the maintenance of an intact spleen capsule. Due to the increased technical difficulty of LS, a capsule may tear during the procedure and splenic tissue may spill, or the retrieval bag may break. A special issue is the risk of cell spilling due to the use of gas-powered devices for hemostasis of a capsule tear (argon beam); in animal experiments, spillage of cells has been observed [4].

In our view, the lateral position is clearly the best. There are no randomized trials comparing anterior and lateral position, but common sense supports the use of the lateral or semilateral position. The spleen is located deep in the left hypochondria and a key maneuver for splenectomy is the mobilization of the organ. The lateral or semi lateral position takes advantage of gravity and avoids spleen grasping and stretching. The full lateral approach with adequate fixation of the patient to the table allows exaggeration of the lateral tilt of the table and better access to the posterior or anterior face of the spleen. A minor drawback of this position is in the case of conversion or the need to change the position to supine in case of simultaneous operation (i.e., cholecystectomy), but the advantages far outweigh these disadvantages. Semilateral or anterior approach may be indicated in rare cases of large spleens in which the medial margin surpasses the midline. A further indication for the semilateral approach is in cases in which hand-assisted techniques are used.

Further technical controversies in laparoscopic splenic surgery in the future may be the feasibility of subtotal or partial splenectomy, the role of LS (if any) in splenic trauma, or the use of robot surgery. The impact of LS on surgical indication for ITP and lymphoma management also merits investigation.

References

1. Targarona EM, Balague C, Trias M. Laparoscopic splenectomy for splenomegaly. In: Katkhouda N, editor; Surgical diseases of the spleen. Problems in general surgery, vol. 19, Soper N, editor-in-chief. Philadelphia: Lippincott, Williams & Wilkins; 2002. pp. 95–101.
2. Targarona EM, Cerdán M, Trias M. Complications of laparoscopic splenectomy. In: Katkhouda N, ed. Surgical diseases of the spleen. Problems in general surgery, vol. 19, Soper N, editor-in-chief. Philadelphia; Lippincott, Williams & Wilkins; 2002., p. 65–72.
3. Balagué C, Targarona EM, Cerdán G, Novell J, Montero O, Bendahan G, et al. Long-term outcome after laparoscopic splenectomy related to hematological diagnosis. Surg Endosc 2004 (in press).
4. Bombuy E, Espert JJ, Targarona EM, Visa J, Trias M. Evaluation of the risk of splenosis during laparoscopic splenectomy in an experimental model in the rat. World J Surg 2001;25:882–5.

Adrenalectomy

AHMAD ASSALIA, MICHEL GAGNER

> ▶ **Key Controversies**
>
> A. Indications
>   - Maximal size of the gland amenable to Laparoscopic Adrenalectomy
>   - Laparoscopic adrenalectomy in malignant lesions
>   - Laparoscopic adrenalectomy in incidentalomas
> B. The choice of endoscopic technique

25.1
Introduction

Since its introduction in 1992 [1], laparoscopic adrenalectomy (LA) has been widely used in the surgical management of virtually all pathologies of the adrenal gland. Worldwide, using different endoscopic approaches, multiple reports demonstrated the well-known benefits of minimally invasive surgery [2–8]. However, beyond shorter recovery and improved cosmesis, attempts were also made to assess the morbidity and mortality of the technique, the clinical outcome of the hormonally active tumors and the long-term results in malignant tumors. Although no prospective randomized studies comparing open adrenalectomy with LA are available, it clearly appears from multiple retrospective analyses [4–10] that while there was no compromise in the functional outcome, LA was associated with less morbidity than open surgery, and it proved to be a cost-effective procedure as well. Even so, after a decade of experience, a few controversies still remain and are discussed below.

25.2
Discussion

25.2.1
Indications

25.2.1.1
The Maximal Size of the Gland Amenable to Laparoscopic Adrenalectomy

While very few surgeons have sporadically described successful LA in large adrenal masses up to 14–15 cm [3, 11, 12], most regarded the maximal size to be laparoscopically resected in the range of 10–12 cm [13–19], because of the technical difficulties and malignant potential associated with these large tumors [18, 20, 21]. Even in the absence of invasion into adjacent structures, such masses make the dissection difficult and are time consuming. The exposure is also problematic because of the limited space available in this area. In addition, these large masses frequently have unusual and numerous retroperitoneal feeding vessels that require tedious dissection and control. It seems that hitherto there is no consensus as to the maximal cutoff in size that makes the mass amenable to LA. Accordingly, the applicability of LA in large masses is dictated mainly by the experience of the individual surgeon. Nevertheless, it appears prudent to advocate that only experienced laparoscopic surgeons should attempt laparoscopic resection of large masses, and for the average hands, laparoscopy is not advisable for lesions greater than 10–12 cm.

25.2.1.2
Role of Laparoscopic Adrenalectomy in Malignant Lesions

The concern that laparoscopy may result in inadequate removal of malignant adrenal tumors, increasing the risk of local and port site recurrences, together with several anecdotal reports describing regional, peritoneal and distant recurrences [22–24], led to the reluctance of many surgeons to adopt laparoscopic surgery in such cases. Taking into consideration the small studies available and the relatively short term follow up, the accumulated data (Table 25.1) shows favorable results that should, however, be interpreted with caution [20, 21, 25–30]. LA proved to be technically feasible, was safe and achieved results comparable with those of LA for benign and small lesions. In addition, tumor-free margins were achieved in all patients, no port-site metastases were reported, and the rate of locoregional recurrence was surprisingly low (3 of 29 cases of primary adrenal cancer – 10.3%). Adrenocortical cancer is a virulent tumor, and even after complete tumor resections recurrences still occur in at least two-thirds of patients [31]. Therefore, it appears that these short-term results are comparable with those of conventional surgery. Laparoscopy offers advantages to the surgeon, in terms of clarity of magnified view and exposure. Consequently, it might be possible that these features of laparoscopy enable this demanding surgery to be carried out with greater precision.

Several authors differentiate between the biologic behavior of adrenal metastasis and primary adrenal cancer as to their suitability for the laparoscopic procedure [30, 32]. Because solitary adrenal metastasis from an extra-adrenal primary is usually small and confined within the adrenal, the laparoscopic approach has considerable appeal for this specific indication [32]. By contrast, adrenal cancer is usually larger and often locally invasive. Since no reliable and accurate preoperative diagnostic test to diagnose adrenal malignancy exists, including fine-needle aspiration [30, 33], it is difficult to determine when an open approach should be used. An initial laparoscopic approach can be used to establish the diagnosis with low morbidity and allows curative resection in many instances [29, 30].

Laparoscopic ultrasound is a simple and effective intraoperative technical adjunct that may be used to evaluate the nature and invasiveness of the suspected adrenal mass. Obviously, in patients who prove to have local invasion during surgery, the laparoscopic approach should be converted to open procedure in order to allow curative wide radical resection. Thus, it appears that a laparoscopic approach is reasonable for metastatic adrenal disease, provided the primary cancer is controlled and there is no evidence of extra-adrenal disease. Similarly, for primary neoplasms, if complete resection is technically feasible, and there is no evidence of local invasion, an initial laparoscopic approach is an acceptable option in experienced hands at selected specialized centers [28, 30, 32].

25.2.1.3
Role of Laparoscopic Adrenalectomy in Incidentalomas

Accepted indications for adrenalectomy included non-functioning lesions larger than 5 cm, hormonally active lesions, and suspicious masses characteristics based on imaging studies and documented increase in size. Traditional teaching usually advocates that a new surgical technique is not supposed to change the indications for the surgical intervention in certain pathology, and some authors even warned that the benefits of the laparoscopic approach should not result in a more liberal policy for excision of clinically silent, benign-appearing adrenal masses [34]. In fact, it appears that after the advent of LA more incidentalomas are being operated upon laparoscopically [17].

Table 25.1. Laparoscopic adrenalectomy in large and malignant tumors. *LTA* lateral trans-abdominal approach, *REA* retroperitoneal endoscopic adrenalectomy approach, *LOS* length of hospital stay, *NR* not recorded.

Study [ref.]	No. of patients/ approach	Malignancy (primary)	Tumor size (range, cm)	Follow-up (months)	Conversion (%)	Operative time (min)	Blood loss (ml)	LOS (day)	Compli- cations (%)	Recurrence
MacGillivray et al. [25]	12 / LTA	3 (2)	8.2 (6–12)	24.5	0	190	100	2	42	1 Systemic metastasis from primary extra-adre nal tumor
Hobart et al. [26]	14 / LTA, REA	8 (7)	8 (NR)	9.9	14.3	205	400	2.4	21.4	0
Propiglia et al. [27]	8 / LTA	8 (4)	NR (5–11)	19	12.5	NR	NR	NR	NR	1 Primary breast cancer
Henry et al. [28]	19 / LTA	6 (6)	7 (6–9)	47	10.5	NR	NR	NR	0	1 Liver metastasis from pri mary adre nal tumor

Table 25.1. *Cotinued*

Study [ref.]	No. of patients/ approach	Malignancy/ (primary)	Tumor size (range, cm)	Follow-up (months)	Conversion (%)	Operative time (min)	Blood loss (ml)	LOS (day)	Compli-cations (%)	Recurrence
Henry et al. [20]	47 / LTA	6 (3)	5.2 (4–12)	24	6.2	129	129	5.1	8.3	0
Valeri et al. [29]	6 / LTA	6 (0)	NR (2.5–6)	19	0	160	260	4	0	3 Systemic metastasis from primary extra-adrenal tumor
Heniford et al. [21]	11 / LTA, REA	12 (1)	5.9 (1.8–12)	8.3	9	181	138	2.3	9	1 Brain metastasis from melanoma
Kebebew et al. [30]	23 / LTA, REA	21 (6)	5.1 (1.5–12)	40	4.3	166	NR	275	12.5	3 Locoregional, 4 systemic metastasis from primary extra-adrenal tumor
Total/Mean	141	70 (29)	6.5 (1.5–12)	24	6.3	171	192	3.1	11.7	

Although, adrenocortical carcinomas are usually seen in masses larger than 6 cm, reports are available of incidentally detected cancer in masses 3–5 cm and even smaller [32, 35]. Another confounding factor is the fact that computed tomography may be associated with approximately 16–40% under-estimation of adrenal tumor size compared with actual size on histopathology [16, 36]. Moreover, needle biopsy is not accurate and can be dangerous (tumor spillage, hemorrhage and pheochromocytoma crisis) [33]. In the light of these facts and the remarkable results of the laparoscopic technique, we and others [32, 33] contend that laparoscopic adrenalectomy is the preferred management for the young and low operative risk patients, with 3- to 5-cm adrenal masses. For older patients with significant comorbidities a threshold of 5 cm was suggested [33]. Another argument against the watchful conservative policy in such cases is the observation that most adrenal nodules increase in size with age [32] and the annual need for imaging and biochemical testing throughout their life. Moreover, the patient will be spared the anxiety, expense and time lost from repeated follow-up appointments and the associated studies needed.

25.2.2
The Choice of Endoscopic Technique

25.2.2.1
Lateral Transabdominal (LTA) Approach

Originally described in 1992 [1, 37], this is the approach of choice practiced by most surgeons [3, 6, 8, 11, 16, 18, 19, 38–40]. Placing of the patient in lateral decubitus position uses gravity to help retract surrounding organs and expose the adrenal glands, resulting in reduced dissection and minimal retraction of adjacent structures.

25.2.2.2
Anterior Transabdominal (ATA) Approach

Very few surgeons have reported LA using this approach [14, 23, 41, 42]. Because more dissection is usually required, it has been claimed to be more demanding and a lengthy procedure [41, 43]. While longer operative time [41, 42], more blood loss, and a trend for slower recovery [42] were cited for this approach compared with the LTA, others [14, 44] found no significant difference.

25.2.2.3
Retroperitoneal Endoscopic Adrenalectomy (REA)

Since the first description of successful REA appeared in 1995 [45], several laparoscopic surgeons [46–50] have advocated this approach. The results of large published series [42, 46–53] indicated that the results with small lesions achieved with this approach are comparable with those of the LTA. The maximal size of resected lesions reported by most authors was 6.5–8 cm.

Proponents of REA claim that a clear advantage of this approach is the avoidance of the peritoneal cavity in patients with previous upper abdominal surgery [47]. However, it should be noticed that the presence of adhesions has been rarely implicated as a reason for conversion to open surgery [3]. Additional non-substantiated claimed advantages include easier dissection in obese patients, especially in the left side, the lack of need for retraction of enlarged liver, the special usefulness of this approach in pregnant women, and the lack of necessity to change the patient position for bilateral exploration [47]. The true drawbacks are the restricted working space available, limiting the usefulness of this approach to tumors not larger than 6 cm, and the inability to explore the abdominal cavity and perform concurrent abdominal procedures. On the other hand, a clear advantage of the transperitoneal approach is that the abdominal cavity, and particularly the liver, can be explored. In addition, opponents of REA, suppose that there are some inherent disadvantages of the retroperitoneal approach which include a lack of familiar anatomic landmarks to most abdominal surgeons and the restricted space available for the conduct of safe dissection in difficult cases. The limited maneuvering ability in this approach, may pose a problem should a vascular injury occur, and conversion to open surgery is more complex than in the transperitoneal approach. However, no reports citing more bleeding problems and conversions do exist and according to Bonjer, turning and re-draping the patients did not require more than 10 min, and conversions could be done either to laparotomy, lumbotomy or thoracolumbotomy [47]. Moreover, the notion that the retroperitoneal space provides fewer anatomical landmarks was disputed by some authors [47, 48], who claim that the lateroconal fascia, the quadratus lumborum muscle and the kidney may provide sufficient guidance to find the adrenal gland. It appears that unlike urologists, who have a preference for the retroperitoneal route because they are more familiar with it [42, 48], most general surgeons prefer the transperitoneal approach. Another concern raised was the occurrence of peritoneal tears, which was reported in up to 30–50% in two series [47, 54]. Although these tears may lead to loss of working space and even conversions [54], others advocated the use of an additional instrument to provide retraction of the peritoneal sac, maintain the working space and thereby obviate conversions [47].

It has been postulated that by avoiding the pneumoperitoneum, this approach might be associated with decreased physiologic impact on the cardiovascular and respiratory systems. This, however, was not supported in two reports specifically addressing this issue [46, 53]. The etiology behind the similar gas absorption during the retroperitoneal route was not elucidated. Perhaps the peritoneal violation, frequently unnoticed, could account for these results [46]. Nevertheless, the available evidence has revealed no apparent difference in patient outcome, morbidity or operative time for the retroperitoneal and transperitoneal approaches [46, 48, 49, 54].

25.2.2.4
Approach in Bilateral Laparoscopic Adrenalectomy

The theoretical advantages of ATA and REA in this setting, where it's unnecessary to change the position of patients, were not substantiated. Using LTA, the 15- to 20-min turnover time usually necessary is offset by easier dissection and better exposure [3]. Therefore, similar to unilateral laparoscopic adrenalectomy, most surgeons prefer this approach for the same reasons [3, 48]. At the present time, no significant differences between different surgical approaches in the setting of bilateral LA are reported [48, 53, 55].

25.3
Summary

— The accumulated evidence indicates that for the average surgeon, LA is not advisable for lesions larger than 10–12 cm.
— The experience with LA in large and malignant tumors is limited and the short-term results are promising, but its role still awaits further definition. At present, an initial laparoscopic approach is acceptable in specialized centers for selected adrenal metastasis and noninvasive primary adrenal cancer.
— In experienced hands and low-risk patients, advocating LA for incidentalomas larger than 3 cm seems to be reasonable.
— Although the lateral transabdominal technique is the preferred and the most practiced, each endoscopic approach has its advantages and drawbacks, and the laparoscopic surgeon should choose the approach he or she are best familiar with, and which is most appropriate for the specific patient and pathology (Table 25.2).

Table 25.2. Endoscopic approaches in laparoscopic adrenalectomy

Approach	Advantages	Disadvantages
Lateral trans-abdominal	Less dissection and better exposure	Change of position in bilateral adrenalectomy
	Appropriate for large tumors	Certain difficulty in cases of peritoneal adhesions
	Other intra-abdominal pathologies may be diagnosed and treated	
	The most practiced approach	
Anterior trans-abdominal	No need for changing position in bilateral adrenalectomy	More dissection is needed and more difficult exposure
	Appropriate for large tumors	Longer operative time?
	Other intra-abdominal pathologies may be diagnosed and treated	More blood loss?
	The least practiced approach	
Retroperitoneal endoscopic adrenalectomy	No need for changing position in bilateral adrenalectomy (with jack-knife position)	The least practiced approach
		Small operative field. Appropriate only for small tumors (<5–6 cm)
	Potential advantage in previous upper abdominal surgery, obese and pregnant patients	Inability to diagnose and treat concurrent intra-abdominal pathology
		Lack of familiar anatomical landmarks to the average abdominal surgeon

References

1. Gagner M, Lacroix A, Bolte E. Laparoscopic adrenalectomy in Cushing's syndrome and pheochromocytoma. N Engl J Med 1992;327:1003.
2. Gagner M, Lacroix A, Prinz RA, et al. Early experience with laparoscopic approach for adrenalectomy. Surgery 1993;114:1120–5.
3. Gagner M, Pomp A, Heniford BT, et al. Laparoscopic adrenalectomy. Lessons learned from 100 consecutive procedures. Ann Surg 1997;226:238–47.
4. Prinz RA. A comparison of laparoscopic and open adrenalectomies. Arch Surg 1995;130:489–94.
5. Brunt LM, Doherty GM, Norton JA, et al. Laparoscopic adrenalectomy compared to open adrenalectomy for benign adrenal neoplasms. J Am Coll Surg 1996;183:1–10.
6. Thompson GB, Grant CS, van Heerden JA, et al. Laparoscopic versus open posterior adrenalectomy: a case- control study of 100 patients. Surgery 1997;122:1132–36.
7. Dudley NE, Harrison BJ. Comparison of open posterior versus transperitoneal laparo-scopic adrenalectomy. Br J Surg 1999;86:656–60.
8. Imai T, Kikumori T, Ohiwa M. A case-controlled study of laparoscopic compared with open lateral adrenalectomy. Am J Surg 1999;178:50–54.
9. Jacobs JK, Goldstein RE, Geer RJ. Laparoscopic adrenalectomy: a new standard of care. Ann Surg 1997;225:495–502.
10. MacGillivray DC, Shichman SJ, Ferrer FA, et al. A comparison of open Vs laparoscopic adrenalectomy. Surg Endosc 1996;10:987–990.
11. Schichman SJ, Sosa RE, Whalen GF, et al. Lateral transperitoneal laparoscopic adrenal-ectomy. World J Urol 1999;17:48–53.
12. Kebebew E, Siperstein AE, Duh QY. Laparoscopic adrenalectomy: the optimal surgical approach. J Laparoendosc Adv Surg Tech 2001;11:409–13.
13. de Canniere L, Michel L, Hamoir E, et al. Multicentric experience of the Belgian group for endoscopic surgery (BGES) with endoscopic adrenalectomy. Surg Endosc 1997;11:1065–1067.
14. Filipponi S, Guerrieri M, Arnaldi G, et al. Laparoscopic adrenalectomy: a report on 50 operations. Eur J Endocrinol 1998;138:548–553.
15. Lezoche E, Guerrieri M, Paganini AM, et al. Laparoscopic adrenalectomy by the anterior transperitoneal approach. Results of 108 operations in unselected cases. Surg Endosc 2000;14:920–5.
16. Pillinger SH, Bambach, Sidhu S. Laparoscopic adrenalectomy: a 6-year experience of 59 cases. Aust N Z J Surg 2002;72:467–70.
17. Miccoli P, Raffaelli M, Berti P, et al. Adrenal surgery before and after the introduction of laparoscopic adrenalectomy. Br J Surg 2002;89:779–82.
18. MacGillivray DC, Whalen GF, Malchoff CD, et al. Laparoscopic resection of large adre-nal tumors. Ann Surg Oncol 2002;9:480–5.
19. Propiglia F, Garrone C, Giraud G, et al. Transperitoneal laparoscopic adrenalectomy: experience with 72 procedures. J Endourol 2002;15:275–9.
20. Henry JF, Defechereux T, Gramatica L, et al. Should laparoscopic approach be pro-posed for large and/or potentially malignant adrenal tumors? Langenbecks Arch Surg 1999;384:366–9.

21. Heniford BT, Arca MJ, Walsh RM, et al. Laparoscopic adrenalectomy for cancer. Semin Surg Oncol 1999;16:293–306.
22. Suzuki K, Ushiyama T, Mugiya S, et al. Hazards of laparoscopic adrenalectomy in patients with adrenal malignancy. J Urol 1997;158:2227.
23. Deckers S, Derdelinclx L, Col V, et al. Peritoneal carcinomatosis following laparoscopic resection of an adrenocortical tumor causing primary hyperaldosteronism. Horm Res 1999;52:97–100.
24. Foxius A, Ramboux A, Lefebvre Y, et al. Hazards of laparoscopic adrenalectomy for Conn's adenoma: when enthusiasm turn to tragedy. Surg Endosc 1999;13:715–7.
25. MacGillivray DC, Whalen GF, Malchoff CD, et al. Laparoscopic resection of large adrenal tumors. Ann Surg Oncol 2002;9:480–5.
26. Hobart MG, Gill IS, Schweizer D, et al. Laparoscopic adrenalectomy for large volume (>5 cm) adrenal masses. J Endourol 2000;14:149–54.
27. Propiglia F, Destefanis P, Fiori C, et al. Does adrenal mass size really affect safety and effectiveness of laparoscopic adrenalectomy? Urology 2002;60:801–5.
28. Henry JF, Sebag F, Iacobone M, et al. Results of laparoscopic adrenalectomy for large and potentially malignant tumors. World J Surg 2002;26:1043–7.
29. Valeri A, Borrelli A, Presenti L, et al. Adrenal masses in neoplastic patients. A role of laparoscopic procedure. Surg Endosc 2001;15:90–3.
30. Kebebew E, Siperstein AE, Clark OH, et al. Results of laparoscopic adrenalectomy for suspected and unsuspected malignant adrenal neoplasms. Arch Surg 2002;137:948–953.
31. Vassilopoulou-Sellin R, Schultz PN. Adrenocortical carcinoma: clinical outcome at the end of the 20th century. Cancer 2001;92:1113–21.
32. Gill IS. The case for laparoscopic adrenalectomy. J Urol 2001;166:429–36.
33. Duh QY. Adrenal incidentalomas. Br J Surg 2002;89:1347–9.
34. Brunt LM, Moley JF. Adrenal incidentaloma. World J Surg 2001;25:905–13.
35. Miccoli P, Raffaelli M, Berti P, et al. Adrenal surgery before and after the introduction of laparoscopic adrenalectomy. Br J Surg 2002;89:779–82.
36. Lau H, Lo CY, Lam KY. Surgical implications of underestimation of adrenal tumor size by computed tomography. Br J Surg 2002;86:385–7.
37. Gagner M, Lacroix A, Bolte E, et al. Laparoscopic adrenalectomy. The importance of a flank approach in the lateral decubitus position. Surg Endosc 1994;8:135–8.
38. Guazzoni G, Cestari A, Montorsi F, et al. Eight-year experience with transperitoneal laparoscopic adrenal surgery. J Urol 2001, 166:820–4.
39. Henry JF, Defechereux T, Raffaelli M, et al. Complications of laparoscopic adrenalectomy: results of 169 consecutive procedures. World J Surg 2000, 24:1342–6.
40. Brunt LM, Moley JF, Doherty GM, et al. Outcome analysis in patients undergoing laparoscopic adrenalectomy for hormonally active tumors. Surgery 2001;130:629–34.
41. Terachi T, Matsuda T, Terai A, et al. Transperitoneal laparoscopic adrenalectomy: experience in 100 cases. J Endourol 1997;11:361–5.
42. Suzuki K, Kageyama S, Hirano Y, et al. Comparison of 3 surgical approaches to laparoscopic adrenalectomy: a non-randomized, background matched analysis. J Urol 2001;166:437–43.
43. Marescaux J, Mutter D, Forbes L, et al. Bilateral laparoscopic adrenalectomy. In: Gagner M, Inabnet B, editors. Minimally invasive endocrine surgery. Philadelphia: Lippincott Williams &Wilkins; 2002. p. 205–16.

44. Lezoche E, Guerrieri M, Felicioti F, et al. Anterior, lateral and posterior approaches in endoscopic adrenalectomy. Surg Endosc 2002, 16:96–9.
45. Mercan S, Seven R, Ozarmagan S, et al. Endoscopic retroperitoneal adrenalectomy. Surgery 1995;118:1071–6.
46. Fernandez-Cruz L, Saenz A, Taura P, et al. Retroperitoneal approach in laparoscopic adrenalectomy: is it advantageous? Surg Endosc 1999;13:86–90.
47. Bonjer HJ, Sorm V, Berends FJ, et al. Endoscopic retroperitoneal adrenalectomy: lessons learned from 111 consecutive cases. Ann Surg 2000;232:796–803.
48. Salomon L, Soulie M, Mouly F, et al. Experience with retroperitoneal laparoscopic adrenalectomy in 115 procedures. J Urol 2001;166:38–41.
49. Siperstein AE, Berber E, Engle KL, et al. Laparoscopic posterior adrenalectomy. Technical considerations. Arch Surg 2000;135:967–71.
50. Walz MK, Pietgen K, Hoermann R, et al. Posterior retroperitoneoscopy as a new minimally invasive approach for adrenalectomy: results of 30 adrenalectomies in 27 patients. World J Surg 1996;20:769–74.
51. Naya Y, Nagata M, Ichikawa T, et al. Laparoscopic adrenalectomy: comparison of transperitoneal and retroperitoneal approaches. BJU Int 2002;90:199–204.
52. Terachi T, Yoshida O, Matsuda T, et al. Complications of laparoscopic and retroperitoneoscopic adrenalectomies in 370 cases in Japan: a multi-institutional study. Biomed Pharmacother 2000;54 Suppl 1:211–4.
53. Fernandez-Cruz L, Saenz A, Benarroch G, et al. Laparoscopic unilateral and bilateral adrenalectomy for Cushing's syndrome. Ann Surg 1996;224:727–36.
54. Takeda M. Laparoscopic adrenalectomy: transperitoneral vs retroperitoneal approaches. Biomed Pharmacother 2000, 54 Suppl 1:207–10.
55. Hsu TH, Gill IS. Bilateral laparoscopic adrenalectomy: retroperitoneal and transperitoneal approaches. Urology 2002;59:184–9.

Commentary

QUAN-YANG DUH

In this chapter Drs. Assalia and Gagner summarized the current consensus and controversies in laparoscopic adrenalectomy using evidence from the published literature. It is a comprehensive review and a well-balanced presentation of areas of active discussion by adrenal surgeons. I agree with the authors' summary and interpretation of the controversies. In this Commentary I will attempt to complement this well written chapter by elaborating on some of the points made by the authors.

There is more consensus than controversy regarding laparoscopic adrenalectomy. Over the past 10 years laparoscopic adrenalectomy has replaced open adrenalectomy for routine treatment of most surgical adrenal diseases. This situation is similar to that for laparoscopic cholecystectomy and it is in contrast to that for laparoscopic hernia repair or laparoscopic colectomy. In addition, these areas of controversies will not likely to be resolved by prospective randomized studies, because adrenal tumors, especially large and malignant ones, are rare, and the choice of surgical technique is usually personal.

Indications

Size

Large adrenal tumors pose two different problems for laparoscopic adrenalectomy. The first is technical. Large tumors are more difficult to manipulate and the surface area increases as the square of the tumor diameter making dissection more time consuming. For example, the surface area of an 8-cm tumor is four times that of a 4-cm tumor, and a 12-cm tumor nine times. Second, the larger the tumor the more likely it is malignant (see Section 25.4.1.2). Thus, for both technical and oncological reasons, laparoscopic adrenalectomy for large tumors can be difficult and is controversial. Laparoscopic adrenalectomy for large adrenal tumors is relatively uncommon. In the University of California, San Francisco experience of 250 consecutive laparoscopic adrenalectomies, most (55%) were performed for tumors between 2 to 6 cm in diameter, 30% were for tumors smaller than 2 cm, and only 15% were for tumors larger than 6 cm. Tumors larger than 6 cm required longer operating time and were more likely to require conversion to open operation.

Hand-assisted laparoscopic adrenalectomy is an option for resecting large adrenal tumors. We have converted three laparoscopic adrenalectomies to hand-assisted operation electively when the dissection was difficult and progress was slow. The recovery time for patients after a hand-assisted laparoscopic adrenalectomy is about half of that after an open adrenalectomy, but twice as long as that after a laparoscopic adrenalectomy.

Malignancy

Laparoscopic resection for cancers is relatively controversial. Preliminary results for laparoscopic resection for colon cancer and renal cell carcinoma are encouraging and support their use. For laparoscopic adrenalectomy for cancer, it is useful to distinguish between adrenal metastases and primary adrenal cortical cancer [1].

Laparoscopic resection for adrenal metastases appears to be relatively safe. It is rare to have positive margins or develop local or port site recurrences, when experienced surgeons perform the operation. The controversy is whether resecting solitary metastasis to the adrenal gland benefits these patients, and how to select the appropriate patients for resection. For melanoma and renal cell carcinoma, metastasectomy is indicated, even when metastases are present elsewhere. For other types of cancers, however, many patients will develop systemic metastasis after resection of an apparently solitary adrenal metastasis. In general, patients with synchronous adrenal metastasis (presenting within 6 months of index cancer) are more likely to develop systemic metastases subsequently than those with metachronous adrenal metastasis. Resection of bilateral adrenal metastases is rarely indicated.

In contrast to metastasis, adrenal cortical cancer presents several problems for laparoscopic adrenalectomy. Adrenal cortical cancer is aggressive and it frequently recurs locally and systemically after resection. A technically well-performed resection may not prevent local or systemic recurrence, but a technically poorly performed operation (fracturing the tumor or breaching the capsule) surely increases the risk of local recurrence. The presentation of adrenal cortical cancer varies; some are obviously malignant, but others are not. Whether a particular tumor is likely to be malignant depends on factors such as size, appearance on imaging studies, secretary profile, etc. Adrenal tumors that are obviously primary adrenal cortical cancers are usually technically difficult to resect laparoscopically because they are usually very large and may be locally invasive and frequently require resecting neighboring organs or lymph nodes. On the other hand, small well-circumscribed tumors, which are unlikely to be cortical cancers, are also technically easier to resect laparoscopically. My opinion is that laparoscopic adrenalectomy is acceptable for the latter if, in the surgeon's judgment, the extent of resection would be no different than if it were performed by an open adrenalectomy.

Incidentalomas

There are several controversies regarding adrenal incidentalomas. A recent National Institutes of Health (NIH) consensus conference was devoted to this topic [2]. The controversial issues include: which diagnostic tests are indicated, when adrenalectomy should be recommended, what type of operation if indicated, and if not operated, what kind of follow-up is required. The consensus statement can be summarized briefly, as "we are not sure, more data are needed". For those that are not hormone secreting, or obviously cancerous by imaging study, the NIH consensus recommended using 4–6 cm as the threshold for resection. Because imaging studies tend to underestimate tumor size compared to surgical specimens, we agree with Assalia and Gagner, and use 3-5 cm as the threshold for resection. We recommend resection for all hormonally active tumors, including those causing only subclinical Cushing syndrome, and all those with imaging characteristics of malignancy [3]. For older patients with comorbidities and shorter life expectancy we use 5 cm, whereas for younger healthy patients we use 3 cm as the threshold to recommend resection.

Techniques – Lateral Transabdominal versus Others

In general, the best laparoscopic adrenalectomy technique is the one the surgeon is most experienced with. Various surgeons have developed or learned different techniques, and have achieved similarly excellent results [4]. Although some surgeons voice strong preferences, the reasons are usually personal preferences. I personally prefer the lateral transabdominal technique, having tried several of the technique described. The lateral transabdominal technique is the most versatile and easiest to teach to general surgery residents and laparoscopic fellows, especially if they also perform laparoscopic splenectomy and colectomy.

Conclusion

Laparoscopic adrenalectomy is the current standard for routine adrenalectomy. Larger tumors are technically difficult to resect and adrenal cortical cancers are likely to recur locally, laparoscopic adrenalectomy for these tumors requires significant experience and surgical judgment. The most versatile technique is the lateral transabdominal technique, but surgeon preference and experience usually dictate the technique used. Laparoscopic resection is an excellent option for resecting adrenal incidentalomas when indicated.

References

1. Kebebew E, Siperstein AE, Clark OH, Duh QY. Results of laparoscopic adrenalectomy for suspected and unsuspected malignant adrenal neoplasms. Arch Surg 2002;137:948–51.
2. Management of the Clinically Inapparent Adrenal Mass (Incidentaloma). National Institutes of Health State-of-the-Science Statement. Draft statement of 4–6 February, 2002 http://consensus.nih.gov/ta/021/021_statement.htm
3. Duh QY. Adrenal incidentalomas. Br J Surg. 2002;89:1347–9
4. Van Heerden, J, Farley D (editors); Duh QY (guest editor). Operative techniques in general surgery. Adrenal surgery, vol. 4, no. 4. Philadelphia: W.B. Saunders; 2002. p. 277–352

26

Donor Nephrectomy

Molly Buzdon, Eugene Cho

▶ **Key Controversies**

A. Indications
  - Should the operation be done?
  - Who should do it?
  - Does the operation increase the volunteer donor pool?
B. Technique
  - Transperitoneal versus retroperitoneal
  - Hand-assisted versus "pure" laparoscopic
  - Right versus left sided donor nephrectomy
  - Is it worth the increased demands on the implant surgeon?

26.1
Introduction

Living donor nephrectomy is the only way to make up for the ever-increasing shortfall of organs for patients with end-stage renal failure and is associated with superior function and longer median survival compared to cadaveric grafts [1]. Unfortunately, the "open" nephrectomy for volunteer renal allograft procurement can be associated with significant morbidity as it usually involves a muscle-dividing flank incision and often removal of a rib [2, 3]. Laparoscopic nephrectomy was first reported in 1991 by Clayman et al. [4], and applied to donor nephrectomy by Ratner et al. in 1995 [5].

26.2
Discussion

26.2.1
Indications

26.2.1.1
Should the Operation Be Done?

Laparoscopic donor nephrectomy itself remains a matter of controversy. In its nascency, presentations of the techniques and results at national scientific meetings were even met with loud catcalls, boos and hisses, so vehement were the concerns of some that the new procedure was no more than a dangerous stunt and a reckless marketing ploy. The fact that the two largest early series were from competing institutions in the same city understandably gave rise to considerable initial skepticism, but the results and conclusions from those early series [6, 7] have since been repeatedly corroborated by other institutions [8–15], including a landmark prospective randomized study from Wolf, Merion and colleagues in 2001 [16], substantiating quicker recovery for donors and equivalent graft function for recipients (Table 26.1). As a result, laparoscopic donor nephrectomy has achieved tentative acceptance as an alternative to open procurement, but remains far from the procedure of choice [17–21]. It is still among the most difficult of laparoscopic procedures and even in the most experienced hands, disaster can occur with alarming rapidity and catastrophic consequences.

Some critics point out that in selected donors (e.g., thin and with no co-morbid conditions), open nephrectomy can be performed through a small, muscle-splitting incision without removal of a rib, and with a hospital stay of 2 days. While the use of volunteer donors who do have co-morbid conditions or who are obese is a controversy in and of itself; if one believes that such persons should be allowed to become donors in the first place, then these are the patients who might benefit most from a minimally invasive approach [22, 23].

Early studies reported both delayed normalization of recipient creatinine levels and significant rates of ureteral complications, and delayed graft function [7, 24, 25], but those same series after technical modifications [26, 27] to minimize trauma to the artery and maximize preservation of ureteral blood supply agree with later series, which are free of these complications and whose authors attribute this freedom to those same technical modifications [25, 28].

Warm ischemia times (defined in our series as the time during which the renal artery is clamped and the kidney has yet to be immersed in cold preservative, NOT to clear effluent of solution from the vein) are not recorded for most open donor nephrectomy series, but during laparoscopic procurement they are certainly longer. Based on data from our series we were unable to find any correlation of warm ischemia times in the range from 40 s to 11 min with recipient creatinine levels [29]. While it is doubtful that warm ischemia time does the graft any good, our data suggest that a longer period of such time would be needed to see a difference in graft function. Others have reported diminished graft function after 10 min of warm ischemia [30] but they imply that significant extraction trauma may have occurred to these kidneys as well. Because the definition varies by institution, meta-analysis becomes problematic.

Laparoscopic insufflation places the kidney in the unnatural environment of positive pressure pneumoperitoneum and concern has been raised regarding damage (possibly ischemic) to the kidney during this time. While decreased urine output during laparoscopy is a well-described observation, no evidence yet exists to suggest that any long-term damage occurs to either donor or recipient kidney function as a result, while at least one well-designed study shows no ill effects at 1 week [31]. Long-term recipient follow-up is needed.

The laparoscopic operation in most centers takes longer and requires expensive specialized equipment. While cost analysis has been attempted, the economic advantage to the donor who returns to work more quickly is extremely difficult to quantify [14, 32, 33]. The earlier return to productive employment may offset the higher cost of the operation in terms of the overall cost to society, but even after the learning curve has optimized operating time, there is no question the laparoscopic operation is more expensive because of the specialized equipment necessary.

26.2.1.2
Who Should Do It?

The application of hand-assisted laparoscopy has dramatically reduced the learning curve for those less familiar with two-handed laparoscopic dissection [34]. With hand-assist technology, there is no reason why any experienced open donor surgeon should not be able to master the procedure, as long as conversion to open surgery is expediently performed in case of trouble. Hand-assist techniques offer far superior control of potentially life-threatening hemorrhage. It has changed the answer to the question "who should perform laparoscopic donor nephrectomy" from surgeons with extensive laparoscopic experience *only* to surgeons who know how to properly handle the kidney for subsequent transplant and can recognize and avoid problems. Whether transplant, urologic or "laparoscopic" surgeon, transplant centers are as a whole moving towards laparoscopic donor nephrectomy. In Finelli

Table 26.1. Comparison of donor nephrectomy procedures (Lap laparoscopic procedure, Hand hand-assisted laparoscopic procedure, Retro hybrid laparoscopic-open retroperitoneal approach, Open open surgical approach)

Study	Procedure	N	OR time (min)	Estimated blood loss (ml)	Warm ischemia time (s)	Conversions (%)	Length of stay (days)	Ureteral complications (%)	Delayed graft function (%)
Cho[a]	Lap	738	202	128	151	1.60	2.2	4.40	2.60
	Open	65	213	408	–	–	3	–	2
Ruiz-Deya et al. [13]	Lap	11	215	–	234	0	1.6	0	–
	Hand	23	165	–	96	1	2	0	–
Yang et al. [41]	Retro	23	165	100	138	0	–	–	–
	Open	95	138	115	132	–	–	–	–
Stifleman et al. [43]	Hand	60	240	82	121	0	3,5	1.60	1.60
	Open	31	265	364	–	–	4,5	3.20	3.20
Troppmann et al. [51]	Lap single[b]	58	304	–	300	5	3	5.10	6.90
	Lap multi[c]	21	345	–	360	1	3	0	0
Kercher et al. [44]	Hand	30	275	99	72	1	3.4	0	0
Wolf et al. [16]	Hand	38	206	156	183	2	1.7	2	2.60
	Open	41	125	216	96	–	2.6	2.4	2.40

Table 26.1. *Continued*

Study	Procedure	N	OR time (min)	Estimated blood loss (ml)	Warm ischemia time (s)	Conversions (%)	Length of stay (days)	Ureteral complications (%)	Delayed graft function (%)
Rawlins et al. [15]	Lap	100	231	–	–	1	3.3	2	–
	Open	50	209	–	–	–	4.7	6	–
Hawasli et al. [12]	Lap	30	180	–	234	–	1.27	0	0
	Open	29	150	–	–	–	4.1	0	0
Montgomery et al. [52]	Lap	200	–	–	288	–	–	6.50	–
	Open	48	–	–	–	–	–	6.20	–
Koffron et al. [9]	Lap	80	–	–	–	–	2.1	0	–
	Open	50	–	–	–	–	3.2	0	–

[a]Unpublished data, [b]Single renal artery, [c]Multiple renal arteries

and colleagues' 2001 survey, 26 of the 31 highest volume transplant centers in the USA had performed some variation of the procedure and only one center had no plans to do so [35].

26.2.1.3
Does the Operation Increase the Volunteer Donor Pool?

Ratner et al. [36] and Schweitzer et al. [37] have each reported that donor evaluations rise significantly when a transplant program offers laparoscopic donor nephrectomy, and others have since agreed [12, 38, 39]. What is not clear is whether these are donors who would not have otherwise volunteered or if they were simply siphoned from another transplant program's list. The answer is likely to be some of each. Because conversion to open may become necessary at any point during the operation, it is of paramount importance that the potential donor understands that the laparoscopic completion of the operation cannot be absolutely guaranteed. As a corollary, the donor surgeon should not agree to operate on a donor who insists that conversion not occur.

Growth in live donation is not limited to laparoscopic donor programs; Barry reported in a well-reasoned discourse against laparoscopic donor nephrectomy that his program had seen its live donor volume double between 1994 and 1999 despite their decision not to offer the laparoscopic option [20].

26.2.2
Technique

26.2.2.1
Transperitoneal versus Retroperitoneal?

Retroperitoneal laparoscopic nephrectomy, first reported by Suzuki et al. in 1997 [40] allows the peritoneal cavity to be left undisturbed, in the same manner as extra peritoneal inguinal herniorraphy, and theoretically avoid intraperitoneal adhesion formation. Adhesions from laparoscopic scars are minimal to begin with, though the extraction incision would be an exception to this.

True retroperitoneoscopy does have some disadvantages: the dissected retroperitoneal space is much smaller than the peritoneal cavity, leaving much less room for maneuvering. Likewise, the ability to gain rapid control of major vessel or organ hemorrhage is poor, the diametric opposite of hand-assist laparoscopy, where this is the most dramatic advantage. Lastly, the extraction incision for a retroperitoneal approach is usually made in the flank, a location both more painful and more likely to result in a difficult-to-repair incisional hernia than a midline extraction site. Nevertheless, series such as Yang and colleagues' [41] describing a hybrid laparoscopic-open retroperitoneal approach where cameras and instruments are used through a small flank incision (6.5 cm) but no insufflation is used, have documented comparable results that bear further investigation.

26.2.2.2
Hand-assisted?

Hand-assist techniques have gained popularity rapidly, and the results of large series are so similar to „total" laparoscopic approaches that they are essentially equivalent in both donor and recipient results [16, 42–44]. They appear to be easier to learn and provide much more confidence to the surgeon without significant laparoscopic experience because his or her hand is able to utilize tactile feedback and apply pressure to control bleeding if needed. Warm ischemia times are generally shorter than for „total" laparoscopic techniques [44], but as mentioned above, it is not clear that this has clinical significance [29].

Since all existing data suggest that hand-assist techniques have no discernable disadvantage compared to total laparoscopic methods and offer some definite advantages, most importantly the ability to rapidly and securely control hemorrhage, hand-assist should be strongly considered as the method of choice to those deciding to perform laparoscopic donor nephrectomy. Those familiar with total laparoscopic manipulation and dissection, and those who have hands large enough that the hand-port incision would be significantly larger than an extraction incision, should consider the various total laparoscopic techniques as well.

26.2.2.3
Right- versus Left-sided Donor Nephrectomy

Critics of laparoscopic donor nephrectomy point out that existing series overwhelmingly favor the left kidney over the right, while open series are for the most part equally divided. Many surgeons performing laparoscopic nephrectomy use the left kidney because they are concerned that the shorter right renal vein will be made even shorter by whatever device is used to ligate and divide the vessel. Most techniques use either a GIA linear stapler and cutter or a TA stapler in combination with shears, hopefully applied to the kidney side of the staple line (which can be hard to see well). Others describe ligating the vessels with locking clip devices, but these have been rumored to catastrophically come off of major vessels during open cases, leading many surgeons to shy away from their use. The open donor surgeon uses clamps to maximize vessel length, cuts above the clamps and then suture-ligates the vessel stumps, but the ideal laparoscopic instrument to achieve this securely without unduly prolonging warm ischemia time has yet to be devised.

Conventional wisdom dictates that the better of the two kidneys should always be left in the donor, and some programs go so far as to test for differential renal function in order to insure this, while others have not and have never placed emphasis on such matters. Regardless of which philosophy one embraces, it is clear that right and left kidneys can be procured laparoscopically with equal safety and efficacy [45–47]. Our own experience with right donor nephrectomy bears this out as well [48]. It suggests that the main reason left kidneys are used so much more often than right in laparoscopic donor nephrectomy is an anticipation of problems with short vessels more than any reality. Moreover, as donor and recipient surgeons become more accustomed to the procedure and as instrument technology catches up to the operation we could see a swing back towards equal use of right and left kidneys.

26.2.2.4
Is It Worth the Increased Demands on the Implant Surgeon?

Laparoscopic donor nephrectomy ends up placing more technical demands on the implanting surgeon. In any technique where staplers are used to divide the vessels, artery and vein length will be lost, and early branching single arteries will be converted by the stapler into two or more arteries. While several authors have looked into this and concluded that this did not cause any significant loss of function in their grafts [49–51], they also admit that more effort than usual was required to avoid suboptimal results, whether that meant additional anastomoses or arterial and/or venous reconstruction prior to implantation. The implication is that while the laparoscopic harvest, or more accurately, the devices currently available to divide the vessels in a laparoscopic environment, can create more work for the implanting surgeon, the competent transplanter should be able to rise to the occasion. The question is still whether the expected increase in volunteer donors and the improved outcomes they have will make the extra effort worthwhile.

26.3
Summary

— Laparoscopic donor nephrectomy continues to gain popularity despite its difficulty, expense and lack of long-term follow-up data.

— Individual programs have documented increases in volunteer donors when laparoscopic donor nephrectomy was offered. This has yet to be shown on a larger scale.

— Hand-assisted laparoscopic methods have markedly eased the learning process and extended the appeal to those surgeons who would not have considered learning the total laparoscopic procedure.

— Retroperitoneal approaches have been described but do not appear to offer decisive advantages over transperitoneal techniques.

— Each surgeon should examine the available data and use the approach that best suits his or her abilities and priorities.

— Right kidneys can and have been procured just as safely and effectively as left kidneys, but many transplant and donor surgeons continue to avoid them for problems more anticipated than real.

— The perfect instrument to safely and quickly divide the renal artery and vein has yet to be produced. Until it is, recipient surgeons face additional challenges in implanting laparoscopically procured living donor kidneys.

— *DO NO HARM!*

— Living donor organ procurement, whichever technique is used, stands alone as a major procedure performed upon a healthy patient who does not need the operation with the only justification the potential to benefit the recipient. It is the only instance in which we as surgeons must modify the credo, "do no harm" to read instead, "do as little harm as possible." It is incumbent upon us to ensure that the trust placed in us by both donor and recipient has been well placed.

References

1. Cecka JM. Living donor transplants. Clinical transplants 1995. Los Angeles: UCLA Tissue Typing Laboratory; 1996. p. 363–77.
2. Dunn JF, Nylander WA, Richie RE, et al. Living related kidney donors. A 14 year experience. Ann Surg 1996;203:637–43.
3. Bay WH, Hebert LA. The living donor in kidney transplantation. Ann Intern Med 1987;106:719–27.
4. Clayman RV, Kavoussi LR, Soper N. Laparoscopic nephrectomy: initial case report. J Urol 1991;146:278–82.
5. Ratner LE, Cisek LJ, Moore RG, et al. Laparoscopic live donor nephrectomy. Transplantation 1995;60:1047–9.
6. Ratner LE, Kavoussi LR, Sroka M, et al. Laparoscopic assisted live donor nephrectomy: a comparison with the open approach. Transplantation 1997;63:229–33.
7. Flowers JL, Jacobs S, Cho E, et al. Comparison of laparoscopic and open live donor nephrectomy. Ann Surg 1997;226:483–90.

8. London E, Rudich S, McVicar J et al. Equivalent renal allograft function with laparoscopic versus open live donor nephrectomies. Transplant Proc 1999;31:258–60.

9. Koffron A, Herman C, Gross O, et al. Laparoscopic donor nephrectomy: analysis of donor and recipient outcomes. Transplant Proc 2001;33):1111.

10. Leventhal JR; Deeik RK; Joehl R Laparoscopic live donor nephrectomy – is it safe? Transplantation 2000;70:602–6

11. Merlin TL, Scott DF, Rao MM, et al. The safety and efficacy of laparoscopic live donor nephrectomy: a systematic review. Transplantation 2000;70:1659–66.

12. Hawasli A, Boutt A, Cousins G, et al. Laparoscopic versus conventional live donor nephrectomy: experience in a community transplant program. Am Surg 2001;67:342–5.

13. Ruiz-Deya G, Cheng S, Palmer E, et al. Open donor, laparoscopic donor and hand assisted laparoscopic donor nephrectomy: a comparison of outcomes. J Urol 2001;166:1270–3.

14. Velidedeoglu E, Williams N, Brayman KL, et al. Comparison of open, laparoscopic and hand-assisted approaches to live-donor nephrectomy. Transplantation 2002;74:169–72.

15. Rawlins MC, Hefty TL, Brown SL, et al. Learning laparoscopic donor nephrectomy safely: a report on 100 cases. Arch Surg 2002;137:531–5.

16. Wolf JS, Merion RM, Leitchman AB, et al. Randomized controlled trial of hand-assisted laparoscopic versus open surgical live donor nephrectomy. Transplantation 2001;72:284–90.

17. Fabrizio MD, Ratner LE, Kavoussi LR. Laparoscopic live donor nephrectomy: pro. Urology 1999;53:665–7.

18. Novick A. Laparoscopic live donor nephrectomy: con. Urology 1999;53:668–70.

19. Ratner LE, Buell JF, Kuo PC. Laparoscopic donor nephrectomy: pro. Transplantation 2000;70:1544–6.

20. Barry JM. Laparoscopic donor nephrectomy: con. Transplantation 2000;70:1546–8.

21. Jacobs SC, Cho E. Laparoscopic donor nephrectomy: why not? Arch Esp Urol 2002;55:714–20.

22. Jacobs,SC, Cho,E, Dunkin,BJ, Bartlett,ST, Flowers JL, Jarrell BE. Laparoscopic nephrectomy in the markedly obese renal donor. Urology 2000;56:926–9.

23. Kuo PC, Plotkin JS, Stevens S, et al. Outcomes of laparoscopic donor nephrectomy in obese patients. Transplantation 2000;69:180–2.

24. Nogueira JM, Cangro CB, Fink JC, et al. A comparison of recipient renal outcomes with laparoscopic versus open live donor nephrectomy. Transplantation 1999;67:722–8.

25. Ratner LE, Montgomery RA, Maley WR, et al. Laparoscopic live donor nephrectomy: the recipient. Transplantation 2000;69:2319–23.

26. Ratner LE, Montgomery RA, Kavoussi LR, et al. Laparoscopic live donor nephrectomy. A review of the first 5 years. Urol Clin North Am 2001;28:709–19.

27. Cho E, Flowers JL. Laparoscopic live donor nephrectomy. In: Zucker KA, ed. Surgical laparoscopy, 2nd edn. St Louis: Quality Medical Publishing; 2001. p. 657–69.

28. Dunkin BJ, Johnson LB, Kuo PC. A technical modification eliminates early ureteral complications after laparoscopic donor nephrectomy. J Am Coll Surg 2000;190:96–7.

29. Buzdon MM, Cho E, Jacobs SC, et al. Warm ischemia time does not correlate with recipient graft function in laparoscopic donor nephrectomy. Surg Endosc 2003;17:746–9.

30. Sasaki TM, Finelli F, Bugarin E, et al. Is laparoscopic donor nephrectomy the new criterion standard? Arch Surg 2000;135:943–7.

31. Hazebroek EJ, de Bruin RW, Bouvy ND, et al. Short-term impact of carbon dioxide, helium, and gasless laparoscopic donor nephrectomy on renal function and histomorphology in donor and recipient. Surg Endosc 2002;16:245–51.

32. Mackey TJ, Flowers JL, Bartlett ST, et al. Cost comparison of laparoscopic versus open donor nephrectomy analyzing provider charges and productivity loss. [Abstract]. J Urol 1997;157 (Suppl):156.

33. Pace KT, Dyer SJ, Phan, et al. Laparoscopic vs open donor nephrectomy: a cost-utility analysis of the initial experience at a tertiary-care center. J Endourol 2002;16:495–508.

34. Bemelman WA, van Doorn RC, de Wit LT, et al. Hand-assisted laparoscopic donor nephrectomy. Ascending the learning curve. Surg Endosc 2001;15:422–4.

35. Finelli FC, Gongora E, Sasaki TM. A survey: the prevalence of laparoscopic donor nephrectomy at large US transplant centers. Transplantation 2001;71:1862–4.

36. Ratner LE, Hiller J, Sroka M, et al. Laparoscopic live donor nephrectomy removes disincentives to live donation. Transplant Proc 1997;29:3402–3.

37. Schweitzer EJ, Wilson J, Jacobs SC, et al: Increased rates of donation with laparoscopic donor nephrectomy. Ann Surg 2000;232:392–400.

38. Kuo PC, Johnson LB. Laparoscopic donor nephrectomy increases the supply of living donor kidneys: a center-specific microeconomic analysis. Transplantation 2000;69:2211–3.

39. Shafizadeh S, McEvoy JR, Murray C, et al. Laparoscopic donor nephrectomy: impact on an established renal transplant program. Am Surg 2000;66:1132–5.

40. Suzuki K, Ushiyama T, Ishikawa A, et al. Retroperitoneoscopy assisted live donor nephrectomy: the initial 2 cases. J Urol 1997;158:1353–6.

41. Yang SC, Ko WJ, Byun YJ, et al. Retroperitoneaoscopy assisted live donor nephrectomy: the Yonsei experience. J Urol 2001;165:1099–102.

42. Buell JF, Alverdy J, Newell KA. Hand-assisted laparoscopic live-donor nephrectomy. J Am Coll Surg 2001;192:132–6.

43. Stifleman MD, Hull D, Sosa RE, et al. Hand-assisted laparoscopic donor nephrectomy: a comparison with the open approach. J Urol 2001;166:444–8.

44. Kercher K, Dahl D, Harland R, et al. Hand-assisted laparoscopic donor nephrectomy minimizes warm ischemia. Urology 2001;58:152–6.

45. Buell JF, Edye M, Johnson M, et al. Are concerns over right laparoscopic donor nephrectomy unwarranted? Ann Surg 2001;233:645–51.

46. Mandal AK, Cohen C, Montgomery RA, et al. Should the indications for laparoscopic live donor nephrectomy of the right kidney be the same as for the open procedure? Anomalous left renal vasculature is not a contraindication to laparoscopic left donor nephrectomy. Transplantation 2001;71:660–4.

47. Lind MY, Hazebroek EJ, Hop WC, et al. Right-sided laparoscopic live-donor nephrectomy: is reluctance still justified? Transplantation 2002;74:1045–8.

48. Swartz DE, Cho E, Flowers JL, Dunkin BJ, Ramey JR, Bartlett ST, Jarrell B, Jacobs SC. Laparoscopic right donor nephrectomy: technique and comparison with left nephrectomy. Surg Endosc 2001;15:1390–4.

49. Kuo PC, Cho E, Flowers JL, et al. Laparoscopic living donor nephrectomy and multiple renal arteries. Am J Surg 1998;176:559–63.

50. Johnston T, Reddy K, Mastrangelo M, et al. Multiple renal arteries do not pose an impediment to the routine use of laparoscopic donor nephrectomy. Clin Transplant 2001;15 (Suppl 6):62–5.
51. Troppmann C, Wiesmann K, McVicar JP, et al. Increased transplantation of kidneys with multiple renal arteries in the laparoscopic live donor nephrectomy era. Arch Surg 2001;136:897–907.
52. Montgomery RA, Kavoussi LR, Su L-M. Improved recipient results after 5 years of performing laparoscopic donor nephrectomy. Transplant Proc 2001;33:1108–10.

Commentary

J. STUART WOLF, JR.

This succinct and insightful chapter summarizes extremely well the pertinent controversies surrounding laparoscopic donor nephrectomy. Buzdon and Cho do an excellent job identifying the actual issues, rather than just the perceived ones. Moreover, they approach the pros and cons in a fresh manner than seems at once both simple and unassailably correct. Without meaning to detract from the authors' own summary, I list below what I feel are their three most important points.

— Much of the concern about recipient graft function and ureteral complications in a laparoscopically harvested kidney is based upon a few of the original series. Not only do updates of these series reassure us as to the equivalence of the open and laparoscopic procedures with regards to these issues, but series from surgeons who had the benefit of starting the procedure in the footsteps of the pioneers report equivalent graft function and ureteral complications as well. In other words, the "learning curve" of laparoscopic donor nephrectomy is not the same as the "inventing curve." The pioneers "inventing" the operation certainly struggled at the outset – but once their technique was improved and then promulgated those surgeons who have only to be concerned about "learning" the procedure start out with a better procedure and obtain excellent results at the outset.

— An adverse effect of pneumoperitoneum and prolonged warm ischemia times on graft viability, although theoretically not unexpected, have not proved to be clinically detectable as long as parameters are in a reasonable range (warm ischemia time <10 min) and precautions are taken (profound hydration and/or diuretics to overcome the effect of pneumoperitoneum on renal blood flow).

— Hand-assistance allows a surgeon skilled at open surgical donor nephrectomy to transfer skills to the laparoscopic procedure with less of a requirement for preliminary laparoscopic expertise. The decision of whether one then moves on to standard laparoscopy or stays with the hand-assisted laparoscopic procedure is simply one of surgeon's choice – the benefits to the donor appear to be essentially the same.

It is most appropriate to end this commentary by quoting from Buzdon and Cho directly. They summarize very well the thoughts that all donor surgeons should carry into the operating room: "Living donor organ procurement ... is the only instance in which we as surgeons must modify the credo, 'do no harm' to read instead, 'do as little harm as possible.' It is incumbent upon us to ensure that the trust placed in us by both donor and recipient has been well placed." Personally, I feel that being able to offer a well-performed laparoscopic donor nephrectomy fits this philosophy perfectly.

27

Pancreatic Surgery

FEDERICO CUENCA-ABENTE, AHMAD ASSALIA, MICHEL GAGNER

▶ **Key Controversies**

A. Value of laparoscopy in the staging and palliation of pancreatic cancer
 – Routine versus selective use
B. Appropriate indications and procedures
C. Technical considerations
 – Distal pancreatectomy – Splenic preservation and management of the pancreatic stump
 – Cyst-gastrostomy – the preferred technique
 – Hand-assisted laparoscopy for the pancreas – is it advantageous?

27.1
Introduction

Laparoscopic surgery for digestive diseases has achieved marked progression over the last decade. However, laparoscopic pancreatic surgery (LPS) is still uncommon because of the anatomic location of the pancreas, technical difficulties of pancreatic resections, relative rarity of surgical pancreatic disorders, the requirements for highly experienced, skilful laparoscopic surgeons, and the necessity of complicated techniques and technological advances. Therefore, the experience worldwide is still very limited, a fact well reflected in the literature describing mainly small series and case reports. In fact, laparoscopic surgery for the pancreas is still considered experimental by many surgeons. Since Gagner and Pomp first described in the early 1990s pancreaticoduodenectomy and distal pancreatectomy for chronic pancreatitis and islet cell tumors [1, 2], various laparoscopic pancreatic procedures have been performed, including laparoscopic distal pancreatectomy (LDP), enucleations (LE), pancreaticoduodenectomy (LPD), cyst-gastrostomy (LCG) and necrosectomy for infected necrosis [3–11]. At the writing of this communication fewer than 130 cases of pancreatic resections (LDP, LPD and LE) were reported in the English literature. It has been demonstrated that certain laparoscopic pancreatic procedures, performed for the correct indications and by experienced surgeons, are feasible, safe and offer the advantages of minimally invasive approach seen in other laparoscopic procedures. This chapter will focus on the main current controversies concerning laparoscopy for pancreatic disease.

27.2
Discussion

27.2.1
Value of Laparoscopy in the Staging and Palliation of Pancreatic Cancer

The role of laparoscopy in staging of pancreatic cancer is still evolving as the number and expertise of laparoscopic surgeons continue to increase as well as the accuracy of modern diagnostic imaging techniques. The rational for implementing laparoscopy in the staging of pancreatic cancer is to detect occult peritoneal and hepatic metastasis missed by preoperative imaging studies, and thus sparing these patients, with dismal prognosis, unnecessary non-therapeutic laparotomies. Pioneering studies in the 1970s by Meyer-Burg et al. [12] and Cuschieri et al. [13], and later in the 1980s by Warshaw et al. [14], have demonstrated the utility of routine laparoscopy in preventing non-therapeutic laparotomies and changing the treatment plan in up to 35% of cases. Patients, after laparoscopy, had fewer complications, short hospital stay, and improved quality of life. This also enabled adjuvant therapies to be given at earlier stages. In addition, improvements in laparoscopic staging techniques [15, 16], the addition of laparoscopic ultrasound [16, 17], and peritoneal cytology [18] have led to increased diagnostic accuracy of laparoscopy. Furthermore, in contrast to some concerns [19], diagnostic laparoscopy was found to be oncologically safe and it did not adversely affect survival of patients [20]. However, recent advances in the quality of dynamic spiral computed tomography (CT) scanning have significantly increased the accuracy of predicting both resectability and unresectability of pancreatic cancer. Therefore, several groups have questioned the earlier conclusions advocating routine laparoscopy in staging algorithms [21–23] and have argued for selective use depending on preoperative parameters. Even though, experienced pancreatic surgeons such as Warshaw [18], Cuschiere [24], as well as others [25, 26], continue to advocate routine use of laparoscopy in the staging process. In order to put this modality in its proper context, recent evidence-based critical reviews of the literature [27, 28] have found that if laparoscopy is performed routinely in patients judged to have resectable disease by high quality CT scans, only 4–13% of them will be spared unnecessary laparotomy. Thus, it seems that the yield of routine laparoscopic staging is relatively low and it cannot be readily justified. On the other hand, selective use is felt to be more cost effective. Based on current data, it is likely that only high risk patients for occult metastasis may benefit from staging laparoscopy. These include cases with ascites, larger primary tumors or those located in the body and tail of the gland, nonfunctioning islet cell tumors, equivocal radiographic findings that may suggest occult disease, and subtle clinical and laboratory findings suggesting more advanced disease [27].

The role of laparoscopy in palliation of unresectable disease is also under debate. Although laparoscopic biliary and gastric bypasses were successfully performed in these circumstances [29, 30], it has been argued that with the availability of endobiliary stenting (albeit sub-optimal), the majority of patients with laparoscopically staged unresectable disease, will not require subsequent biliary or gastric bypass [31]. Additional theoretical advantage of diagnostic laparoscopy is the possibility for pain palliation in the form of celiac block. However, to date, this was reported only in a porcine model [32] and no reports in humans have been described.

27.2.2
Appropriate Indications and Procedures

In order to determine the suitability of certain pathology to laparoscopic pancreatic surgery, one should evaluate whether the specific procedure performed for this indication is readily feasible, safe and reproducible. In addition, the results in terms of cure of the disease process (lack of recurrence) should be ascertained.

Although clinical experience with LPS remains limited, an early consensus seems to have emerged [3]. Several surgeons have noted that LDP for benign and low grade malignant (or pre-malignant) disease of the body and tail of the pancreas offers adequate clinical outcome in terms of morbidity and recovery [3–5, 8–10, 33–35]. Long-term follow-up is still lacking. Reported indications in decreasing order of frequency, included insulinomas, mucinous and serous cystadenomas, chronic pancreatitis, pseudocysts, and other neuro-endocrine and islet cell tumors. Serous and mucinous cystic neoplasms appear to be suitable for laparoscopic approach based on the frequent location in the body and tail and high frequency of these neoplasms being benign or pre-malignant [4]. The final pathological diagnosis revealed several cases of malignancy not known preoperatively. Although in early series, conversion rates as high as 36% were reported [9], with increased experience conversions rates of 8–15% are cited in several available relatively large series [3–5, 8]. Furthermore, no deaths were reported so far and the complications of LDP compared favorably with those of open surgery [3, 4, 8, 34]. Pancreatic fistula appears to be less frequent than previously thought and will be discussed later. It seems that in particular, benign islet cell tumors [3, 4, 7, 34, 35], chronic pancreatitis [6] and cystic neoplasms [3, 4, 34] are suitable for laparoscopic pancreatic resections because they require neither regional lymphadenectomy nor reconstruction.

Laparoscopic enucleations (LE) for benign solitary small tumors (<2 cm) located on the surface of the pancreas and not in contact with splenic vessels or main pancreatic duct, have achieved good results both in terms of morbidity and cure [4, 8, 34, 36]. If these conditions are not met, a distal pancreatectomy is the best choice. The indications included mainly insulinomas but gastrinoma, cystadenoma, cysts and multiple endocrine neoplasia (type I) were also reported [34]. The experience gained with laparoscopic resections for malignancies is scant and in many cases the diagnosis was confirmed postoperatively. At present, it is generally felt that laparoscopy may compromise the principles of surgical oncology in that it is rather difficult to achieve radical operations with sufficient lymphadenectomy and adequate margins [33]. Most importantly, however, in the very limited experience to date with *laparoscopic pancreaticoduodenectomy* [9, 37], patients appeared to have derived no benefits when compared to those on open surgery. The conversion rate was high (40%), operative time was prolonged (averaged 8.5 h) and the postoperative stay averaged almost 3 weeks [9]. Furthermore, a high complication rate in the order of 50% was seen and the issue of recurrence of disease was assessed only for the short term. Although the hand-assisted approach enabled the procedure to be performed more easily with shorter operative time [9], at present, this operation should not be considered or offered to patients [3, 9].

Using different techniques and approaches, laparoscopic cyst-gastrostomy (LCG) for the treatment of pancreatic pseudocyst (PP) has been performed successfully in several reports with adequate clinical outcome regarding complications, recovery and recurrence as well [3, 29, 38–40]. Although no comparisons with endoscopic internal drainage techniques has been done to date, the results compare favorably with them as well as with open surgery [3], offering the patients short recovery and comparable success rates.

Laparoscopic (or laparoscopic-assisted) necrosectomy (LN) of infected pancreatic necrosis (IPN) has been also described in several communications [41–47]. Various techniques were utilized to approach the infected necrosis and to install systems of drainage and lavage: laparoscopic retrogastric-retrocolic [42], laparoscopic trans-gastric [42, 48], laparoscopic infra-colic [43], endoscopic retroperitoneal [42, 44, 49, 50] and laparoscopic intracavitary drainge using either percutaneous drains as guides [45] or alternatively performed during open surgery for internal drainage of pseudocysts [47]. In addition, sinus tract endoscopy was also reported to be successfully carried out [49]. The incentive of minimally invasive surgery in this setting was to lessen the stress of surgical intervention in the already compromised patient with IPN. In spite of the advances in surgical technique and intensive care, morbidity and mortality in this subset of patients remains significant with open surgery. Less activation of the systemic inflammatory response by minimally invasive techniques, provided they will be equally efficacious in controlling the local sepsis, is supposed to reduce the "second hit" phenomenon and, thus, lead to a better outcome. Moreover, it has been argued that, if necessary, repeated laparoscopic interventions could be carried out with much less physiological impact on the critically ill patient than traditional surgery. Therefore, in an institution with advanced laparoscopic pancreatic surgeon, it seems that the occasional patient with the late well-defined IPN, or pancreatic abscess not amenable to percutaneous drainage, may be a candidate for minimally invasive intervention. However, although the initial results are encouraging, the experience is still too small and comparison with open surgery and endoscopic management [51] is still pending.

27.2.3
Technical Considerations

27.2.3.1
Laparoscopic Distal Pancreatectomy (LDP)

To Preserve the Spleen or Not? Which Technique to Use? As with open surgery, splenic preservation is encouraged whenever is technically feasible, provided the procedure will not oncologically compromise the outcome. In cases of malignancy, especially if the tumor involves the hilum of the spleen, or with hilar fibrosis and scarring due to past inflammation or abscess formation, splenic preservation should be avoided [52] and laparoscopic en-bloc pancreatico-splenectomy is the safest technique. This has the advantage of giving an adequate lymph node sampling and avoids the high risk of bleeding during the dissection of the upper edge of the pancreas [2]. In the largest series to date reporting 25 LDPs by Park and Heniford [3], it was noted that also insulinomas that were in close proximity to the splenic vein frequently have intense desmoplastic reaction, making the separation from the vessels difficult, and may cause significant bleeding, thus precluding preservation of the spleen. In most of the series of LDP, splenic salvage was successfully achieved in 50–100% of patients [3–5]. The two techniques known from open surgery were adopted in laparoscopic pancreatic surgery: *LDP with splenic vessels preservation* and *LDP with splenic vessel ligation*. The former requires longer operative time and laparoscopic surgical expertise [4, 5, 34]. The magnified view using laparoscopy facilitates separation of the splenic vessels from the pancreas and the dissection, ligation and division of branching arteries and veins into the pancreas [3, 4]. The splenic-preserving distal pancreatectomy with splenic vessel ligation requires the ligation and transection of the splenic vessels at both the level of pancreatic section and at the splenic hilium. The spleen subsequently receives vascular supply from the short gastric vessels. This technique is applied in cases of malignancy (adequate lymph-node sampling) and during uncontrollable bleeding from the splenic vessels along the upper edge of the pancreas. The experience gained to date with this technique showed that it has a low risk of splenic infarction and several advantages regarding duration of surgery and blood loss. In fact, only two splenic infarctions and one abscess were reported in the literature [4, 34].

Management of the Pancreatic Stump. Pancreatic fistula is a potentially serious complication of both distal pancreatectomy and pancreatic enucleation. It is the most common complication after LDP and can course asymptomatically or be devastating. In a review of the literature summarizing 47 cases of LDP [34], the reported overall incidence was 6.4%. Another recent two series, of 11 and 25 cases each, reported an occurrence of 9% and 4.3%, respectively [3, 5]. Fernandez-Cruz in his last communication describing 11 patients with LDP and 4 with enucleation, has documented a high incidence of 27.7% [4]. However, the course of these fistulas was benign and they were treated conservatively with drainage in the vast majority of cases. Therefore, the contention that laparoscopic surgery carries higher risk for fistulas is not substantially supported. To date, no "magic bullet" does exist for the prevention of pancreatic fistulas. Several maneuvers were described but none is proven as "the best" and notwithstanding all these methods, pancreatic fistula still occurs. The way in which the surgeon approaches the pancreatic transection seems to be important. A useful ergonomic consideration is that the stapler used to transect the pancreas has to be introduced through a trocar that is far away from the pancreas [8] (left paramedian location). This may avoid disruption of the gland, which could happen if the stapler approximating the pancreas is in a perpendicular position. Oversewing of the stapled end of the stump with a non-absorbable suture is one of those "preventive" measure intends to secure the staple line [3, 35, 53]. Using this method, Park and Heniford in their series of 25 LDPs have encountered just one fistula [3]. Some authors feel that if the pancreatic parenchyma is too thick and fibrotic, dividing the isthmus with ultrasonic shears and separately suturing the pancreatic duct would be helpful [5]. Others do that routinely if they visualize the duct after transaction [8].

Pre-operative somatostatin analogs have been described as another method for preventing fistula formation or accelerating its closure when administrated postoperatively [8]. Even so, the administration of this drug has not statistically proved to be helpful [54, 55]. Despite the lack of strong confirmatory evidence, some authors [35, 56] have used fibrin glue as an additional method to prevent fistula formation. The recent use of staple line reinforcement novel materials needs further evaluation.

27.2.3.2
Laparoscopic Cystgastrostomy (LCG)

The Procedure of Choice? LCG may be carried out using a variety of approaches [3]. *The lesser sac (or posterior approach)* avoids the anterior gastrostomy done with other techniques, while preserving the benefit of the generous stapled anastomosis [3]. Occasionally, inflammation may result in obliteration of the lesser sac precluding this approach.

LCG can also be achieved through an *anterior transgastric approach*. The procedure may be accomplished with creation of a gastrotomy on the anterior gastric wall and the communication between the cyst and the posterior wall of the stomach is then created with different instruments (linear stapler, electrocautery or ultrasonic shears). This technique carries potential complications involving the anterior gastrostomy. More frequently, however, and in order to minimize the trauma to the stomach, it combines the insertion of a gastroscope in order to inflate the stomach and to enable the introduction of trocars inside it and allow intragastric laparoscopic surgery to be performed [3, 29, 38–40]. Intragastric laparoscopic intervention may be accomplished either with 12-mm balloon-tipped trocars, allowing transgastric introduction of a stapler device [40], or with needlescopic (2-mm) instruments, obviating the need for pneumoperitoneum, creating less operative trauma and avoiding the closure of the anterior gastric puncture sites [57].

When the bulge of the pseudocyst is seen mainly through the transverse mesocolon, LCG or laparoscopic cyst-jejunostomy were reported to be readily accomplished using the *infracolic approach* [3, 4].

Obviously, several techniques are feasible and the preliminary experience appears to be safe and effective. Each surgeon has to choose the technique he or she is most accustomed to, according to his or her preference and the local expertise.

27.2.3.3
Hand-assisted Laparoscopic Surgery (HALS) for the Pancreas

Is It Advantageous? HALS provides assistance from the surgeon's non-dominant hand and is reported to have advantages in terms of exposure and safety over the total laparoscopic technique for major surgery of the pancreas [10, 53, 58, 59]. The procedure is mostly recommended for cases involving large tumors, massive intraoperative bleeding, dense adhesions, malignancy and in obese patients. It can also be used at the outset or as an intermediary step, when the surgeon faces intraoperative difficulty [8]. The advantages include: assistance of the hand for dissection, direct tactile sensation, (especially important in the pancreas), retraction, mobilization of organs, the use of small instruments that can be introduced through the hand-assisted device, protection of the wound during extraction of malignant specimens and the utilization of the fingers to rapidly stop unexpected bleeding. With HALS, operative time, bleeding and costs may be reduced [10, 58] and difficult cases that otherwise would not be performed laparoscopically, can be completed. However, as with many laparoscopic procedures of the pancreas, the reported experience is very limited and formal evaluations are not yet available.

27.3
Summary

— The field of laparoscopic pancreatic surgery is slowly evolving and still is in its infancy. The experience is very limited in every perspective. Many issues remain to be clarified and long-term follow-up is still lacking. Therefore, much more experience is required before definitive recommendations are made and wide applications for the average surgeon are adopted.
— Selective staging laparoscopy is cost effective and has a definite role in patients in whom occult metastasis are still suspected in spite of preoperative high quality spiral CT scan. The routine used is debatable as well as the role in palliation.
— Acceptable indications for laparoscopic pancreatic resections (distal pancreatectomy and enucleations), include chronic pancreatitis and small benign and pre-malignant tumors of the body and tail of the gland. Laparoscopy for malignant lesions is not advised and pancreaticoduodenectomy is not recommended at the present time.
— Patients with large pancreatic pseudocysts or those not amenable to endoscopic drainage should be considered candidates for laparoscopic internal drainage.
— Pancreatic fistula after LDP occurs less than was previously estimated. It is mostly self-limited, but is still common. None of the techniques described for prevention has proved to successfully achieve this goal.
— Laparoscopic pancreatic surgery should be performed only in selected centers and by surgeons experienced both in open pancreatic and advanced laparoscopic surgery.

References

1. Gagner M, Pomp A. Laparoscopic pylorus-preserving pancreatoduodenectomy. [Abstract]. In: Second Annual Congress, Canadian Society for Endoscopic and Laparoscopic Surgery, Ottawa, Canada, 10–11 September 1992. pp. 26–9.
2. Gagner M, Pomp A, Herrera MF. Early experience with laparoscopic resections of islet cell tumors. Surgery 1996;120:1051–4.
3. Park A, Heniford BT. Therapeutic laparoscopy of the pancreas. Ann Surg 2002;236:149–58.
4. Fernandez-Cruz L, Saenz A, Astudillo E, Martinez I, Hoyos S, Pantoja JP, Navarro S. Outcome of laparoscopic pancreatic surgery: endocrine and non-endocrine tumors. World J Surg 2002;26:1057–65.
5. Fabre JM, Dulucq JL, Vacher C, Lemoine MC, Wintringer P, Nocca D, Burgel JS, Domergue J. Is laparoscopic left pancreatic resection justified? Surg Endosc 2002;16:1358–61.
6. Fernandez-Cruz L, Saenz A, Astudillo E, et al. Laparoscopic pancreatic surgery in patients with chronic pancreatitis. Surg Endosc 2002;16:996–1003.
7. Fernandez-Cruz L, Herrera M, Saenz M, et al. Laparoscopic pancreatic surgery in patients with neuroendocrine tumors: indications and limits. Best Pract Res Clin Endocrinol Metab 2001;15:161–75.
8. Patterson EJ, Gagner M, Salky B, Inabnet WB, Brower S, Edye M, Gurland B, Reiner M, Pertsemlides D. Laparoscopic pancreatic resection: single-institution experience of 19 patients. J Am Coll Surg 2001;193:281–7.
9. Gagner M, Pomp A. Laparoscopic pancreatic resection: is it worthwhile ? J Gastrointest Surg 1997;1:20–6.
10. Cuschieri A. Laparoscopic hand-assisted surgery for hepatic and pancreatic disease. Surg Endosc. 2000;14:991–6.
11. Cuschieri A, Jakimowicz JJ, Spreeuwel J. Laparoscopic distal 70% pancreatectomy and splenectomy for chronic pancreatitis. Ann Surg 1996;223:280–5.
12. Meyer-Burg J, Ziegler U, Palme G. Zur supragastralen Pankreaskopie: Ergebnisse aus 125 Laparoskopien. Dtsch Med Wochenschr 1972;97:1969–71.
13. Cuschieri A, Hall AW, Clark J. Value of laparoscopy in the diagnosis and management of pancreatic carcinoma. Gut 1978;19:672–7.
14. Warshaw AL, Tepper JE, Shipley WU. Laparoscopy in the staging and planning of therapy for pancreatic cancer. Am J Surg 1986;151:76–80.
15. Conlon KC, Dougherty E, Klimsra DS, et al. The value of minimal access surgery in the staging of patients with potentially resectable peripancreatic malignancy. Ann Surg 1996;223:134–40.
16. Kwon AH, Inui H, Kamiyama Y. Preoperative laparoscopic examination using surgical manipulation and ultrasonography for pancreatic lesions. Endoscopy 2002;34:464–8.
17. Taylor AM, Roberts SA, Manson JM. Experience with laparoscopic ultrasonography for defining tumor resectability in carcinoma of the pancreatic head and periampullary region. Br J Surg 2001;88:1077–83.
18. Jimenez RE, Warshaw AL, Fernandez-Del Castillo. Laparoscopy and peritoneal cytology in the staging of peritoneal cancer. J Hepatobiliary Pancreat Surg 2000;7:15–20.

19. Ridgway PF, Ziprin P, Jones TL, et al. Laparoscopic staging of pancreatic tumors induces increased invasive capacity in vitro. Surg Endosc 2003;17:306–10.

20. Urbach DR, Swanstrom LL, Hansen PD. The effect of laparoscopy on survival in pancreatic cancer. Arch Surg 2002;137:191–9.

21. Gloor B, Todd KE, Reber HA. Diagnostic workup of patients with suspected pancreatic carcinoma: The University of California-Los Angeles approach. Cancer 1997;79:1780–6.

22. Rumstadt B, Schwab M, Schuster K, et al. The role of laparoscopy in the preoperative staging of pancreatic carcinoma. J Gastrointest Surg 1997;1:245–50.

23. Nieveen van Dijkum EJM, Romijn MG, Terwee CB, et al. Laparoscopic staging and subsequent palliation in patients with peripancreatic carcinoma. Ann Surg 2003;237:66–73.

24. Cuschieri A. Role of video-laparoscopy in the staging of intra-abdominal lymphomas and gastrointestinal cancer. Semin Surg Oncol 2001;20:167–72.

25. Brooks AD, Mallis MJ, Brennan MF, et al. The value of laparoscopy in the management of ampullary, duodenal and distal bile duct tumors. J Gastrointest Surg 2002;6:139–46.

26. Vollmer CM, Drebin JA, Middleton WD, et al. Utility of staging laparoscopy in subsets of peripancreatic and biliary malignancies. Ann Surg 2002;235:1–7.

27. Pisters PWT, Lee JE, Vauthey JN, et al. Laparoscopy in the staging of pancreatic cancer. Br J Surg 2001;88:325–37.

28. Hennig R, Tepia-Caliera AA Hartel M, et al. Staging laparoscopy and its indications in pancreatic cancer patients. Dig Surg 2002;19:484–8.

29. Taragona EM, Pera M, Martinez J, et al. Laparoscopic treatment of pancreatic disorders: diagnosis and staging, palliation of cancer and treatment of pancreatic pseudocyst. Int Surg 1996;81:1–5.

30. Underwood RA, Soper NJ. Current status of laparoscopic surgery of the pancreas. J Hepatobiliary Pancreat Surg 1999;6:154–64.

31. Yoshida T, Matsumoto T, Morii Y, et al. Staging with helical computed tomography and laparoscopy in panctreatic head cancer. Heapatogastroenterology 2002;49:1428–31.

32. Underwood RA, Wu JS, Cohen MS, et al. Laparoscopic approach to neurolitic celiac plexus block. Surg Endosc 1998;12:487.

33. Park A, Schwartz R, Anvari M. Laparoscopic pancreatic surgery. Am J Surg 1999;177:158–63.

34. Tagaya N, Kasama K, Suzuki N. et al. Laparoscopic resection of the pancreas and review of the literature. Surg Endosc 2002;17:201–6.

35. Gramatica L, Herrera MF, Mercado-Luna A, et al. Videolaparoscopic resection of insulinomas: experience in two institutions. World J Surg 2002;26:1297–300.

36. Brendes FJ, Cuesta MA, Kazemier G, et al. Laparoscopic detection and resection of insulinomas. Surgery 2000;128:386–91.

37. Uyama I, Ogiwara H, Iida S, et al. Laparoscopic minilaparotomy pancreaticoduodenectomy with lymphadenectomy using an abdominal wall-lift method. Surg Laparosc Endosc 1996;6:405–10.

38. Atabek U, Meyer D, Amin A, et al. Pancreatic cystgastrostomy by combined upper endoscopy and percutaneous transgastric instrumentation. J Laparoendosc Surg 1993;3:501–4.

39. Gagner M. Laparoscopic transgastric cystgastrostomy for pancreatic pseudocyst. [Abstract]. Surg Endosc 1994;8:239.

40. Trias M, Taragona EM, Balague C, et al. Intraluminal stapled laparoscopic cystgastrostomy for treatment of pancreatic pseudocyst. Br J Surg 1995;82:403.

41. Gagner M. Laparoscopic treatment of acute necrotizing pancreatitis. Semin Laparosc Surg 1996;3:10–4.

42. Pamoukian VN, Gagner M. Laparoscopic necrosectomy for acute necrotizing pancreatitis. J Hepatobiliary Pancreat Surg 2001;8:221–3.

43. Cuschieri A, JakimowiczJJ, Stultiens G. Laparoscopic infracolic approach for complications of acute pancreatitis. Semin Laparosc Surg 1998;5:189–94.

44. Horvath KD, Kao LS, Wherry CA, et al. A technique for laparoscopic assisted percutaneous drainage of infected pancreatic necrosis and pancreatic abscess. Surg Endosc 2001;15:1221–5.

45. Alverdy J, Vargish T, Desai T, et al. Laparoscopic intracavitary debridement of peripancreatic necrosis: preliminary report and description of the technique. Surgery 2000;127:112–4.

46. El Yassini AE, Hoebeke Y, Keuleneer RD. Laparoscopic treatment of secondary infected pancreatic collection after an acute pancreatitis: two cases. Acta Chir Belg 1996;96:226–8.

47. Oria A, Ocampo C, Zandalazini H, et al. Internal Drainage of giant acute pseudocysts, The role of video-assisted pancreatic necrosectomy. Arch Surg 2000;135:136–40.

48. Ammori BJ. Laparoscopic transgastric pancreatic necrosectomy for infected pancreatic necrosis. Surg Endosc 2002;16:1362.

49. Ross Carter C, McKay CJ. Imrie CW. Percutaneous necrosectomy and sinus tract endoscopy in the management of infected pancreatic necrosis: an initial experience. Ann Surg 2000;232:175–80.

50. Slavin J, Ghaneh P, Sutton R, et al. Initial results with a minimally invasive technique of pancreatic necrosectomy. Br J Surg 2001;88:476.

51. Baron TH, Thaggard WG, Morgan DE, et al. Endoscopic therapy for organized pancreatic necrosis. Gastroenterology 1996;111:755–64.

52. Warshaw A. Conservation of the spleen with distal pancreatectomy. Arch Surg. 1988;123:550–3.

53. Shinchi H, Takao S, Noma H, Mataki Y, Iino S, Aikou T. Hand-assisted laparoscopic distal pancreatectomy with mini-laparotomy for distal pancreatic cystadenoma. Surg Laparosc Endosc Percutan Tech 2001;11:139–43.

54. Holloran CM, Ghanch P, Bossennet L, et al. Complications of pancreatic cancer resection. Dig Surg 2002;19:138–46.

55. Bassi C, Falconi M, Salvia R, Caldiron E, Butturini G, Pederzoli P. Role of octreotide in the treatment of external pancreatic pure fistulas: a single institution prospective experience. Langen Arch Surg 2000. 385:10–3.

56. Matsumoto T, Kitano S, Yoshida T, Bandoh T, Kakisako K, Ninomiya K, Tsuboi S, Baatar D. Laparoscopic resection of a pancreatic mucinous cystadenoma using laparoscopic coagulation shears. Surg Endosc 1999;13:172–3.

57. Klinger P, Hinder R, Menke DM, Smith S. Hand-assisted laparoscopic distal pancreatectomy for pancreatic cystadenoma. Surg Laparosc Endosc 1998;8:180–4.

58. Fugino Y, Shimomura K, Hashimoto D, et al. Hand-assisted laparoscopic distal pancreatectomy in pigs using our original hand device (Lap Disc). Surg Today 2002;32:663–5.

59. Gagner M, Gentileschi P. Hand-assisted laparoscopic pancreatic surgery. Semin Laparosc Surg 2001;8:114–25.

Commentary

PETER KIENLE, MARKUS BÜCHLER

This chapter by Cuenca-Abente, Assalia and Gagner adequately summarizes the scarce data available on minimal invasive pancreatic surgery. The role of laparoscopy for staging of pancreatic cancer has been put into the right perspective in the last years.

Diagnostic Laparoscopy

Data from several groups including our own [1] have documented that only a small minority of patients actually benefit from diagnostic laparoscopy and, assuming further progress in other non-invasive diagnostic modalities such as high resolution computed, magnetic resonance and positron emission tomography, we expect the indications for this procedure to be narrowed down further. Certainly, in agreement with the authors' conclusions, high-risk patients demonstrating clinical signs suspicious for generalized disease such as ascites are still good candidates for diagnostic laparoscopy.

Pancreatic Fistulas

The authors write "the contention that laparoscopic surgery carries higher risk for fistulas is not substantially supported". However, this assumption has also not been refuted. Most patients included in the published, limited series were actually highly selected and in the wake of this a fistula rate of 4% to up to 30% seems unacceptably high even if these fistulas are unproblematic in their management and seldom require reoperation. In our own institution the fistula rate is 9% in a series of over 50 distal pancreatic resections performed in the last 20 months, which is comparable to the fistula rate in other large conventional series. Our concept to prevent fistulas is to cover the stapled stump with gastric wall or small bowel whenever it can be easily accomplished; at least the suturing of the dorsal aspect of the stump seems technically difficult via laparoscopy. It may be true that the efficacy of somatostatin analogs for preventing fistula or leakage has not yet been proven. However, six randomized controlled trials have actually shown a statistically significant reduction of the overall complication rate in the treatment group, whereas only one single-center randomized trial has failed to do so [2, 3]. Therefore the situation, if anything, remains unclear. On the basis of the available data, we generally use octreotide perioperatively in patients undergoing elective pancreatic resection.

Acute Pancreatitis

It is difficult to imagine a role for minimal invasive surgery in acute pancreatitis in the present time as the incidence of surgical intervention has continuously receded over the recent years. The consensus now is that only severe cases with infected necrosis should undergo surgery [4]. These are probably not patients that can be adequately explored laparoscopically. The promising results reported in the literature may at least partially be explained by questionable patient selection. Horvarth et al., for example, treated six patients with acute pancreatitis. One of the treated patients was able to leave the hospital on the first postoperative day, hardly a patient generally considered for surgery at all [5]. Zhu et al. successfully treated 10 patients with acute pancreatitis by laparoscopic necrosectomy and drainage, but all patients were operated within 72 h of diagnosis [6]. Again, in most of these patients the indication for surgery is probably debatable. On the basis of the assumption that the new, minimal invasive techniques are less traumatizing, the indications for surgery are somewhat expanded.

Pseudocysts

This also holds true for the concept of cystogastrostomy or cystojejunostomy. This operation is very rare at least in our large experience in pancreatic surgery. Most of the pancreatic cysts are not adequately managed with the above procedures; in the case of suspected malignancy resection is mandatory, and in the case of cysts on the basis of chronic or recurrent acute pancreatitis duodenum-preserving pancreatic head resection is the treatment of choice for good long-term results, at least in our hands. For the occasional cyst, not caused by obstruction in the proximal pancreatic duct, laparoscopic cystogastrostomy may indeed be a viable option.

Hand Assisted?

There is evidence that hand-assisted laparoscopic techniques are safer and faster for performing complex gastrointestinal procedures such as pancreatic resections; however, it remains to be shown whether the remaining advantages over conventional techniques will make this approach worthwhile. As Targarona et al. write in a recent review "there is not enough evidence-based data available to know exactly the final outcome of this technique in general surgery" [7].

Conclusions

The main problem of laparoscopic pancreatic surgery and for that case for most of minimal invasive surgery is that scientific evidence is still lacking. Randomized controlled trials have not yet been conducted for any aspect of laparoscopic pancreatic surgery and therefore laparoscopic pancreatic surgery still has to be considered as experimental. Obviously many minimal invasive laparoscopic operations are technically feasible, but are they indeed advantageous for the patient and are they cost-effective in times of limited financial resources? Only very few indications in pancreatic surgery in selected patients are probably suitable for minimal invasive techniques, distal pancreatectomy maybe being one of them, especially in the context of innovative robotic techniques. Laparoscopic pancreatic surgery has probably not yet overcome its learning curve; therefore randomized controlled trials will not be available for some time. But the specialized centers performing these kinds of operations will have to plan and conduct these trials in order to define the future role of laparoscopic pancreatic surgery.

References

1. Friess H, Kleef J, Silva JC, Sadowski C, Baer HU, Büchler MW. The role of diagnostic laparoscopy in panreatic and periampullary malignancies. J Am Coll Surg 1998;186: 675–82.
2. Berberat PO, Friess H, Kleef J, Uhl W, Büchler MW. Prevention and treatment of complications in pancreatic cancer surgery. Dig Surg 1999;16:327–36.
3. Gouillat C. Somatostatin for the prevention of complications following pancreatoduodenectomy. Digestion 1999;60:59–63.
4. Uhl W, Warshaw A, Imrie C, et al. International Association of Pancreatology: IAP guidelines for the surgical management of acute pancreatitis. Pancreatology 2002;2: 565–73.

5. Horvath KD, Kao LS, Wherry CA, et al. A technique for laparoscopic assisted percutaneous drainage of infected pancreatic necrosis and pancreatic abscess. Surg Endosc 2001;15:1221–5.
6. Zhu JF, Fan XH, Zhang XH. Laparoscopic treatment of severe acute pancreatitis. Surg Endosc 2001;15:146–8.
7. Targarona EM, Gracia E, Rodriguez M, Cerdan G, Balague C, Garriga J, Trias M. Hand-assisted laparoscopic surgery. Arch Surg 2003;138:133–41.

Colorectal Surgery

Antonio M. Lacy, Homero Rivas, Salvadora Delgado

> ▶ **Key Controversies**
>
> A. Patient issues – are all patients candidates for laparoscopy?
> B. Pathology issues – benign versus malignant diseases.
> C. Surgeon issues – who should perform laparoscopic colorectal surgery?

28.1
Introduction

If one would want to debate about the existing controversies in laparo-scopic surgery, the use of minimal access surgery for the management of colorectal diseases will be the most controversial topic. More than a decade after the first laparoscopic colon resection was reported [1], there continues to be some reluctance to adopt minimal access techniques for the management of colorectal diseases.

To better understand the possible benefits or hazards of such approach, an equation, with three denominators being "patient – pathology – surgeon", may be useful. These different factors may be crucial to understand whether open or laparoscopic techniques would be ideal for the treatment of colorec-tal disorders. In general, the type of disease, benign or malignant, would be the cornerstone of major controversy.

28.2
Discussion

28.2.1
Patient Issues

There is little controversy that minimal access surgery in general offers many advantages to patients over conventional open techniques. Overall, there are several well-known benefits distinctive to laparoscopy such as a lower surgical trauma, less immunosuppression, faster recovery of pulmonary function, shorter length of stay, fewer postoperative complications, and better cosmetic results, among others. Some of these results appear more dramatic early after surgery.

Generally, minimal access techniques maintain the same principle of treatment, regardless of the pathology to treat, which is to utilize the least trauma necessary to perform an operative technique which otherwise may require a greater degree of surgical insult. In the case of colo-rectal resections, this may become substantial, and it results intuitive to believe that the use of laparoscopy would translate in similar or better results due to a lesser insult to the patient.

Indeed, patients may have similar outcomes with either approach, however as patients may have higher operative risks, the short-term benefits from laparoscopic surgery will become more evident [2]. Even when high-risk patients are more frequently excluded from laparoscopic surgery, paradoxically they may benefit the most from it. This is where the first denominator of the eluded equation takes place. Are all patients suited for laparoscopy? This is a point of great controversy, with a favorable answer to minimal access surgery.

Elderly, obese, transplant recipients, cirrhotic, among other high-risk patients, all have more associated comorbidities that may worsen more easily with the more trauma they may be exposed to [2–4]. All of these patients would have to tolerate an open procedure, which may render them with a more complex and lengthier postoperative period than the otherwise improved one of minimal access surgery. Our experience, along with several prospective and retrospective series, indicates that, indeed, high-risk patients receive greater advantages from laparoscopic surgery, and therefore they should not be excluded as part of contraindications of this type of surgery.

28.2.2
Pathology Issues

- Benign disease
    - Diverticular disease
    - Inflammatory bowel disease
    - Familial adenomatous polyposis syndromes
    - Rectal prolapse
    - Others
- Malignant disease
    - Colorectal cancer

The type of pathology represents the next denominator in the equation. There is a dichotomy into benign and malignant disorders. There is not much controversy regarding the use of laparoscopy for the management of benign colonic disease, and in fact, generally it is well accepted that experienced surgeons in advanced laparoscopic techniques may perform this type of surgery outside investigational clinical trials [5, 6]. At the present time, oncologic colon resections have been limited to open conventional techniques, and only less than 2% of colorectal malignances undergo laparoscopic assisted resection.

The most common benign conditions that have been managed with laparoscopic techniques include diverticular disease, inflammatory bowel disease, familial adenomatous polyposis, rectal prolapse, etc. [7–21]. The level of present evidence to base any benefit from laparoscopic surgery in benign colonic disease, is as limited as with any other surgical entity. Only a few prospective, randomized studies are available [15–18]; however, numerous independent series continue to report beneficial results inherent to laparoscopic techniques [7–14, 19–21]. This latter situation is the case of diverticular disease, where most of the available data is only retrospective. Indeed, when comparing this approach to open conventional techniques, the benefits appear to be relevant; however, there are no randomized controlled trial (RCTs) to probe such believes. Our institution is one of the expert centers of an ongoing Dutch RCT evaluating laparoscopic colon resections for diverticular disease. In general our experience and the preliminary results indicate a clear difference, with superiority of laparoscopy over conventional open techniques.

Initially, surgeons were reluctant to apply laparoscopic techniques to inflammatory bowel disease, and especially to Crohn's disease because of concerns over evaluating and excising inflamed tissue using laparoscopic methods [15]. These concerns rapidly vanished, soon after improved results from minimal access techniques were obtained at different centers. In spite of these results, there are only few RCTs that have evaluated this [15, 16], and most evidence is based on single institutional series [7–14]. In our view, laparoscopic surgery offers substantial benefits to patients with Crohn's disease when compared to open resections. Most affected patients start with the disease while being young, and the great majority of them (up to 75%) would require throughout their lives more than one surgical procedure. Opposite to what was initially believed, previous abdominal surgeries, presence of an abscess, phlegmon, or recurrent disease at the previous ileocolic anastomosis do not represent a contraindication for laparoscopic surgery, especially in this patient group [12, 14]. Many times, only very minimal incisions from laparoscopy may be necessary to resolve a problem. Also, in laparoscopic-assisted bowel resections, where a Pfannenstiel incision may be used, this would not only be attractive to the young population affected by Crohn's, but also such incision would preserve fresh tissue in the lower quadrants in the event that reoperation or stoma placement are required in the future owing to recurrent disease [7]. The improved body image and cosmesis results correlate strongly with a better quality of life after comparisons have been evaluated among patients with Crohn's undergoing laparoscopic versus open procedures [10].

This same phenomenon is seen with patients with ulcerative colitis [16, 19, 20], who may require extensive colectomies (subtotal or total colectomies). Restorative proctocolectomy with ileal pouch anal anastomosis is one of the most commonly used procedures for elective treatment of patients with mucosal ulcerative colitis and familial adenomatous polyposis. These multiquadrant surgical procedures would require extensive incisions, which otherwise may be avoided with the use of laparoscopic techniques. There is very little doubt of the great benefits laparoscopy has to offer to these patients, especially when some of the steps, such as creation of the ileal pouch, or the ileal pouch anal anastomosis, are performed by conventional open techniques [16, 20].

The main subject of controversy in laparoscopic colorectal surgery evolves around the management of oncologic disease. This surgery remains controversial since its beginning, mainly due to initial reports on port-site metastases emerging in an otherwise potentially curable disease [22, 23]. These reports caused major concern, and since then laparoscopic-assisted colectomies for cancer have been subject of intense investigation and at the present time, only less than 4% of colorectal malignances undergo laparoscopic- assisted resection [24–29].

Although studies with large numbers of patients now suggest that the incidence of port-site metastases (0.6–0.68%) [24–29] is comparable with the incidence of wound metastases in open surgery (~1%) [30–32], the pathogenesis of these recurrences remains unclear. Experimental studies and one randomized clinical trial indicate that laparoscopic surgery might even result in lower recurrence rates. In spite of this well founded evidence, this rare entity continues to be a concern and a topic of controversy, and is especially quoted by non-laparoscopic surgeons in an effort to ban laparoscopic bowel resections for colorectal cancer.

Several studies have suggested that laparoscopic assisted colectomies in patients with colon cancer are associated with lower surgical trauma, less immunosuppression, fewer postoperative complications, faster postoperative recovery, and also with a very low risk for wound metastasis [24–29]. In addition, some of them have shown that this approach does not compromise the number of resected lymph nodes or the margins of resection, as compared with the standard open colectomies.

We have completed the first prospective randomized trial comparing open conventional techniques and laparoscopy in colon cancer in terms of tumor recurrence and survival [24]. This study demonstrated improved 3-year cancer related survival following laparoscopic surgery compared to open surgery (91% versus 74%, respectively). The observed benefit could mainly be attributed to lower tumor recurrence and a longer overall survival of patients with stage III colonic cancer. We concluded that laparoscopic colectomy is preferred to open colectomy in patients with colonic cancer.

The improved survival experienced by stage III patients who underwent laparoscopic surgery could only be explained by different theories. Although unproven, these results may be arise from better preservation of immunological and physiological status after surgery due to a lesser surgical stress in patients who underwent laparoscopic-assisted resections [33–39]. In an experimental animal environment, data suggests that laparotomy is associated with significantly increased rates of tumor growth and metastasis formation. Open surgery suppress cell-mediated immunity more than laparoscopy in animal and human beings. The more immune-suppressed a patient may be after a surgical procedure, the higher the morbidity and mortality would be expected to be. Also, cancer response can be correlated with more immune-suppression [40]. A patient undergoing a laparoscopic procedure would likely experience less surgical stress, and therefore less immunosuppression, and a lesser cancer response, than someone who would have the same procedure done open. Results of our study have to be interpreted with great care because they represent a single institution experience with a relatively small number of patients. Results of large multicenter trials will have to be awaited. Interim analysis of these randomized trails has not shown significant differences of recurrence rate so far, as none of the trials have ceased including new patients for this reason.

Several ongoing randomized trials will report their results in the near future: COST (USA trial), COLOR (European trail), CLASSIC (UK trial) and an Australian trial. Should the rest of these trials confirm these results, then there will be different subjects of debate such as whether technical issues involved in laparoscopic surgery may contribute or not to better outcomes. We foresee that laparoscopic surgery for rectal cancer will mimic the results that are being experienced in colon cancer. Also, new techniques such as robot-assisted surgery and intraoperative enhanced imaging will contribute a great deal to the management of colorectal cancer in the near future.

28.2.3
Surgeon Issues

Lastly, but of quintessential importance, is the controversy of who would be the best type of surgeon to perform these procedures. This problem may have no right answer, since either general laparoscopic surgeons or trained colorectal surgeons should not be excluded, and, ideally if possible, they both should work in integrated teams. Interestingly, up to now, most large colorectal laparoscopic series have been published by general surgeons with great expertise in minimal access surgery [24, 25, 28, 29].

Laparoscopic colorectal surgery requires advanced skills in minimal access surgery. As opposed to other types of laparoscopic procedures, it often involves multiple abdominal quadrants. When performing these operations it is crucial to follow well-organized steps, especially in the case of oncological procedures, where further considerations should be taken. It has been suggested that standardization of these procedures would be beneficial for their widespread acceptance [41].

We believe these procedures are safe under experienced hands, and their results to be reproducible; however a steep learning curve is required. Surgeons who would engage in these type of procedures should be experienced in open colorectal resections, and if their background in minimal access surgery is limited, they should master their laparoscopic dexterity in the animal or cadaveric laboratory before experiencing it in the operating room [5, 41, 42]. Opposite to what is advised, we believe that the new laparoscopic colorectal surgeon may find complicated diverticular disease much more difficult to treat laparoscopically than even non-metastatic colon cancer. A prudent approach should always be taken with a proper patient selection, especially early in the learning curve.

Should the rest of ongoing trials confirm that laparoscopic surgery for colon cancer is an adequate cancer operation compared with open procedures, this will encourage the medical community to include eligible candidates outside clinical trials for laparoscopic-assisted colectomies. This, in addition to well informed patients demanding more minimally invasive procedures, will inevitably multiply the already great need for surgeons performing these techniques.

In an effort to avoid the scenario of inexperienced surgeons being pressured by the patient demand and driven by market forces, it is essential to integrate even more, the training of advanced minimal access techniques, not only in colorectal and laparoscopic fellowships, but especially in general surgery residency programs. Also credentialing must be taken seriously and an inexperienced start to "try out" the procedure without adequate training or proctoring must be avoided.

28.3
Summary

— Laparoscopic colorectal surgery remains controversial. More and more evidence indicates that minimal access surgery is safe and may offer more benefits than those foreseen initially.
— The numerous well-known advantages of laparoscopy are shared by laparoscopic colon resections of benign disease, and there is well-founded evidence that this would include as well colorectal cancer.
— For oncological disease, the initial results seem promising, and may prove to give better survival outcomes unique to laparoscopy. This could be a result of a preserved immunity due to minimal levels of surgical stress.
— Colorectal surgery requires advanced laparoscopic techniques, complex in nature, which may only be attained after a steep learning curve. The results of laparoscopic surgery are however reproducible under experienced laparoscopic surgeons.
— There is very little doubt, that in the near future, open conventional techniques may appear as a thing of the past, and new motives of controversy will arise.

References

1. Jacobs M, Verdeja JC, Goldstein HS. Minimally invasive colon resection (laparoscopic colectomy). Surg Laparosc Endosc 1991;1:144–50.
2. Delgado S, Lacy AM, Garcia Valdecasas JC, Balague C, Pera M, Salvador L, Momblan D, Visa J. Could age be an indication for laparoscopic colectomy in colorectal cancer? Surg Endosc 2000;14:22–6.
3. Detry O, Defraigne JO, Chiche JD, Meurisse M, Joris J, Honore P, Jacquet N, Limet R. Laparoscopic-assisted colectomy in heart transplant recipients. Clin Transplant 1996;10:191–4.
4. Yeh CN, Chen MF, Jan YY. Laparoscopic cholecystectomy in 226 cirrhotic patients. Experience of a single center in Taiwan. Surg Endosc 2002;16:1583–7.
5. Young-Fadok TM. Raising the bar. Laparoscopic resection of colorectal cancer. Surg Endosc 2001;15:911–2.
6. Ortega AE, Beart RW, Steele GD, Winchester DP, Greene FL. Laparoscopic bowel surgery registry: preliminary results. Dis Colon Rect 1995;38:681–685.
7. Greene AK, Michetti P, Peppercorn MA, Hodin RA. Laparoscopically assisted ileocolectomy for Crohn's disease through a Pfannenstiel incision. Am J Surg 2000;180:238–40.
8. Bemelman WA, Slors JF, Dunker MS, van Hogezand RA, van Deventer SJ, Ringers J, Griffioen G, Gouma DJ. Laparoscopic-assisted vs. open ileocolic resection for Crohn's disease. A comparative study. Surg Endosc 2000;14:721–5.

9. Alabaz O, Iroatulam AJ, Nessim A, Weiss EG, Nogueras JJ, Wexner SD. Comparison of laparoscopically assisted and conventional ileocolic resection for Crohn's disease. Eur J Surg 2000;166:213–7.

10. Dunker MS, Stiggelbout AM, van Hogezand RA, Ringers J, Griffioen G, Bemelman WA. Cosmesis and body image after laparoscopic-assisted and open ileocolic resection for Crohn's disease. Surg Endosc 1998;12:1334–40.

11. Shore G, Gonzalez QH, Bondora A, Vickers SM. Laparoscopic vs conventional ileocolectomy for primary Crohn disease. Arch Surg 2003;138:76–9.

12. Evans J, Poritz L, MacRae H. Influence of experience on laparoscopic ileocolic resection for Crohn's disease. Dis Colon Rectum 2002;45:1595–600.

13. Canin-Endres J, Salky B, Gattorno F, Edye M. Laparoscopically assisted intestinal resection in 88 patients with Crohn's disease. Surg Endosc 1999;13:595–9.

14. Wu JS, Birnbaum EH, Kodner IJ, Fry RD, Read TE, Fleshman JW. Laparoscopic-assisted ileocolic resections in patients with Crohn's disease: are abscesses, phlegmons, or recurrent disease contraindications? Surgery 1997;122:682–8.

15. Milsom JW, Hammerhofer KA, Bohm B, Marcello P, Elson P, Fazio VW. Prospective, randomized trial comparing laparoscopic vs. conventional surgery for refractory ileocolic Crohn's disease. Dis Colon Rectum 2001;44:1–8.

16. Marcello PW, Milsom JW, Wong SK, Hammerhofer KA, Goormastic M, Church JM, Fazio VW. Laparoscopic restorative proctocolectomy: case-matched comparative study with open restorative proctocolectomy. Dis Colon Rectum 2000;43:604–8.

17. Braga M, Vignali A, Gianotti L, Zuliani W, Radaelli G, Gruarin P, Dellabona P, Di Carlo V. Laparoscopic versus open colorectal surgery: a randomized trial on short-term outcome. Ann Surg 2002;236:759–67.

18. Solomon MJ, Young CJ, Eyers AA, Roberts RA. Randomized clinical trial of laparoscopic versus open abdominal rectopexy for rectal prolapse. Br J Surg 2002;89:35–9.

19. Garbus JE, Potenti F, Wexner SD. Current controversies in pouch surgery. South Med J 2003;96:32–6.

20. Schmitt SL, Cohen SM, Wexner SD, Nogueras JJ, Jagelman DG. Does laparoscopic-assisted ileal pouch anal anastomosis reduce the length of hospitalization? Int J Colorectal Dis 1994;9:134–7.

21. Dwivedi A, Chahin F, Agrawal S, Chau WY, Tootla A, Tootla F, Silva YJ. Laparoscopic colectomy vs. open colectomy for sigmoid diverticular disease. Dis Colon Rectum 2002;45:1309–14.

22. Alexander RJ, Jaques BC, Mitchell KG. Laparoscopically assisted colectomy and wound recurrence. Lancet 1993;341:249–50.

23. Berends FJ, Kazemier G, Bonjer HJ, Lange JF, Subcutaneous metastases after laparoscopic colectomy. Lancet 1994;344:58.

24. Lacy AM, Garcia-Valdecasas JC, Delgado S, Castells A, Taura P, Pique JM, Visa J. Laparoscopy-assisted colectomy versus open colectomy for treatment of non-metastatic colon cancer: a randomised trial. Lancet 2002;359:2224–9.

25. Hazebroek EJ; COLOR Study Group. COLOR: a randomized clinical trial comparing laparoscopic and open resection for colon cancer. Surg Endosc 2002;16:949–53.

26. Weeks JC, Nelson H, Gelber S, Sargent D, Schroeder G; Clinical Outcomes of Surgical Therapy (COST) Study Group. Short-term quality-of-life outcomes following laparoscopic-assisted colectomy vs open colectomy for colon cancer: a randomized trial. JAMA 2002;287:321–8.

27. Milsom JW, Bohm B, Hammerhofer KA, Fazio V, Steiger E, Elson P. A prospective randomized trial comparing laparoscopic versus conventional techniques in colorectal cancer surgery: a preliminary report. J Am Coll Surg 1998;187:46–54.

28. Poulin EC, Mamazza J, Schlachta CM, Gregoire R, Roy N. Laparoscopic resection does not adversely affect early survival curves in patients undergoing surgery for colorectal adenocarcinoma. Ann Surg 1999;229:487–92.

29. Franklin ME, Kazantsev B, Abrego D, Diaz EJ, Balli J, Glass L. Laparoscopic surgery for stage III colon cancer: long term follow up. Surg Endosc 2000;14:612–6.

30. Reilly WT, Nelson H, Schroeder G, Wieand HS, Bolton J, O'Connell MJ. Wound recurrence following conventional treatment of colorectal cancer. Dis Colon Rectum 1996;39:200–7.

31. Hughes ESR, McDermott FT, Polglase AL, Johnson WR. Tumor recurrence in the abdominal wall scar after large bowel cancer surgery. Dis Colon Rectum 1983;26:571–2.

32. Hoffman G, Baker J, Fitchett C, Vansant J. Laparoscopic-assisted colectomy. Initial experience. Ann Surg 1994;219:732–43.

33. Allendorf JD, Bessler M, Horvath KD, Marvin MR, Laird DA, Whelan RL. Increased tumor establishment and growth after open vs laparoscopic surgery in mice may be related to differences in postoperative T-cell function. Surg Endosc 1999;13:233–5.

34. Allendorf JD, Bessler M, Kayton ML, Oesterling SD, Treat MR, Nowygrod R, Whelan RL. Increased tumor establishment and growth after laparotomy vs laparoscopy in a murine model. Arch Surg 1995;130:649–53.

35. Bouvy ND, Marquet RL, Jeekel J, Bonjer HJ. Laparoscopic surgery is associated with less tumor growth stimulation than conventional surgery: an experimental study. Br J Surg 1998;84:358–61.

36. DaCosta ML, Redmond HP, Finnegan N, Flynn M, Bouchier-Hayes D. Laparatomy and laparoscopy differentially accelerate experimental flank tumor growth. Br J Surg 1988;85:1439–42.

37. Delgado S, Lacy AM, Filella X, Castells A, Garcia-Valdecasas JC, Pique JM, Momblan D, Visa J. Acute phase response in laparoscopic and open colectomy in colon cancer: randomized study. Dis Colon Rectum 2001;44:638–46.

38. Vittimberga FJ Jr, Foley DP, Meyers WC, Callery MP. Laparoscopic surgery and the systemic immune response. Ann Surg 1998;227:326–34.

39. Whelan RL. Laparotomy, laparoscopy, cancer, and beyond. Surg Endosc 2001;15:110–5.

40. Cole WH. The increase in immunosuppression and its role in the development of malignant lesions. J Surg Oncol 1985;30:139–44.

41. Greene FL. Standard setting for laparoscopic resection of colorectal cancer. Surg Endosc 2001;15:109.

42. Schlachta CM, Mamazza J, Seshadri PA, Cadeddu M, Gregoire R, Poulin EC. Defining a learning curve for laparoscopic colorectal resections. Dis Colon Rectum 2001;44:217–22.

Commentary

PER-OLOF NYSTRÖM

New techniques and new ideas in surgery can be rated by their capacity for change. The change may be measured according to whether the new method is easier, faster and cheaper, or provides a better result. To be different the new method must make a difference that can be observed in the overall result. It means that the advantage of the new method applies not only to a small segment of the patients with a particular diagnosis but to sufficiently large numbers that the benefit will improve the overall result. I will rate laparoscopic colorectal surgery accordingly.

In the chapter by Drs. Lacy, Rivas and Delgado, an "inside" view to gauge the merit of minimal invasive surgery is applied. They use three denominators, viz., the patient, the pathology, and the surgeon. It is claimed that because the trauma is less with the minimal invasive method patients are likely to gain from the smaller operation. The controversy is whether all patients are suited for laparoscopy. Here they claim that most patients are suitable and those with limited physiological reserves or more comorbidities are indeed the true beneficiaries of the lesser surgical trauma. With respect to pathology it is claimed that there is little controversy about benign pathology but the controversy is with colorectal cancer. The surgeon should be an expert with the tools used for the operation and knowledgeable about the pathology and anatomy. This applies, of course, to both open and laparoscopic surgery. The difficulty here is the availability of suitable cases to train colorectal surgeons to become expert in using the laparoscopic instruments. That difficulty becomes acute with the authors statement that no more than 2–4% of colonic cancers are currently operated with laparoscopic technique.

Why Are Closed and Open Operations any Different?

This question needs to be repeatedly asked because if an element of one technique is superior then that element should be transferred to the technique of the other. Such an outset assumes that neither technique has reached its peak performance. The only difference in the end would be that the operation is performed through the ports in closed operations but through the coeliotomy in the open operation. The same instruments and methods for dissection, resection and anastomosis would apply equally. Only then would it be possible to identify if the closed method has advantages that surpass the open operation [1]. It might even be possible to find out whether it is the type of surgeon that makes the difference.

We attempted such an approach for right and left colectomy for cancer, having the same surgeons perform both techniques. The essential result was an important but similar reduction of the operation time for both the open and closed operation. The open operation remained about 45 min faster but the operation time for the closed operation became identical to the historical open operation time.

Is Minimal Invasive Surgery Easier?

Once the instrumentation and the steps of the operation have been mastered, it is the particular pathology and anatomy that determines the ease of the operation. The overall situation is that the open operation will be successfully completed in nearly every case while the closed operation will increasingly fail with increasing proportions attempted. The relationship is not linear but appears to be exponential and asymptotically approaches 100% failure at some point of complex anatomy [2]. To some extent the point of conversion reflects the surgeon's skill and experience in what is generally referred to as the learning curve [3, 4].

Patient selection is the key to successful colorectal laparoscopic surgery. Patients with smaller, mobile tumors are preferred, and those with palpable tumors or scarred abdomens are avoided. We adopted a simple guiding rule, meaning that once the ports had been placed and the camera inserted we should be able to identify the tumor, the distal and proximal resection margins and the origin of the vascular pedicle. In such cases the completeness of the laparoscopic operation was certain while the failure rate increased sharply with each missing observation. Completeness means that all intended steps of the operation were accomplished through the ports with no need for additional mobilization through the coeliotomy.

Is Minimal Invasive Surgery Faster?

It is the dissection and resection parts of the closed operation that are more difficult and therefore take longer time. In our measurements, the time needed for those parts of the colectomy for cancer is about double that of the open operation when comparing operations rated by the surgeon as of average complexity or simpler. It is a general observation that resection of bowel, as in cancer, diverticulitis or Crohn's disease, needs longer time with the laparoscopic method. For extensive resection, such as total colectomy for ulcerative colitis, or restorative proctectomy, the operation time is substantially prolonged and may approach twice that needed for the open counterpart [5–8].

Long operations for the same diagnosis are often associated with worse outcome. This is easily understood as the prolonged operation usually marks a more severe anatomical complexity and hence a greater surgical trauma. It is an interesting thought that the potential benefit of minimal invasive surgery may be abrogated by minimal duration open surgery.

Is Minimal Invasive Surgery Cheaper?

The closed operation needs more expensive instruments and takes longer time to complete. The extra cost incurred is expected to be counterbalanced by the lesser trauma that makes up for a shorter hospital stay and convalescence. The calculations usually incorporate only the direct costs to the hospital. A requisite for an even balance, or gain with the closed operation, is the earlier discharge [9]. The expense for the instruments is real while the gain in the hospital stay is fictive as long as the beds and staff are not reduced or productivity can be increased.

In a Swedish sub-protocol to the COLOR trial the total cost incurred to society with both the laparoscopic and open operations was measured in 210 patients equally randomized to either operation. Ten hospitals participated in this study, which attempted to measure total costs up to 3 months postoperatively. As expected the operating room cost for the closed operation was substantially higher but also the hospital cost exceeded the cost for an open operation. Reasons for this were the similar hospital stay (9 days) and the reoperation rate was higher in the laparoscopic group. The total costs to society at 3 months remained nominally higher for the closed operation but were no longer statistically different [10]. Henrik Kehlet in Copenhagen conducted a randomized study of segmental colectomy blinding the ward staff to the operative method and using his accelerated recovery program. Median hospital stay was 2 days in both operations (Kehlet, personal communication 2004). Such carefully conducted prospective studies question perceptions of an overall cheaper closed operation.

Is the Result Better with Minimal Invasive Surgery?

Dr Lacy and co-authors find that the result can be better in some operations. The main interest is centered on outcome in cancer surgery. The Barcelona group reported that stage III colorectal cancer had a better survival after the laparoscopic operation. Recently the result of the COST study was published and showed similar rate of recurrence and no survival benefit after laparoscopic surgery, neither overall nor for stage III cancer [11]. A meta-analysis of the 3-year disease-free survival from the three main multicenter trials (COLOR, CLASSIC and COST trials) is underway to confirm or refute the survival benefit of minimal invasive surgery for colorectal cancer.

There is little doubt that minimal invasive surgery provides benefits in some respects to some patients as outlined in the chapter. I raise the question of whether these benefits are big enough and can be conferred on sufficiently large numbers of patients with colorectal disease to change the overall result. A better result became evident for laparoscopic cholecystectomy with 70–80% penetration but remains uncertain for laparoscopic colorectal surgery with much lesser penetration [12]. In hospitals under severe cost restraints it is also uncertain if young surgeons can achieve expertise in minimal invasive colorectal surgery.

Summary

The conclusion is firm that minimal invasive surgery for colorectal disease is not easier, not faster, probably not cheaper and the improvement of the overall result is not obvious. It is my impression that laparoscopic colorectal surgery is no longer industry driven, not even patient driven, but remains active in a small number of hospitals. Minimal invasive surgery as a new concept certainly boosted interest in surgical technique and conduct of operations. Maybe open surgery has improved to the extent that the difference has become too small to be measured.

References

1. Mathur P, Seow-Choen F. The difference between laparoscopic and keyhole surgery. Br J Surg 2003;90:1029–30.
2. Vargas HD, Ramirez RT, Hoffman GC, Hubbard GW, Gould RJ, Wohlgemuth SD, et al. Defining the role of laparoscopic-assisted sigmoid colectomy for diverticulitis. Dis Colon Rectum 2000;43:1726–31.
3. Schlachta CM, Mamazza J, Seshadri PA, Cadeddu M, Gregoire R, Poulin EC. Defining a learning curve for laparoscopic colorectal resections. Dis Colon Rectum 2001;44:217–22.
4. Gervaz P, Pikarsky A, Utech M, Secic M, Efron J, Belin B, et al. Converted laparoscopic colorectal surgery: a meta-analysis. Surg Endosc 2001;15:827–32.
5. Dunker MS, Bemelman WA, Slors JF, van Hogezand RA, Ringers J, Gouma DJ. Laparoscopic-assisted vs open colectomy for severe acute colitis in patients with inflammatory bowel disease (IBD): a retrospective study in 42 patients. Surg Endosc 2000;14:911–4.
6. Seshadri PA, Poulin EC, Schlachta CM, Cadeddu MO, Mamazza J. Does a laparoscopic approach to total abdominal colectomy and proctocolectomy offer advantages? Surg Endosc 2001;15:837–42.

7. Hasegawa H, Watanabe M, Baba H, Nishibori H, Kitajima M. Laparoscopic restorative proctocolectomy for patients with ulcerative colitis. J Laparoendosc Adv Surg Tech A 2002;12:403–6.

8. Marcello PW, Milsom JW, Wong SK, Brady K, Goormastic M, Fazio VW. Laparoscopic total colectomy for acute colitis: a case-control study. Dis Colon Rectum 2001;44:1441–5.

9. Delaney CP, Kiran RP, Senagore AJ, Brady K, Fazio VW. Case-matched comparison of clinical and financial outcome after laparoscopic or open colorectal surgery. Ann Surg 2003;238:67–72.

10. Jansson M, Björkholt I, Carlsson P, Haglind E, Henriksson M, Lindholm E, et al. Randomized clinical trial of the costs of open and laparoscopic surgery for colonic cancer. Br J Surg 2004;91:409–17.

11. The Clinical Outcomes of Surgical Therapy Study Group (COST). A comparison of laparoscopically assisted and open colectomy for colon cancer. N Engl J Med 2004;350:2050–9.

12. Mavrantonis C, Wexner SD, Nogueras JJ, Weiss EG, Potenti F, Pikarsky AJ. Current attitudes in laparoscopic colorectal surgery. Surg Endosc 2002;16:1152–7.

29

Appendectomy

David R. Urbach

▶ **Key Controversies**

A. Is laparoscopic appendectomy "better" than open appendectomy?
B. Does the use of laparoscopic appendectomy affect the risk of surgical infection?
C. Should a laparoscopic appendectomy be done for a perforated appendix?
D. Should the appendix be ligated or stapled during a laparoscopic appendectomy?
E. Should a normal-appearing appendix be removed during a laparoscopic appendectomy for suspected appendicitis?
F. Should laparoscopic appendectomy be done in pregnant women?

29.1
Introduction

Acute appendicitis is a common disease in North America, with an annual incidence of approximately 250,000 cases in the USA, accounting for an estimated 1 million days of hospitalization per year. Appendicitis is most common in the second decade of life, and is 40% more common in males than in females [1]. The diagnosis of acute appendicitis is frequently difficult, especially in young women [2]. Recent increases in the use of diagnostic modalities such as abdominal ultrasonography and computed tomography [3] do not appear to have improved the diagnostic accuracy of appendicitis at the population level [4]. The use of laparoscopic appendectomy varies considerably in North America. In fact, the most important determinant of whether an open or laparoscopic appendectomy is done appears to be the preference of the surgeon who treats the patient [5]. There are several important controversies regarding the use of laparoscopic appendectomy. These include the issues discussed below.

29.2
Discussion

29.2.1
Is Laparoscopic Appendectomy "Better" than Open Appendectomy?

Whether or not laparoscopic appendectomy is "better" than open appendectomy depends on what outcome measure is being compared. Various outcomes can be assessed: resource consumption measures, such as duration of the operation and the cost of hospitalization, and postoperative recovery measures, such as the length of the hospital stay, the time to return to activity, and postoperative pain. Many randomized controlled trials comparing laparoscopic with open appendectomy with respect to one or more of these measures have been published.

The Cochrane Library published a systematic review of randomized controlled trials comparing laparoscopic with open appendectomy in 2003 [6]. Although there was substantial heterogeneity in outcome measures between some of the trials, this meta-analysis provides the best synthesis of the literature available to date. Overall health resource consumption was similar for laparoscopic and open appendectomy. Although open appendectomy tended to have a shorter duration of surgery (by 14.3 min, 95% confidence interval 9.9–18.8) and decreased cost for the operation, there was little difference in cost associated with the hospital stay, presumably due to a reduction in the duration of hospitalization for patients having laparoscopic appendectomy. Laparoscopic appendectomy was superior to open appendectomy in regard to measures of postoperative recovery, such as pain reduction on a 10 cm visual-analogue scale (by 0.8 cm, 95% confidence interval 1.3–0.3), shorter length of hospital stay (by 0.7 days, 95% confidence interval 1.0–0.4), and reduced time to return to normal activity (by 6.0 days, 95% confidence interval 7.8–4.2).

Although the randomized controlled trials comparing laparoscopic and open appendectomy are plagued by several biases, and it is difficult to interpret the importance of some outcome measures (such as pain on the visual-analogue scale), they represent the best evidence currently available. At this time it appears that laparoscopic appendectomy has a small but important benefit over open appendectomy for postoperative recovery, with no associated overall increase in health resource use.

29.2.2
Does the Use of Laparoscopic Appendectomy Affect the Risk of Surgical Infection?

One of the principal advantages of laparoscopy over open surgery is the decreased incidence of wound complications after laparoscopy [7]. This is of special importance in the case of appendectomy, where postoperative surgical site infection accounts for a substantial burden of postoperative complications [8]. As compared with conventional surgery, the smaller incisions used for laparoscopic surgery reduce the exposure of subcutaneous tissues to contaminated intra-abdominal contents. In contrast, the use of pneumoperitoneum, dependent positioning, and increased duration of surgery with laparoscopic appendectomy, may increase the risk of developing intra-abdominal infection as compared with that of open surgery [9].

Many published randomized controlled trials have compared open and laparoscopic appendectomy with respect to surgical infection. The Cochrane systematic review of 34 trials found a substantial reduction in the risk of wound infection with laparoscopic appendectomy (pooled odds ratio 0.47, 95% confidence interval 0.36–0.62), and an increase in the risk of abdominal abscess (pooled odds ratio 2.77, 95% confidence interval 1.61–4.77) [6].

Do the conflicting effects on surgical site infection and intra-abdominal infection found in meta-analyses cancel each other out? I do not believe so. First, among the clinical trials, the prevalence of wound infection (5.7%) was much greater than abdominal abscesses (1.2%). Use of laparoscopic surgery would be expected to prevent more surgical site infections than it would promote intra-abdominal infections. Second, the modern management of intra-abdominal infection, including percutaneous abscess drainage and the use of effective antibiotics, has substantially reduced the morbidity of abdominal abscess after appendectomy [10]. Finally, the pooled analysis was highly influenced by one large study [10] that accounted for 30% of all the intra-abdominal abscesses, and included more subjects with gangrenous or perforated appendix in the laparoscopic group than in the open group (130 versus 100 subjects).

29.2.3
Should a Laparoscopic Appendectomy Be Done for a Perforated Appendix?

While many patients are found to have a perforated appendix only after the peritoneal cavity has been examined by laparoscopy or open exploration, some have preoperative evidence that is highly suggestive of gross perforation, such as generalized peritonitis, signs of the systemic inflammatory response syndrome, or radiological findings [11] suggesting gross perforation. When a surgeon has a high suspicion that a patient already has a perforated appendix, is it appropriate to proceed with laparoscopic appendectomy?

The increased risk of abdominal abscess associated with laparoscopic appendectomy principally occurs if there is appendiceal perforation [10] (the status of the appendix – perforated or non-perforated – provides a nice example of a biologic "interaction," where the risk of postoperative abscess associated with laparoscopic appendectomy varies according to whether the appendix is perforated or not). In light of this, I believe that some consideration should be given to avoiding laparoscopy in these patients. In the presence of gross perforation and generalized peritonitis, it is desirable to minimize the operative time, and peritoneal toilet may be more effective with open surgery than with laparoscopy. Further, in contrast to a patient with simple appendicitis, the recovery of a patient with gross peritonitis depends more on the resolution of the intra-abdominal process than the effect of the abdominal wall incision. Patients with perforation have a longer length of hospital stay regardless of whether laparoscopy is used [12].

Having said that, when a perforated appendix is discovered unexpectedly during a laparoscopic appendectomy, the surgeon should certainly complete the operation laparoscopically if feasible, and not "convert" to an open operation. Also, eschewing laparoscopic appendectomy in patients suspected of having a gross perforation would not confer the benefit of a reduced risk of wound infection associated with laparoscopy.

29.2.4
Should a Normal-Appearing Appendix Be Removed During a Laparoscopic Appendectomy for Suspected Appendicitis?

Since a normal-appearing appendix will occasionally be identified during laparoscopic appendectomy (including up to 45% of cases in young women) [1], a surgeon should be prepared for dealing with this situation. Historically, surgeons have removed normal-appearing appendices during open appendectomy, on the assumption that physicians would assume that a patient with a right-lower quadrant incision has already had his or her appendix removed, and miss the diagnosis of appendicitis should it occur in the future. Since port-site incisions may not be interpreted as evidence of prior appendectomy, the use of laparoscopic appendectomy potentially alters this approach, and the question of whether the normal-appearing appendix should be removed at laparoscopic appendectomy has become controversial.

In some cases, there is obvious evidence of a pathologic process other than appendicitis that can explain the patient's presentation, such as acute sigmoid diverticulitis, inflammation of an epiploic appendage, pelvic inflammatory disease, endometriosis, or ovarian torsion. In these cases, the operation should be modified in light of the unexpected findings (in some circumstances, this includes conversion to a laparotomy). Appendectomy is unnecessary in most of these circumstances.

A more difficult decision arises when another cause of pain is not obvious at laparoscopy, or when there is uncertainty as to whether or not the appendix is actually diseased. In some cases of viral gastroenteritis or mesenteric adenitis, there may be free intra-abdominal fluid, mild vascular congestion and hyperemia of the appendiceal wall, and thickening of the mesentery in the ileocecal region that may arouse suspicion that the appendix is in fact inflamed. My preference is to complete a laparoscopic appendectomy in the absence of another explanation for abdominal pain, for several reasons. There may be pathologic inflammation even if the appendix appears grossly normal [13]. Adequate inspection of the appendix often requires substantial dissection and mobilization, which may cause some trauma and make it inadvisable to leave the appendix *in situ*. To adequately examine the appendix, the placement of additional trocars has usually already been done to facilitate manipulation, countering the argument that avoiding appendectomy makes additional port-site incisions unnecessary. Appendectomy for a normal appendix is usually a quick and uncomplicated operation [14]. Finally, in the absence of a plausible explanation for the presentation of a patient with suspected appendicitis at laparoscopic exploration, patients may continue to have similar episodes of pain in the future, with the same diagnostic uncertainty if an appendectomy is not performed. In one study, 7 of 44 patients (16%) with a normal appendix not removed at laparoscopy returned to the emergency department because of recurrent abdominal pain after a median time of 8 months [15].

29.2.5
Should the Appendix Be Ligated or Stapled During a Laparoscopic Appendectomy?

There are two ways of dividing and ligating the base of the appendix: division with a linear cutting stapler, or ligation with a ligature device (such as an Endo-loop). The principal advantage of using a stapler instead of loop ligation is the ability to divide the appendiceal mesentery and appendix in a single maneuver, even in the presence of severe inflammation and thickening of the mesoappendix. The principal disadvantages of a stapler include the increased cost and the requirement of a larger trocar site. A randomized trial comparing stapled and ligated appendectomy found that the operative time was the same regardless of whether a stapler or ligature was used [16]. An interesting (and still unexplained) finding of this trial was the observation that ligated appendectomy was associated with a higher incidence of vomiting and ileus than was stapled appendectomy.

Several considerations may guide the choice of method for appendiceal division. Because an uninflamed appendix is so easily devascularized and divided with endo-loops, the added expense of a linear stapler likely does not justify its use in most instances where a normal appendix is removed. However, in the presence of severe inflammation, thickening of the mesoappendix and appendiceal base, use of a stapler can greatly facilitate the operation. Care should be taken to ensure hemostasis in the stapled appendiceal mesentery (especially if a vascular cartridge is not used), and that important structures such as the terminal ileum, right ureter, or gonadal vessels are not included in the jaws of the stapler. When there is inflammation of the base of the appendix and cecum, careful application of the stapler across the uninvolved cecum (taking care to avoid narrowing of the ileocecal valve) may provide more reliable management of the appendiceal stump.

29.2.6
Should Laparoscopic Appendectomy Be Done in Pregnant Women?

Pregnant women with acute abdominal conditions are at risk for fetal loss through spontaneous abortion in the first trimester, and premature labor in the third trimester [17]. While abdominal surgery in pregnant women should be deferred until after the pregnancy whenever possible, acute appendicitis is an emergency that requires urgent surgical intervention, and delay in treatment resulting in appendiceal perforation and intra abdominal infection may have catastrophic consequences.

Concerns were raised early about the safety of laparoscopic surgery in pregnancy due to the potential effects of pneumoperitoneum and increased intra-abdominal pressure on uterine blood flow, fetal acidosis, and the risk of uterine injury from peritoneal access and trocar placement [18]. Subsequent case reports from a variety of centers have suggested that laparoscopic appendectomy can be done in pregnant women, with a low incidence of fetal loss [19–21]. It is important to recognize that there is almost certainly a strong publication bias in favor of studies supporting the safety of laparoscopic appendectomy in pregnancy. In the absence of long-term prospective studies, surgeons should be judicious in the use of laparoscopic appendectomy in pregnancy. During the informed consent process, it is especially important for surgeons to emphasize the potential risks of laparoscopic surgery to the pregnancy, since the risk of adverse pregnancy outcomes with an acute abdomen is high regardless of the underlying disease process and therapeutic approach [17]. For example, some women with suspected appendicitis in pregnancy will have an unappreciated small placental abruption. Not only will these women have a "normal" appendix, but they also have a high likelihood of fetal loss.

I believe that laparoscopy is a reasonable approach in pregnant women with suspected appendicitis, with several caveats and modifications in technique. An obstetrical consultation should be obtained to exclude obstetric causes of acute abdominal pain, and to guide appropriate fetal and maternal monitoring. An open technique of peritoneal access should be used, especially after the first trimester, because of the risk of uterine puncture with a Veress needle [22]. Laparoscopy may not be feasible at all in the presence of a grossly enlarged uterus in the third trimester of pregnancy. To minimize the risk of decreased uterine blood flow and fetal hypercarbia, pneumoperitoneum pressures should be kept as low as possible. In light of the increased risk of thromboembolic disease in pregnancy, prophylaxis of deep venous thrombosis should be used.

29.3
Summary

— Based on the available evidence, laparoscopic appendectomy has several important advantages over open appendectomy. Laparoscopic appendectomy is well tolerated by patients, is not associated with increased overall cost, and reduces the risk of postoperative wound infection.
— The risk of postoperative intra-abdominal abscess may be higher after laparoscopic appendectomy in the setting of appendiceal perforation.
— In most cases, a normal appendix that is identified at laparoscopic appendectomy for suspected appendicitis should be removed.
— Caution should be exercised in the use of laparoscopic appendectomy in pregnant women and in patients who present with clear evidence of gross perforation.

References

1.   Addiss DG, Shaffer N, Fowler BS, Tauxe RV. The epidemiology of appendicitis and appendectomy in the United States. Am J Epidemiol 1990;132:910–25.
2.   Wen SW, Naylor CD. Diagnostic accuracy and short-term surgical outcomes in cases of suspected acute appendicitis. CMAJ 1995;152:1617–26.
3.   Rao PM, Rhea JT, Novelline RA, Mostafavi AA, McCabe CJ. Effect of computed tomography of the appendix on treatment of patients and use of hospital resources. N Engl J Med 1998;338:141–6.

4. Flum DR, Morris A, Koepsell T, Dellinger EP. Has misdiagnosis of appendicitis decreased over time? A population-based analysis. JAMA 2001;286:1748–53.

5. Cervini P, Smith LC, Urbach DR. The surgeon on call is a strong factor determining the use of a laparoscopic approach for appendectomy. Surg Endosc 2002;16:1774–7.

6. Sauerland S, Lefering R, Neugebauer EAM. Laparoscopic versus open surgery for suspected appendicitis (Cochrane Review). In: The Cochrane Library, Issue 1, 2003. Oxford: Update Software, 2003.

7. Holzman MD, Purut CM, Reintgen K, Eubanks S, Pappas TS. Laparoscopic ventral and incisional hernioplasty. Surg Endosc 1997;11:32–5.

8. Andersen BR, Kallehave FL, Andersen HK. Antibiotics versus placebo for prevention of postoperative infection after appendectomy. Cochrane Database Syst Rev 2001;3: CD001439.

9. Balague Ponz C, Trias M. Laparoscopic surgery and surgical infection. J Chemother 2001;13 Spec No 1:17–22.

10. Pedersen AG, Petersen OB, Wara P, et al. Randomised controlled trial of laparoscopic versus open appendicectomy. Br J Surg 2001;88:200–5.

11. Horrow MM, White DS, Horrow JC. Differentiation of perforated from nonperforated appendicitis on CT. Radiology 2003;227:45–51.

12. Piskun G, Kozik D, Rajpal S, Shaftan G, Fogler R. Comparison of laparoscopic, open, and converted appendectomy for perforated appendicitis. Surg Endosc 2001;15:660–2.

13. Grunewald B, Keating J. Should the 'normal' appendix be removed at operation for appendicitis? J R Coll Surg Edinb 1993;38:158–60.

14. Greason KL, Rappold JF, Liberman MA. Incidental laparoscopic appendectomy for acute right lower quadrant abdominal pain. Its time has come. Surg Endosc 1998;12:223–5.

15. van den Broek WT, Bijnen AB, De Ruiter P, Gouma DJ. A normal appendix found during laparoscopic appendectomy should not be removed. Br J Surg 2001;88:251–4.

16. Ortega AE, Hunter JG, Peters JH, Swanstrom LL, Schirmer B; Laparoscopic Appendectomy Study Group. A prospective, randomized comparison of laparoscopic appendectomy with open appendectomy. Am J Surg 1995;169:208–12; discussion 212–3.

17. Al-Fozan H, Tulandi T. Safety and risks of laparoscopy in pregnancy. Curr Opin Obstet Gynecol 2002;14:375–9.

18. Amos JD, Schorr SJ, Norman PF, et al. Laparoscopic surgery during pregnancy. Am J Surg 1996;171:435–7.

19. Buser KB. Laparoscopic surgery in the pregnant patient – one surgeon's experience in a small rural hospital. J Soc Laparoendosc Surg 2002;6:121–4.

20. Lyass S, Pikarsky A, Eisenberg VH, et al. Is laparoscopic appendectomy safe in pregnant women? Surg Endosc 2001;15:377–9.

21. de Perrot M, Jenny A, Morales M, Kohlik M, Morel P. Laparosocpic appendectomy during pregnancy. Surg Laparosc Endosc Percutan Tech 2000;10:368–71.

22. Friedman JD, Ramsey PS, Ramin KD, Berry C. Pneumoamnion and pregnancy loss after second-trimester laparoscopic surgery. Obstet Gynecol 2003;99:512–3.

Commentary

E. Patchen Dellinger

Dr. Urbach's well-presented review of this topic has covered the literature in a thorough manner and addressed all of the relevant topics carefully. As in most areas of medicine and surgery, examination of the available data still leaves many areas where knowledge of the specific circumstances of the individual patient and the experience, abilities, and preferences of the individual surgeon will be required to determine management. Dr. Urbach concludes that laparoscopic appendectomy takes slightly longer in the operating room, results in slightly shorter hospital stays, and results in a more rapid recovery of the patient than open appendectomy. In summary statistics, the operative time difference is measured in minutes, the reduced hospital stay is less than a day, and the recovery is improved by a week. For individual patients and surgeons these differences may or may not hold. In our practice, young healthy patients usually stay in hospital less than a day for unperforated appendicitis after open appendectomy, and, in a thin patient, an open appendectomy can be accomplished while the laparoscopic equipment is being set up. The differences here between open and laparoscopic procedures can disappear. The more rapid recovery may well hold up, but this is strongly influenced by local custom and the messages given to the patient by the surgical team. In the case of young women, or patients of either sex with an uncertain diagnosis, the value of laparoscopy for evaluation of the remainder of the abdomen in the presence of a normal appendix appears self-evident. Unmentioned by Dr. Urbach, and perhaps unstudied, is the subjective advantage of the laparoscopic approach in very obese patients. The open approach in these patients can require an extended incision, extra time in the operating room, and an increased risk of wound complications.

The data on infection are intriguing. The data are overwhelming that the laparoscopic approach reduces the risk of incisional surgical site infection for a wide range of procedures [1, 2]. Unexpected is the reported increase in right lower quadrant intra-abdominal abscesses reported after the laparoscopic approach to perforated appendicitis. I am puzzled and not entirely convinced by these data. I agree with Dr. Urbach that if a perforated appendix is found during laparoscopy I would continue and complete the appendectomy laparoscopically. Further, if one has a patient with a high likelihood of perforation who also has a relative indication for the laparoscopic approach such as morbid obesity, it is quite reasonable to proceed laparoscopically. The potential small increased risk of abscess, which could be managed by percutaneous drainage, is outweighed by the substantial morbidity of a surgical site infection in the morbidly obese patient and by the increased difficulty and large incision needed for open appendectomy in these patients. I am not entirely convinced that peritoneal toilet would be better with an open appendectomy than with the laparoscopic approach as suggested by Dr. Urbach. In fact, my personal observation is that I can see more and debride and/or irrigate more efficiently away from the right lower quadrant with laparoscopy than through a McBurney incision. Regardless, there are, in fact, no objective data relating the quality of peritoneal toilet to subsequent intra-abdominal infectious complications.

I agree with Dr. Urbach that it is sensible to proceed with appendectomy when a normal appendix is found at laparoscopy, but I would not criticize a surgeon who did not. It seems impossible to be dogmatic about this issue. In regard to the patient who has other identifiable pathology such as endometriosis or ovarian torsion I would probably proceed with appendectomy as well. Once the ports are in and the appendix identified the removal is simple, safe, and rapid. Endometriosis is often chronic and an ovary may twist again. Each surgeon will have to decide based on the circumstances faced at the time. However, I see no reason to discourage appendectomy in this setting. Dr. Urbach's discussion of stapling versus ligation of the appendix and of the approach to pregnant women is well stated, and I have nothing to add.

References

1. Gaynes RP, Culver DH, Horan TC, Edwards JR, Richards C, Tolson JS. Surgical site infection (SSI) rates in the United States, 1992–1998: the National Nosocomial Infections Surveillance System basic SSI risk index. Clin Infect Dis 2001;33:S69–77.
2. Chang L, Dellinger EP. Impact of laparoscopy on surgical-site infections. Semin Infect Control 2002;2:102–107.

Incisional and Ventral Hernia Repair

Karl A. LeBlanc

▶ **Key Controversies**

A. Choice of prosthetic biomaterial to repair the hernia
B. Fixation method of the prosthetic biomaterial
C. Management of the hernia repair following intestinal injury
D. Seroma management

30.1
Introduction

The laparoscopic approach to the repair of incisional and ventral hernias was first reported in 1993 [1]. Since that time there has been a slow acceptance of this procedure because of the improvement recovery of the patient, the decrease in the wound complications and the notable decline in the recurrence compared with that of the open techniques. In general, all of the significant operative aspects of the operation do not differ but there are several areas of contention regarding several aspects that impact the outcomes of the procedure. The most controversial of these are presented below.

30.2
Discussion

30.2.1
Choice of Prosthetic Biomaterial to Repair the Hernia

The original description of this procedure used an early form of expanded polytetrafluoroethylene (ePTFE). Currently there are several different products that are designed to be used specifically for this procedure (Table 30.1). In the vast majority of centers, this procedure is performed entirely in the intraperitoneal position. Because of this, the biomaterial will contact the intestinal contents. The use of ePTFE is preferred in the majority of reported series because it is much less prone to the development of adhesions to itself.

Table 30.1. Biomaterials for use in laparoscopic incisional and ventral hernioplasty

Product type	Product and manufacturer
ePTFE	DualMesh, W.L. Gore and Associates, Flagstaff, AZ, USA DualMesh Emerge, W.L. Gore and Associates DualMesh Plus, W.L. Gore and Associates DualMesh Plus Emerge, W.L. Gore and Associates DualMesh with Holes, W.L. Gore and Associates DualMesh Plus with Holes, W.L. Gore and Associates Dulex, C.R. Bard, Inc., Cranston NJ, USA
Composite	Composix, C.R. Bard, Inc. Composix EX, C.R. Bard, Inc. Paritex Composite, Sofradim International, Villfranche-sur-Saône, France Paritene Composite, Sofradim International Sepramesh, Genzyme Corporation, Cambridge, Massachusetts, USA Glucamesh, Brennen Medical, Inc., St. Paul, MN, USA Glucatex 3D, Brennen Medical, Inc.
Collagen matrix	Surgisis ES, Cook Surgical, Inc., Bloomington, IN, USA Surgisis Gold, Cook Surgical, Inc. FortaPerm, Organogensis Inc., Canton MA, USA FortaGen, Organogensis Inc. Permacol, Tissue Science Laboratories plc, Covington, GA, USA Alloderm, Lifecell, Inc., Branchburg, NJ, USA

There are those that believe that the parietal ingrowth that occurs with that product will be insufficient to repair the hernia adequately. For this reason, they have chosen to use a polypropylene product instead [2, 3]. The risk to the patient is the potential for the development of significant adhesions with their attendant risk of an enterocutaneous fistula. In Franklin's series [3], only one-third of the re-operated patients had no adhesions. The risk of adhesions and the complications related to them may take many years to become manifest [4, 5]. Therefore, longer-term follow-up will be needed to fully assess the use of these and other biomaterials.

All of the DualMesh products are single component patches that have a rough "parietal" surface and a smooth "visceral" surface. The manufacture of these biomaterials results in interstices that penetrate through the entire material. This is in contrast to that of the Dulex, which is laminated. The ingrowth of the latter will not be throughout the entire prosthesis. The DualMesh Plus products are impregnated with silver and chlorhexidine, which are antimicrobial agents. The benefit of this is the potential to decrease the risk of infection but, additionally, the silver in the product imparts a brown color to the patch. This reduces the glare of the prosthesis when used laparoscopically. These have been very effective in the repair of incisional hernias [6–9].

Other newer materials have tried to address some of the issues that are raised regarding the ingrowth and ease of use of the ePTFE biomaterials. These are composite products that combine two different products in one form or another (Table 30.1). The Composix and Composix EX products are similar in that they both have polypropylene mesh (PPM) that is attached with a thin layer of ePTFE. The former has two PPM layers with ePTFE that is heat sealed onto it. The latter has one PPM that is sewn to the ePTFE layer. Both are attempting to incur the significant scarification that is known to occur with PPM and shield the viscera with the use of the ePTFE. There has been only one study that has shown that this can be used with laparoscopic incisional and ventral hernioplasty (LIVH) [10]. There have been reports of pain and adhesions that are quite significant with the use of these biomaterials [11]. One laboratory showed that the use of ePTFE over PPM does not appear to be protective against adhesions [12].

The Parietex and the Parietene composite products combine polyester and polypropylene biomaterials with a layer of a mixture of oxidized atelocollagen type I, polyethylene glycol and glycerol. This collagen is absorbed within 14 days, which prevents the development of adhesions to the biomaterial. There is only a very few reports of the use of these products in the repair of the incisional hernias at this time [13]. The early clinical reports of the use of this biomaterial seem favorable but there are few laboratory studies involving these and the materials that are described below. Of concern is the fact that the long-term consequences of the implantation of these products have been shown to predispose to the development of complications such as fistulization [4]. Therefore, the use of these absorbable products cannot be an absolute assurance of the prevention of these long-term complications, whether or not they adequately repair the hernia defect.

The very recent release of the latter composite biomaterials, Glucamesh and Glucamesh 3D, have not allowed the clinical evaluation that results from the use in the repair of incisional hernias either open or laparoscopically. The concept is rather new in that these products are coated with oat -glucan, which is absorbed to leave the polypropylene or polyester mesh to repair the hernia defect permanently. The effectiveness of this in both the prevention of intra-abdominal adhesions and the repair of the hernia has yet to be confirmed in the clinical setting.

None of the collagen matrix biomaterials has a long-term follow-up that will verify the effectiveness of either the entire class of these products or the results of any individual prosthesis. These are based upon the non-cellular collagen of either the porcine small intestinal submucosa or dermal collagen model or the human cadaver dermis. It is the intent of these biomaterials that the native collagen of the patient will penetrate and replace the collagen fibrils of the implanted material so that a "neofascia" is created to repair the defect in the fascia. This is anecdotally reported to be particularly effective in the presence of an active infection. Clinical trials are still lacking to confirm these claims.

The choice of the biomaterial to repair any hernia is of paramount importance because of the proven efficacy of the products. The laparoscopic repair has resulted in a heightened awareness of the risk of adhesion formation that may occur with this repair because of the necessary of the placement of the biomaterial in the intraperitoneal position in the majority of patients. There are only a few centers that are using an extraperitoneal mesh to repair these hernias [14].

There are many choices of biomaterials to repair the incisional hernias laparoscopically. The difficulty is in the understanding of the characteristics of these materials in the healing process that actually repair the hernia. Most surgeons do not understand the cellular physiology of the prosthetic biomaterials and use these products on information that is based upon the handling characteristics rather than the long-term data that may or may not be available for these products. A thorough understanding of them and a complete description of them are beyond the scope of this chapter. The controversial point of the choices of biomaterials is the products themselves. The published literature will provide short- and long-term data upon which to base the use of any of these products. This, as well as sufficient laboratory testing, should be used in the decision-making process regarding the choice of biomaterial to repair hernia rather than the unsubstantiated evidence of the manufacturer's representative.

30.2.2
Fixation Method of the Biomaterial

The choice of the fixation of the biomaterial that is selected for the repair of the incisional hernia is also a frequent area of controversy. The majority of the published reports of this procedure employ the use of transfascial sutures in addition to one of the different types of metal fixation devices. Park and colleagues first popularized the use of sutures in 1996 [15]. The benefits of the additional use of these sutures have been shown in several papers. The longest reported series of patients that underwent this procedure was able to evaluate the differences in the result of the patients that had and those that did not have the use of these sutures. In that study, in the patients that did not have the use of the transfascial sutures, the recurrence rate was 13% compared with zero in those that did [16]. During this initial experience we modified our methodology to include the placement of transfascial nonabsorbable sutures that were spaced approximately 5 cm apart. This change has eliminated placement as a source of recurrence. In the largest series published to date, there were 14 recurrences [7]. Of these, six were subsequent to the lack of transfascial suture placement. During the course of this study, the participants adopted the use of transfascial sutures in all cases. They, and we, continue to do so.

There have been several studies that contrasted the results of the open versus laparoscopic repair of incisional hernias. One of two recurrences that were seen in Ramshaw's series occurred without the use of these sutures. The other recurrence appeared to be related to a trocar-site hernia. He modified his technique to place sutures as others have done [17]. In Holzman's comparison using polypropylene and a hernia stapler, there were two recurrences in that group of patients. These were stated to be "due to insufficient stapling of one edge of the mesh". He did not elaborate what would have constituted adequate stapling of the mesh [18]. It would seem, at least in these two studies that the use of additional points of fixation, such as sutures, would be preferred given the results that were noted.

The majority of authors recommend a large overlap of the prosthetic biomaterial. As noted earlier, however, the view that sutures are mandatory with this procedure is an additional point of controversy with this operation. Carbajo and colleagues have extensive experience with LIVH in which they utilize a "double-crown" technique [8]. They place two concentric rows of tacks along the periphery of the DualMesh Plus with holes (WL Gore & Associates, Flagstaff, AZ, USA). This product is 1.5 mm thick and has perforations throughout the prosthesis. Whether this has any significant bearing on their results is not known but their recurrence rate is 4.4% with a mean follow-up period of 44 months.

Gillian et al. has used a composite mesh of polypropylene and ePTFE without the use of suture fixation [10]. They believe that the use of the polypropylene material eliminates the need for transfascial sutures. They, too, fix the biomaterial with two rows of tacks with a 3–5 cm overlap. They report the use of this technique in 100 patients over a 27-month period with only one recurrence. This is stated to be due to an inadequate overlap of the biomaterial. The average length of follow-up was not given but longer observation will be needed to adequately assess these findings.

Rosen presented the results of 100 ventral hernia repairs from 4 to 65 months of experience. The average follow-up was 30 months, and 17 recurrences were noted. In these patients, tacks alone were used in six, sutures and tacks in ten and sutures alone in one patient. According to this analysis, there was no statistical difference in the outcomes based upon fixation. However, these repairs were in the early experience of several different surgeons and there was no standardized technique in this institution. Therefore, it is rather difficult to draw firm conclusions based upon these data.

Finally, there has been a laboratory evaluation of the use of these fixation methods. This study found that suture fixation was always stronger than tacks alone. They determined that the ideal number of fixation points per diameter of mesh could be determined by the formula of $(2r/7)(3)$. They also stated that based upon the findings of their experiments that "the addition of transabdominal sutures should be preferred" [19].

Based upon the available evidence, it appears that the use of transfascial sutures is preferred. Further clinical studies are needed to accurately assess the possibility of the elimination of the points of fixation. Perceived advantages include a decrease in the incidence of persistent postoperative pain, a more rapid operative procedure and conceivably a reduced cost. More time will be needed to evaluate these claims. The possibility of newer prosthetic biomaterials may enhance this concept. It is incumbent upon the surgeon to use the method that is the best in his or her hands.

30.2.3
Management of the Hernia Repair Following Intestinal Injury

This is a significant event and one that occurs with some frequency. The serosal injury that occurs during the dissection of the intestine can be managed as one would during any bowel surgery. If the lumen has not been violated, one may elect to leave this injury untouched or the surgeon can close this either with sutures or with the application of endoscopic staples. There does not appear to be any benefit or adverse events associated with any of these choices [6].

A recognized enterotomy is a known complication of both the open and laparoscopic operations. The reported incidence of this complication varies significantly. Most series report an absence of this complication but in some reports the incidence of this complication are as high as 6 and 14.3% [20, 21]. Generally, however, the actual number of patients that have incurred an enterotomy is approximately 1–3% [6, 8, 22–24].

The management of a recognized enterotomy is currently somewhat controversial. In many centers, if this event occurs, the hernia procedure is terminated. The surgeon will repair the injury either laparoscopically or by a conversion to the open operation [16]. If the open option is selected, the bowel injury will be repaired or resected, whereupon the hernia can either be repaired using a tissue repair or this can be deferred if the hernia is very large necessitating a prosthesis to adequately repair the defect. Alternatively, the intestine can be repaired laparoscopically followed by a planned return to the operative suite 2–4 days later. At that time, the delayed laparoscopic hernioplasty can be performed. This delay will allow any contamination to be eliminated and this short time span will not allow the formation of dense adhesions subsequent to the intra-abdominal procedure. Some will delay for several weeks but this is not recommended unless there was a significant amount of spillage of intraluminal contents.

More recently, there have been reports that have shown that the repair of this recognized injury to the small bowel and completion of the intended hernia repair may be safe. This enterotomy must not be associated with significant spillage of the intestinal contents. Some published series have repaired this injury and proceeded to repair the hernia in the intended manner including the laparoscopic insertion of a prosthetic biomaterial [7, 8]. Others have resected gangrenous bowel and completed the hernia repair [25]. In these few reports, there does not appear to be an adverse consequence to this decision. However, if the intestinal necrosis that may occur with an electrosurgical injury is underestimated when the injury is oversewn, there may be an extension of the necrosis and subsequent development of an intra-abdominal abscess. This can then require laparotomy, resection of the intestine, and removal of the prosthesis at the time that this is recognized [22].

An injury to the colon carries a much greater potential for infectious complications if the hernia repair is completed as planned with the insertion of the prosthetic biomaterial. Therefore, the majority of surgeons will simply repair the injury and repair the hernia by a laparotomy without a prosthetic product. Some, however, have carried out the hernia repair with a simultaneous colon resection as a preplanned operation with an adequately prepared colon [8]. An alternative that may be considered is the use of one of the nonsynthetic collagen based biomaterials that are currently available. However, there are no reports that describe this use at this time.

The current recommendations for the treatment of an recognized bowel injury could be:

— **Serosal injury.** No treatment or closure by any method; completion of the hernia repair as planned with a prosthetic biomaterial.
— **Small intestinal intraluminal injury.** Primary closure by any method; completion of the hernia repair as planned *if* a laparoscopic enterorrhaphy is secure and there has been minimal or no spillage of the intestinal contents. If there has been significant spillage and/or the surgeon is not facile with the laparoscopic repair of the injury, the procedure should be converted to a laparotomy and the hernia repaired with sutures alone at that time. A return to the operating suite at a later planned time following the repair of the injury can also be chosen.

— **Colonic injury.** Primary closure by any method, open or laparoscopic; a non-prosthetic open repair could be done simultaneously with an open procedure. Alternatively, the colon could be closed only and the patient could be returned to operation at a later time for a laparoscopic prosthetic repair.

30.2.3.1
An Unrecognized Enterotomy

An unrecognized enterotomy is a significant complication that occurs in up to 6% of the patients. However, it is usually less that 1% [7, 17, 20, 22, 23]. This enterotomy can occur either as a traction injury from one of the grasping instruments that are used in the procedure or may result from a burn that is incurred during the use of an energy source to lyse the adhesions. In either case, the injury will not be manifest in the initial hours following the procedure, in most instances. The usual postoperative course of LIVH patients is a rapid discharge from the hospital, usually less than 24–48 h [6, 7, 8]. Therefore, increasing pain, fever, and abdominal distension should be evaluated with laboratory testing and computed tomography scanning if the patient does not appear to exhibit an acute surgical abdomen. Following the LIVH, there should not be any significant accumulation of intraperitoneal fluid. Free air should have been resorbed before the third postoperative day [26]. If there is ascites or free air within the abdominal cavity, the patient should be laparoscoped to assess the abdomen if there is even a slight suspicion of an unrecognized enterotomy. If the findings appear to eliminate the concern of an intestinal injury, then no further therapy is needed. If significant contamination is found, open laparotomy will generally be required with resection of the involved intestine and excision of the prosthesis. One must also inspect all of the intestinal contents to insure that there are no simultaneous injuries. The abdomen could be closed primarily with or without retention sutures. However, if there is a concern of an abdominal compartment syndrome, the prosthesis could be left in place to allow the expansion of the abdomen. The status of the biomaterial should be closely monitored and removal of this could be electively planned as the condition of the patient stabilizes.

30.2.4
Seroma Management

The development of a seroma is so common after this procedure that many surgeons do not believe it to be a real complication. This occurrence should be expected because the peritoneum within the hernia sac is not removed. The fluid that will be secreted by the peritoneal membrane surface will result in a fluid collection that will be contained by the prosthetic biomaterial that is used to repair the hernia. There has been one series of patients that were evaluated by ultrasonic study found that the incidence of this event was 100% in all of the patients that were followed [27]. With this data, it is surprising that the incidence of seroma that is reported in the literature is not significantly greater.

This apparent disparity is related to the definition of the seroma. Many authors do not list this as a complication unless the fluid collection persists beyond 6 weeks [7, 28]. Others, such as this author, believe that the seroma must persist for longer than 8–12 weeks. Additionally, this should be associated with symptoms such as pain or this mass should be clinically obvious for it to be considered as a complication. The incidence of this varies widely and ranges from 0–43% [6, 8, 17, 28–30]. An overall review of the current literature summarizes the incidence of clinically significant seromas to average roughly 4–5% in patients subsequent to LIVH.

The prevention and treatment of these seromas is not fully delineated by the experts that have reported this problem. For most, however, it is acknowledged that it is virtually impossible to prevent these with certainty. Kirshtein and colleagues attempted to pierce the biomaterial with the Veress needle but found that omitting this step did not have any appreciable effect upon the incidence of seromas [8, 31]. Others have used the prosthetic DualMesh with holes (WL Gore & Associates) but this did not eliminate the condition because the seromas that were associated with these patients occurred in 11.8% of them postoperatively [8]. Therefore, it does not appear that perforation of this product offers any benefit to the prevention of these seromas. This is probably related to the fact that the cellular ingrowth and collagen deposition is so rapid that these small openings are sealed rather quickly while the fluid production persists. Other biomaterials that are known to have macroporous structures, such as polypropylene, do not eliminate the occurrence of these fluid collections [2, 10, 32].

Some surgeons have attempted to use pre-emptive measures to prevent this problem. Simple measures such as the application of an abdominal binder on these patients have significantly reduced this complication [2, 6]. The argon beam coagulator has been used at the initial procedure to scarify the peritoneum of the hernia sac to diminish the seromas postoperatively. The application of the electrocautery and the ultrasonic scalpel with the use of a single suture in the center of the hernia defect to fixate the prosthetic biomaterial has been reported. A prospective randomized study used a central suture in one group of patients and added the application of the energy source in a second group. The seroma rate was statistically significantly different in the second group (25% versus 4%). This study, however, did not evaluate any hernias that were larger than 100 cm^2, which are the hernias that are the most likely to develop notable fluid accumulations postoperatively [33]. Nevertheless, this may be a useful technique. There is a potential risk of the excessive application of the electrosurgical energy to the thin area of the tissue covering the hernia itself, which could result in a full thickness necrosis of the thin subcutaneous tissue and skin. This could result in slough of the tissue and exposure of the prosthetic biomaterial, which will increase the risk of infection. There have been no reported events such as this that have been reported to date, however.

In an effort to inhibit or diminish the development of these known problems, many surgeons will place an abdominal binder on the patient while he or she is still on the operating table. This will be worn for 3–14 days depending upon the initial size of the protruding hernia. The size of the binder, the length of time that its use is recommended, and whether a bulky dressing is applied have not been standardized. There has not been any prospective randomized trials to evaluate the effectiveness of this maneuver but the experience, such as that of this and other authors, appears to suggest that there is a decrease in both the size and duration of the seromas that are clinically significant by as much as 50% [2, 6].

Once the seroma is confirmed, the management of this problem is controversial. Many surgeons believe that it will resolve if allowed the time for the fluid to be absorbed. This will usually occur within 12 weeks [16, 30, 31, 34]. Not all authors agree, however. Carbajo and associates aspirated seromas of all of the 11.8% that occurred in their recent series without any complication [8]. I do not attempt to aspirate seromas unless the patient remains symptomatic for longer than 6 months and the ultrasound evaluation fails to demonstrate any significant resolution of the seroma. If the patient is obviously symptomatic with a degree of pain, this will be necessary earlier than that time. One or two aspirations will usually suffice. This occurs in less than 1% of my patients, however.

Aspiration is not free of risk. Bacteria can be introduced into the fluid collection with a resulting infection. This has been noted in a few series [16, 29]. Therefore, strict sterile technique is mandatory to minimize this occurrence. It is recommended that the patient undergo an ultrasound examination of the fluid collection to ensure that a recurrent hernia is not misdiagnosed so that the intestine will not inadvertently punctured during the aspiration procedure. These tests will also identify the presence of a multiloculated fluid collection that will be difficult to aspirate in its entirety. If this is found, ultrasonically directed aspiration or even incision and drainage would be needed to adequately treat this seroma. This is rarely necessary, however.

A computed tomography scan can also be used to evaluate the hernia sac. This can be another effective tool to verify whether the content of the former hernia site is a recurrent hernia or a seroma. Interestingly, one study noted that some of the postoperative fluid collections contained air as late as 6–12 days postoperatively [32]. This can mimic either a recurrent hernia or an abscess. None of the cases in which this was discovered required any intervention and all resolved. Therefore, clinical and laboratory correlation is important.

One author has reported the use of the argon beam to scarify the hernia sac subsequent to the development of a postoperative seroma [35]. This was used successfully in three patients. A three trocar technique using 5- and 10-mm trocars was used to suction the contents of the fluid collection. An argon beam coagulator was then used to scarify the entire surface of the lining of the seroma cavity. This was followed by the instillation of a slurry of talc (4 g) and 30 cc bupivacaine to promote sclerosis while providing postoperative analgesia. These patients were placed in abdominal binders subsequent to this procedure. Two of these three patients had complete and permanent resolution of the seroma. The third required a single aspiration as an office procedure 6 months postoperatively. Further evaluation of this technique may reveal that this is an appropriate option for the patients with a persistent seroma.

The fact that seromas develop with this procedure seems to be an accepted occurrence. The methods of prevention and treatment are still not firmly established. There is significant disagreement amongst the experts in this field currently. One should recognize the method that appears to lessen this occurrence in one's own patients and survey the literature to identify any new options that are under evaluation. Possibly the future will afford the surgeon new biomaterials and techniques that further diminish or eliminate this problem.

30.3
Summary

— Biomaterials should be used that are allow sufficient ingrowth and ease of handling.
— Fixation of these biomaterials should include the use of transfascial sutures in addition to a metal fixation device.
— Repair of the hernia may be completed if there is minimal spillage of intestinal contents following small bowel injury but must be avoided if the colon is injured.
— Seromas are expected and can be managed expectantly in most cases.

References

1. LeBlanc KA, Booth WV. Laparoscopic repair of incisional abdominal hernias using expanded polytetrafluoroethylene: preliminary findings. Surg Laparosc Endosc 1993;3:39–41.
2. Chowbey PK, Sharma A, Khullar R, et al. Laparoscopic ventral hernia repair. J Laparoendosc Adv Surg Tech 2000;10:79–84.
3. Franklin ME, Dorman JP, Glass JL, Balli JE, Gonzales JJ. Laparoscopic ventral and incisional hernia repair. Surg Laparosc Endosc 1998;8:294–9.
4. Leber GE, Garb JL, Alexander AI, Reed WP. Long-term Complications associated with prosthetic repair of incisional hernias. Arch Surg 1998;133:378–82.
5. Losanoff JE, Richman BW, Jones JW. Entero-colocutaneous fistula: a late consequence of polypropylene mesh abdominal wall repair: case report and review of the literature. Hernia 2002;6:144–7.
6. LeBlanc KA, Whitaker JM, Bellanger DE, Rhynes VK. Laparoscopic incisional and ventral hernioplasty: lessons learned from 200 patients. Hernia 2003;7:118–24.
7. Heniford TB, Park A, Ramshaw BJ, Voeller G. Laparoscopic ventral and incisional hernia repair in 407 patients. J Am Coll Surg 2000;190:645–50.
8. Carbajo MA, Martín del Olmo JC, Blanco JI, Toledano M, et al. Laparoscopic approach to incisional hernia. Surg Endosc 2003;17:118–22.
9. Wright BE, Niskanen BD, Peterson DJ, Ney AL, et al. Laparoscopic ventral hernia repair: are there comparative advantages over traditional methods of repair? Am Surg 2002;68:291–6.
10. Gillian GK, Geis WP, Grover G. Laparoscopic incisional and ventral hernia repair (LIVH): an evolving outpatient technique. JSLS 2002;6:315–22.
11. LeBlanc KA, Whitaker JM. Management of chronic postoperative pain following incisional hernia repair with Composix mesh. Hernia 2002;6:194–7.
12. Naim JO, Pulley D, Scanlan K, et al. Reduction of postoperative adhesions to Marlex mesh using experimental adhesion barriers in rats. J Laparoendosc Surg 1993;3:187–90.
13. Balique JG, Alexandre JH, Arnaud JP, Benchetrit S, et al. Intraperitoneal treatment of incisional and umbilical hernias: intermediate results of a multicenter prospective clinical trial using an innovative composite mesh. Hernia 2000;4 [Suppl]:S10–6.
14. Roll S, Marujo W, Cohen R. Laparoscopic preperitoneal hernioplasty of incisional and ventral hernias. In: LeBlanc KA, editor. Laparoscopic hernia surgery: an operative guide. London: Arnold Medical; 2003.
15. Park A, Gagner M, Pomp A. Laparoscopic repair of large incisional hernias. Surg Laparosc Endosc 1996;6:123–8.
16. LeBlanc KA, Booth WV, Whitaker JM, Bellanger DE. Laparoscopic incisional and ventral herniorraphy in 100 patients. Am J Surg 2000;180:193–7.
17. Ramshaw BJ, Escartia P, Schwab J, Mason EM, Wilson RA, Duncan TD, Miller J, Lucas GW, Promes J. Comparison of laparoscopic and open ventral herniorraphy. Am Surg 1999;65:827–32.
18. Holzman MD, Purut CM, Reintgen K, Eubanks S, Pappas TN. Laparoscopic ventral and incisional hernioplasty. Surg Endosc 1997;11:32–35.

19. van't Riet M, de Vos van Steinwijk PJ, Kleinrensink GJ, et al. Tensile strength of mesh fixation methods in laparoscopic incisional hernia repair. Surg Endosc 2002;16:1713-6.
20. Koehler RH, Voeller G. Recurrences in laparoscopic incisional hernia repairs: a personal series and review of the literature. JSLS 1999;3:293-304.
21. Chari R, Chari V, Eisenstat M, Chung R. A case controlled study of laparoscopic incisional hernia repair. Surg Endosc 2000;14:117-9.
22. Berger D, Bientzle M, Müller A. Postoperative complications after laparoscopic incisional hernia repair. Surg Endosc 2002;16:1720-3.
23. Bageacu S, Blanc P, Breton C, Gonzales M, et al. Laparoscopic repair of incisional hernias. Surg Endosc 2002;16:345-8.
24. Rosen M, Brody F, Ponsky J, Walsh RM, et al. Recurrence after laparoscopic ventral hernia repair. Surg Endosc 2003;17:123-8.
25. Voeller G. Laparoscopic repair in the emergent setting. In: LeBlanc KA, editor. Laparoscopic hernia surgery: an operative guide. London: Arnold Medical; 2003;111-114.
26. Feingold DL, Widmann WD, Calhoun SK, Teigen EL, et al. Persistent post-laparoscopy pneumoperitoneum. Surg Endosc 2003;17:296-9.
27. Susmallian S, Gewurtz G, Ezri T, Charuzi I. Seroma after laparoscopic repair of hernia with PTFE patch: is it really a complication? Hernia 2001;5:139-41.
28. Park A, Birch DW, Lovrics P. Laparoscopic and open incisional hernia repair: a comparison study. Surg 1998;124:816-22.
29. DeMaria EJ, Moss JM, Surgerman HJ. Laparscopic intraperitoneal polytetrafluoroethylene (PTFE) prosthetic patch repair of ventral hernia. Surg Endosc 2000;14:326-9.
30. Parker HH, Nottingham JM, Bynoc RP, Yost MJ. Laparoscopic repair of large incisional hernias. Am Surg 2002;68:530-4.
31. Kirshtein B, Lantsberg L, Avinoach E, Bayma M, et al. Laparoscopic repair of large incisional hernias. Surg Endosc 2002;16:1717-9.
32. Lin BHJ, Vargish T, Dachman AH. CT findings after laparoscopic repair of ventral hernias. Am J Rad 1999;172:389-92.
33. Tsimoyiannis EC, Siakas P, Glantzouissis G, Koulas S, et al. Seroma in laparoscopic ventral hernioplasty. Surg Laparosc Endosc Percutan Tech 2001;11:317-21.
34. Park A, Heniford BT, LeBlanc KA, Voeller GR. Laparoscopic repair of incisional hernias. Part 2: surgical technique. Contemp Surg 2001;57:225-38.
35. Lehr SC, Schuricht AL. A minimally invasive approach for treating postoperative seromas after incisional hernia repair. JSLS 2001;5:267-71.

Commentary

Abdalla E. Zarroug, Michael G. Sarr

LeBlanc provides an insightful, fair, and comprehensive discussion of several of the most controversial aspects of repair of ventral and incisional abdominal wall hernias via a laparoscopic, minimal access technique. Our discussion will address these as yet unsolved dilemmas from a somewhat different aspect – we acknowledge that our remarks are complimentary to those of LeBlanc, represent largely our opinion, and are equally based not on level 1 evidence-based studies, but rather on our opinion, of course, biased by personal experience.

Choice of Prosthetic Biomaterial

As our understanding of the genomic control of the biology of hernia formation increases, we realize that incisional hernias in most patients have their origin in some abnormality in collagen metabolism – thus, the interest in prosthetic-based repair. LeBlanc discusses the various prostheses available– polypropylene, ePTFE, composite prostheses of both ePTFE and polypropylene, polypropylene covered with an absorbable collagen-based coating, and more recently the collagen biomaterial-based technology.

Laparoscopic repair of ventral hernias, as opposed to inguinal hernia repair, lacks ready access to a significant preperitoneal space that would isolate the prosthesis used from direct contact with the intra-abdominal viscera. This necessity for intra-abdominal placement of the laparoscopically placed prosthesis leads to problems with adhesion between mesh and viscera. Having struggled through too many re-operations on patients who have had previous intraperitoneal polypropylene, we can see no justification for its use when ePTFE can be used. This latter prosthetic forms a pseudocapsule between the ePTFE and the viscera, thereby preventing visceral adhesion. Whether use of the „protected" polypropylene meshes coated or interwoven with a bioabsorbable barrier will prove truly effective in humans is yet to be proven. Until then, we feel strongly that some form of ePTFE should be used for the visceral side. Whether the collagen-based biomaterials Alloderm (LifeCell, Branchburg, NJ, USA), Surgisis® (Cook Surgical, Bloomington, IN, USA), or Permacol (Tissue Science Laboratories, Covington, GA, USA) will prove as viable options needs well-planned studies. We remain a bit skeptical of their reliability to serve as a permanent foundation upon which a new, fully functional, strong „neo-abdominal" wall will be formed for the following reason. Many or most patients with an incisional hernia have an underlying defect in collagen metabolism even if not diagnosed with a formal disorder – thus, reliance on endogenous mechanisms of adequate wound healing is why the incisional hernia formed in the first place!

Fixation of Prosthesis

LeBlanc clearly points out the compelling findings that some form of transfascial (versus intraperitoneal, staple-like fixation or „drilling") is superior. A question not addressed (and also not resolved) is whether the suture used should be a permanent suture or an absorbable one. This controversy is especially pertinent if just ePTFE is used, where there is *no* ingrowth into the prosthesis to "fix" it in place, as occurs with the woven or knitted polypropylene. Even the use of the composite grafts (ePTFE on visceral side, polypropylene on abdominal wall side) are not proven to allow ingrowth from the parietal peritoneum into the polypropylene of adequate enough strength to fully immobilize the prosthesis to effect a durable, permanent repair, as occurs when polypropylene is positioned within the abdominal wall as with the Rives-Stoppa technique [1, 2].

Finally, another concept of prosthetic-based repairs has surfaced, i.e., the concept of extrudability. Some materials are more easily extruded or pushed up through a defect, raising the concept of the mechanics (not the *bio*mechanics) of the mesh construction. This idea of flexibility, extradurability, stretchability and shrinkage, in addition to biomaterial, mesh size, fiber size, etc., has become of considerable interest to bioengineers involved in the design of prosthetic materials.

Enterotomy at Time of Proposed Laparoscopic Ventral Herniorrhaphy

Undoubtedly, the solution to this dilemma is preventive. Careful preoperative selection [based on review of previous operative note(s) describing multiple adhesions or known presence of intraperitoneal polypropylene] and *early* conversion to open repair are the keys to prevention. While we are all (or we think we are) good laparoscopic surgeons, virtually all large series show both recognized and unrecognized enterotomies. Experience with open surgery with placement of prosthetic mesh at the time of gastrointestinal surgery (even clean-contaminated procedures) shows a higher (and in our opinion, unacceptable) rate of prosthetic infection. These data question the approach of placing non-bioabsorbable prosthetic mesh concomitantly at the time of any enterotomy. We would urge the laparoscopist to fix the enterotomy, postpone the repair, and come back at a later date (maybe even within the week), especially if a laparoscopic repair is the ultimate goal. Should the enterotomy be made in the presence of multiple adhesions, is not an open repair indicated, especially if it can be accomplished extraperitoneally? We think so; abandonment of a laparoscopic repair is not and should not be considered a "failure" by the surgeon.

Seroma Formation

We have no real insight into preventing seroma formation, but readily second LeBlanc's caution to obtain an ultrasonography before puncturing the "mass". Abdominal binders may prove to be beneficial in the prevention of large hernias. Repeated aspirations rather than early placement of an indwelling drain (a drain is a two-way tract for bacteria) seem most prudent. A rare persistent seroma (probably better termed pseudobursa) will require open excision of the mesothelial wall of the cavity. We have no experience with a topical sclerosant like talc, but it seems a logical alternative.

Summary

Laparoscopic ventral herniorrhaphy is here to stay. But, just like most other minimal access procedures, patient selection is paramount. Currently, laparoscopic repair requires intraperitoneal prosthetic material as a "patch." Repair of a congenital 2-cm umbilical hernia should not be undertaken with this approach (one end of the spectrum) nor should a multiply recurrent incisional hernia in a patient with known, severe intraperitoneal adhesions. The best approach requires good patient selection, honest acknowledgement of one's own laparoscopic skills, lack of a cavalier cowboyish attitude as the surgeon, and the insight that conversion to open repair is not a failure.

References

1. Stoppa RE. Treatment of complicated groin and incisional hernias. World J Surg 1989;18:545–54.
2. Temudom T, Siadati M, Sarr MG. Repair of complex giant or recurrent ventral hernias by using tension-free intraparietal prosthetic mesh (Stoppa technique): lessons learned from our initial experience (fifty patients). Surgery 1996;120:738–44.

Inguinal Hernia Repair

E. Matt Ritter, C. Daniel Smith

> ▶ **Key Controversies**
>
> A. The role of the laparoscopic approach to inguinal hernia repair
> B. The choice of laparoscopic technique
> C. The role of mesh fixation

31.1
Introduction

Since the "modernization" of hernia surgery by Bassini in the late nineteenth century [1] no area of surgery has been more steeped in dogma and controversy than the repair of groin hernias. The search for the "best" way to repair this common condition has produced a vast number of solutions, whose staunch supporters readily sing the praises of their chosen approach. Fuel was added to the debate in the early 1990s with the introduction of the laparoscopic approach for inguinal hernia repair [2]. The refinement of the laparoscopic techniques to the now widely accepted transabdominal preperitoneal (TAPP) approach [3] and the totally extraperitoneal (TEP) technique [4] has established a sound basis for the laparoscopic approach to the repair of groin hernias.

As with all new techniques, laparoscopic inguinal hernia surgery has its own unique set of controversies. The major issues currently being debated include determining the exact role for the laparoscopic approach for the repair of groin hernias, the choice of laparoscopic technique, and whether or not fixation of the prosthetic mesh is required. These controversies will be objectively evaluated and discussed below.

31.2
Discussion

31.2.1
The Role of the Laparoscopic Approach
to Inguinal Hernia Repair

The controversy most central to laparoscopic inguinal hernia repair is the fundamental question of where does laparoscopy fit into the already crowded milieu of herniorrhaphy techniques? Since laparoscopic inguinal hernia repair is based on the open preperitoneal techniques described by Stoppa, Nyhus, and Wantz [5–7], the common benefits of avoiding previous surgical fields and the ability to address all types of groin hernia recurrences has lead to the laparoscopic approach being *readily accepted for the repair of recurrent and bilateral inguinal hernias.* This acceptance is supported by large series reporting low complication and recurrence rates similar to those reported in series of open preperitoneal repairs [8, 9]. While the two randomized trials comparing the open preperitoneal techniques with laparoscopic repair for recurrent hernias [10, 11] demonstrated patient benefits with the laparoscopic approach, both report recurrence rates in the laparoscopic groups that is much higher than most current series, and likely reflects the authors' learning curve. As for the issue of bilateral inguinal hernias, a single prospective randomized trial compared the laparoscopic preperitoneal approach with the anterior tension free Lichtenstein repair [12]. While there was no significant difference in short-term recurrence, the patients repaired laparoscopically had less pain and returned to work significantly faster than the open surgery group.

The application of the laparoscopic approach to unilateral primary inguinal hernias has not been met with the same enthusiasm that is seen for recurrent or bilateral hernias. There are several reasons for this. Several large studies including randomized multicenter trials [13] as well as a meta-analysis of over 30 randomized trials [14] show benefit for laparoscopic herniorrhaphy when compared with non-mesh conventional repairs with regard to postoperative pain and recurrence rates, but the shift away from open native tissue repairs to open tension-free mesh repairs dilutes the importance of these findings. Several recent series, however, have compared laparoscopic herniorrhaphy with open tension free mesh repairs and have shown benefit for the laparoscopic approach [11, 15–19]. These reports are summarized in Table 31.1. The benefits of the laparoscopic techniques studied center around patients experiencing a faster and more comfortable early postoperative recovery and lower rates of long-term groin pain. These benefits are balanced by an increased rate of serious complications with laparoscopy in addition to greater cost of laparoscopic approaches, and no difference in recurrence rates. The continued success of the open tension-free mesh repairs has made it difficult for many surgeons to justify the time and expense required to learn a new and technically challenging procedure such as laparoscopic inguinal hernia repair (LIH).

Anesthesia concerns also factor into the decision to employ a laparoscopic approach to inguinal hernia repair. While the totally extraperitoneal approach can be performed under regional or even local anesthesia, laparoscopic herniorrhaphy is most commonly performed under general anesthesia. The risks associated with general anesthesia make the laparoscopic approach less attractive for elderly or comorbid patients, especially with primary, unilateral inguinal hernias.

Procedural costs are another issue. Since all herniorrhaphies are typically performed in an outpatient setting, laparoscopic herniorrhaphy cannot compensate for increased procedural costs by yielding decreased hospital stay as was seen for laparoscopic cholecystectomy. Additionally, the costs per procedure are highly variable and depend on the type of instrumentation, use of a dissecting balloon, use of a fixation device, and the surgeon's ability to perform the procedure in a timely fashion. Swanstrom has shown that cost savings can be realized by reducing dependence on single use instruments, avoiding mesh fixation (discussed in Sect. 31.2.3) and improving operating room efficiency to shorten operating times [20]. Additionally, direct costs may be balanced by socioeconomic analysis taking into account the reduction of time out of work after a laparoscopic repair. This type of cost analysis is very difficult to carry out and will depend on the practice setting of the individual surgeon. Given this degree of variability, it is difficult to come to a definitive conclusion on the issue of cost for laparoscopic inguinal herniorrhaphy. There is little debate however, that based solely on direct costs, laparoscopic herniorrhaphy is generally more costly than more conventional open herniorrhaphy.

Finally, there remains an issue regarding complications unique to LIH. Several studies have reported a higher rate of significant complication such as bowel and vascular injury with LIH than with open hernia repair [18]. In most of these studies, these complications occurred early in a series of LIH or from groups without much experience with LIH suggesting that this is more a reflection of the learning curve for performance of safe LIH that being inherent to the procedure itself. Also, most of these potential complications can be eliminated by proper selection of the laparoscopic approach to use (see Sect. 31.2.2).

So should we be performing laparoscopic herniorrhaphy on primary unilateral hernias when, compared with anterior tension-free repair, the only benefits appear to be less pain, faster recovery, and fewer problems with long-term groin pain, all with an increased cost and potential for significant complications not typically seen in open herniorrhaphy? The answer is yes,

Table 31.1. Outcomes of laparoscopic inguinal hernia (LIH) repair. *PRCT* prospective randomized controlled trial, *PRT* prospective randomized trial, *MC* multicenter, *TAPP* transabdominal preperitoneal approach, *TEP* totally extraperitoneal approach

Author, year [ref.]	Study type	Findings
Johansson et al., Ann Surg 1999 [15]	PRT, MC TAPP vs open preperitoneal mesh	1-year follow-up LIH: less pain, faster recovery, greater cost and complications No difference in recurrence
Beets et al., Surg Endosc 1999 [11]	PRT Recurrent hernias TAPP vs open preperitoneal mesh	3-year follow-up LIH: less pain, faster recovery, greater recurrence rate No difference in cost
Douek et al., BMJ 2003 [19]	PRT, MC TAPP vs open anterior mesh	5-year follow-up LIH: less permanent groin pain and paresthesias No difference in recurrence
Andersson et al., Surgery 2003 [17]	PRCT TEP vs open anterior mesh	1-year follow-up LIH: less pain, faster recovery, greater cost, more recurrences (2/81 vs 0/87) No difference in complications
McCormack et al., Cochrane Database Syst Rev 2003 [18]	Systematic literature review of PRCTs LIH vs open mesh	1.5–36 months follow-up LIH: less pain, faster recovery, more serious complications (bowel & vascular), longer operative time No difference in recurrence

Table 31.1. *Continued*

Author, year [ref.]	Study type	Findings
Bringman et al., Ann Surg 2003 [16]	PRT	20 months follow-up
	TEP vs open anterior mesh vs mesh plug	LIH: less pain, faster recovery, longer operative time
		No difference in recurrence

PRCT prospective, randomized, controlled trial, *PRT* prospective, randomized trial, *MC* multicenter, *TAPP* transabdominal perperitoneal, *TEP* totally extraperitoneal

especially in patients where the benefits of rapid recovery will be significant and justified (e.g., young manual laborer). While this may seem surprising in light of the information presented, understanding this position requires us to re-examine the issue of recurrent hernias. Accepting that a laparoscopic approach is better for recurrent hernias, these hernias are frequently very challenging as the addition of scar tissue to the preperitoneal dissection often masques landmarks and distorts anatomy.

If the average surgeon reserves the laparoscopic approach only for these difficult hernias, the likelihood of success will be low and the likelihood of frustration high. Acquisition and maintenance of experience and skills through performance of laparoscopic herniorrhaphy for less demanding primary hernias in low-risk patients who may potentially benefit from the more rapid return to activity or modest decreases in postoperative pain will allow the surgeon to be adequately equipped to tackle more difficult recurrent and bilateral cases as they arise. Also, more experience with a technique will minimize complications, operating time, and subsequently cost. The bottom line is that to offer a patient optimal care, a surgeon should be skilled in both open *and* laparoscopic techniques, and performing LIH in select unilateral hernias will best allow a surgeon to achieve this goal.

31.2.2
The Type of Laparoscopic Approach

Once the decision is made that the laparoscopic approach is indicated, the controversy shifts to the choice of laparoscopic approach. As previously mentioned, laparoscopic inguinal hernia repair is based on the principles of the open preperitoneal repair developed by Stoppa, Nyhus, and Wantz [5–7]. While the open repairs all enter the preperitoneal space through an anterior abdominal wall incision, the preperitoneal space of Bogros is typically approached laparoscopically in one of two ways: by first entering the peritoneal cavity and then opening the peritoneum (transabdominal preperitoneal or TAPP) or by staying totally extraperitoneal (TEP). Benefits of the TAPP approach include easier visualization of the inguinal anatomy, direct visualization of the contents of the hernia sac, and facilitated management of large scrotal or incarcerated hernias as the hernia sac can be divided and left in place without consequence. The benefits of being intraperitoneal also bring with them potential consequences. Entering the peritoneal cavity with trocars and instruments can lead to vascular or hollow viscus injury and these complications have been reported with this approach [18, 21–23]. Reperitonealization to completely cover the mesh, if incomplete, can also lead to complications such as mesh erosion or bowel obstruction from internal herniation. By avoiding the peritoneal cavity, the TEP approach eliminates many of these complications. By remaining totally extraperitoneal, bowel or major vascular injury should be minimized and peritoneal closure is not required. However, staying extraperitoneal and the resulting limited working space makes use of larger mesh more challenging than in a TAPP approach, as is identification of anatomic landmarks. Also, tears in the peritoneum during TEP can lead to pnuemoperitoneum which will encroach on the preperitoneal space adding further challenge to this approach. This most commonly occurs in patients with previous lower abdominal or preperitoneal surgery such as prostatectomy, or in patients with incarcerated or large scrotal hernias necessitating division of the hernia sac. If the peritoneal defect is large or the preperitoneal space cannot be maintained, conversion to TAPP or open repair may be required.

While there has been no prospective randomized trial comparing the two approaches, several authors have retrospectively compared TEP and TAPP [22, 24]. In nearly all studies, recurrence, perioperative complications and return to work were similar for the two repairs. Intra-abdominal complications such as bowel and vascular injuries from trocar insertion or dissection, and bowel obstruction were reported more frequently in the TAPP group than in the TEP. The TAPP complications, however, typically occurred early in a group's experience suggesting a learning curve effect.

So which of these approaches is the best for laparoscopic herniorrhaphy? The answer is, there is no one "best" approach. As stated earlier, surgeons performing inguinal herniorrhaphy should be facile with both open and laparoscopic approaches, and this should include both the TAPP and TEP techniques. Our approach is to employ the TEP technique for patients who have not had previous preperitoneal dissection, as we feel that avoidance of the

Table 31.2. Risk/benefits of totally extraperitoneal (TEP) and trans-abdominal preperitoneal (TAPP) approaches to laparoscopic inguinal hernia repair

TEP (totally extraperitoneal)	TAPP (trans-abdominal preperitoneal)
Anatomical landmarks difficult	Anatomical landmarks easy
Wide dissection easy	Wide dissection more challenging
Peritoneal tear may lead to conversion	Peritoneum can be divided at will (but must eventually be closed)
Avoids bowel/vascular injury	Bowel/vascular injury more likely
Avoids intraperitoneal adhesions	Minimizes exposure to extraperitoneal adhesions

peritoneal cavity is beneficial. However, for those patients with previous extraperitoneal surgery (e.g., prior LIH or lower midline incision in which scar obliterates the preperitoneal space), we will preferentially utilize a TAPP approach. Potential benefits for each approach are summarized in Table 31.2.

31.2.3
The Role of Mesh Fixation

No matter what the indication or the operative approach, one issue that must be addressed by all surgeons performing laparoscopic herniorrhaphy is whether to fixate the mesh. The debate over whether to employ fixation is focused on two main issues: whether lack of fixation leads to higher recurrence rates, and whether use of fixation leads to increased rates of chronic pain and neuralgias. A secondary issue relates to cost; if mesh fixation is eliminated the cost of the procedure is reduced. Proponents of mesh fixation cite concerns over mesh migration, rolling or shrinking leading to hernia recurrence as the basis for fixation. These concerns are based on case reports of mesh migration [25] as well as animal studies showing higher degrees of mesh displacement and shrinkage when fixation is not employed [26, 27]. This position is also supported by several reports focusing on causes of recurrence following laparoscopic inguinal herniorrhaphy [28–30]. All of these papers identified inadequate fixation as a major cause of recurrence. In fact, a multicenter study reported that up to 65% of all recurrences were in some way related to inadequate fixation [30]. While these recurrences were often confounded by deficiencies in mesh size, each author concluded that adequate mesh fixation to prevent or reduce mesh displacement was essential to reduce hernia recurrences.

Those advocating no mesh fixation cite the excellent results reported by Nyhus, Stoppa, and others [5, 6] with the open preperitoneal approach utilizing no mesh fixation. This group argues that mesh size is more important than fixation in the prevention of recurrence, and that adequate exposure and the use of mesh in the 10–15 cm × 10–15 cm range will yield recurrence rates similar to the open series quoted above. They contend that while mesh migration and shrinkage occurs, it can be compensated for with adequate mesh size alone.

With respect to neuralgia or chronic pain, advocates of no fixation cite a myriad of papers implicating staples or tacks as the cause of the pain [21, 22, 31]. While most acknowledge that exercising care in the location of fixation, especially avoiding the area dorsal to the iliopubic tract lateral to the internal ring, there can be considerable variability in the lumbar plexus anatomy [32, 33], resulting in aberrancies of the cutaneous nerves. When present, these aberrant nerves are more susceptible to injury from tacks or staples placed anywhere. However, elimination of fixation does not completely eliminate neuralgia and groin pain [13, 34]. There are large series utilizing anatomically guided careful mesh fixation that report low nerve injury rates equivalent to series with no fixation at all [35].

In an attempt to definitively define the role of mesh fixation in laparoscopic inguinal herniorrhaphy, two prospective randomized studies have been undertaken [36, 37]; one employed the TAPP approach, and the other the TEP. Neither study showed a statistically significant difference between the fixed and non-fixed mesh with respect to hernia recurrence or postoperative neuralgia. The TEP study actually reported no recurrences or neuralgia with or without fixation. On the surface this would seem like overwhelming support for not fixating mesh, but these studies are not without flaw. Each study suffers from small numbers, and short and inadequate follow-up. More subjects and longer follow up is necessary before these studies can definitively answer the question about mesh fixation.

The application of mesh fixation may not be an all or none phenomenon as illustrated by a study that attempted to calculate the optimal mesh overlap in a theoretical ex vivo model. This study showed that for defects up to 2 cm, a 2-cm overlap was adequate to prevent recurrence and fixation was not required. However, for defects greater than 4 cm, the anatomy of the inguinal region prevented adequate overlap, and fixation was recommended to prevent recurrence [38]. Thus, use of fixation only in the setting of large or multiple defects may prove to be the essential compromise. This concept must be demonstrated clinically before the issue of the effect of defect size on the need for fixation can be addressed.

The controversy over whether to fix mesh in inguinal hernia repair has yet to be resolved. It is our position that until hernia recurrence rates without mesh fixation are definitively shown to be equivalent to recurrence rates with fixation, mesh fixation should be performed in laparoscopic inguinal herniorrhaphy. Careful fixation technique should be employed to avoid injury to the cutaneous nerves of the lumbar plexus, specifically the ilioinguinal, lateral femoral cutaneous, and genitofemoral nerves. No fixation should be placed below or even near the level of the iliopubic tract lateral to the internal ring as the variability of the nerve anatomy results in nerves frequently passing through the iliopubic tract. We feel that this careful use of fixation will minimize both recurrence and neuralgia and result in optimal long term results.

31.3
Summary

— Laparoscopic inguinal hernia repair is clearly indicated for bilateral and recurrent inguinal hernias and should be offered to select unilateral primary inguinal hernia patients.
— In patients without previous preperitoneal dissection, the totally extraperitoneal (TEP) approach is the approach of choice due to avoidance of the peritoneal cavity and the resultant potential for fewer major complications. However, the transabdominal preperitoneal (TAPP) repair should be employed without hesitation for TEP difficulties requiring conversion, or when previous preperitoneal dissection is present.
— A large (>100 cm²) piece of mesh should be used with adequate, carefully placed fixation to minimize both chronic pain and recurrence.

References

1. Bassini E. Nuovo metodo sulla cura radicale dell' ernia inguinale. Arch Soc Ital Chir 1887;4:380.
2. Ger R, Monroe K, Duvivier R, Mishrick A. Management of indirect inguinal hernias by laparoscopic closure of the neck of the sac. Am J Surg 1990;159:370–3.
3. Corbitt JDJ. Transabdominal peritoneal herniorrhaphy. Surg Laparosc Endosc 1993;3:328–32.
4. McKernan J, Laws H. Laparoscopic repair of inguinal hernias using a totally extraperitoneal prosthetic approach. Surg Endosc 1993;7:26–8.

5. Nyhus L, Pollack R, Bombeck C, Donohue P. The preperitoneal approach and prosthetic buttress repair for recurrent hernia. Ann Surg 1988;208:722–7.

6. Stoppa R, Rives J, Walamount C, Palot J, Verhaege P, Delattre J. The use of Dacron in the repair of hernias of the groin. Surg Clin North Am 1984;64:269–85.

7. Wantz GE. Properitoneal hernioplasty with unilateral giant prosthetic reinforcement of the visceral sac. Contemp Surg 1994;44:83–9.

8. Felix E, Michas C, Gonzalez MJ. Laparoscopic repair of recurrent hernia. Am J Surg 1996;172:580–4.

9. Frankum CE, Ramshaw BJ, White J, Duncan TD, Wilson R, Mason EM, Lucas GW, Promes J. Laparoscopic repair of bilateral and recurrent hernias. Am Surg 1999;65:839–43.

10. Champault G, Rizk N, Cathrine G, Barrat C, Turner R, Boutelier P. Inguinal hernia repair: totally preperitoneal laparoscopic approach versus Stoppa operation: a randomized trial 100 cases. Hernia 1997;1:31–6.

11. Beets G, Dirksen C, Go P, Geisler F, Baeten C, Kootstra G. Open or laparoscopic preperitoneal mesh repair for recurrent inguinal hernia. A randomized control trial. Surg Endosc 1999;13:323–7.

12. Sarli L, Iusco D, Sansebastiano G, Costi R. Simultaneous repair of bilateral inguinal hernias: a prospective, randomized study of open, tension-free versus laparoscopic approach. Surg Laparosc Endosc Percutan Tech 2001;11:262–7.

13. Liem MSL, Van Der Graaf Y, Van Steensel CJ, Boelhouwer RU, Clevers G-J, Meijer WS, Stassen LPS, Vente JP, Wedema WF, Schrijvers AJP, Van Vroonhovern T. Comparison of conventional anterior surgery and laparoscopic surgery fro inguinal-hernia repair. N Engl J Med 1997;336:1541–7.

14. Collaboration EHT. Laparoscopic compared with open methods of groin hernia repair: systematic review of randomized controlled trials. Br J Surg 2000;87:860–7.

15. Johansson B, Hallerback B, Glise H, Anesten B, Smedberg S, Roman J. Laparoscopic mesh versus open preperitoneal mesh versus conventional technique for inguinal hernia repair. A randomized multicenter trial (SCUR Hernia Repair Study). Ann Surg 1999;230:224–31.

16. Bringman S, Ramel S, Heikkinen T-J, Englund T, Westman B, Anderberg B. Tension free inguinal hernia repair: TEP versus mesh-plug versus Lichtenstein. Ann Surg 2003;237:142–7.

17. Andersson B, Hallen M, Leveau P, Bergenfelz A, Westerdahl J. Laparoscopic extraperitoneal inguinal hernia repair versus open mesh repair: a prospective randomized controlled trial. Surgery 2003;133:464–72.

18. McCormack K, Scott N, Go P, Ross S, Grant A; EU Hernia Trialists Collaboration. Laparoscopic techniques versus open techniques for inguinal hernia repair. Cochrane Databasef Syst Rev 2003;1:CD001785.

19. Douek M, Smith G, Oshowo A, Stoker D, Wellwood J. Prospective randomized controlled trial of laparoscopic versus open inguinal hernia mesh repair: five year follow-up. BMJ 2003;326:1012–3.

20. Swanstrom LL. Laparoscopic hernia repairs. the importance of cost as an outcome measurement at the century's end. Surg Clin North Am 2000;80:1341–51.

21. Phillips E, Arregui M, Carroll B, Corbitt J, Crafton W, Fallas M, Filipi CJ, Fitzgibbons RJJ, Franklin M, McKernan B, Olsen D, Ortega A, Payne JHJ, Peters J, Rodriquez R,

Rosette P, Schultz L, Seid A, Sewell R, Smoot R, Toy F, Waddell R, Watson S. Incidence of complications following laparoscopic hernioplasty. Surg Endosc 1995;9:16–21.

22. Felix EL, Michas C, Gonzalez MJ. Laparoscopic hernioplasty. TAPP vs TEP. Surg Endosc 1995;9:984–9.

23. Cohen RV, Alvarez G, Roll S, Garcia M, Kawahara N, Schiavon C, Dan Schaffa T, Pereira PR, Margarido N, Rodrigues A. Transabdominal or totally extraperitoneal laparoscopic hernia repair? Surg Laparosc Endosc 1998;8:264–8.

24. Ramshaw BJ, Tucker JG, Conner T, Mason EM, Duncan TD, Lucas GW. A comparison of the approaches to laparoscopic herniorrhaphy. Surg Endosc 1996;10:29–32.

25. Hume R, Bour J. Mesh migration following laparoscopic inguinal hernia repair. J Laparoendosc Surg 1996;6:333–5.

26. Katkhouda N, Mavor E, Friedlander MH, Mason RJ, Kiyabu M, Grant SW, Achanta K, Kirkman EL, Narayanan K, Essani R. Use of fibrin sealant for prosthetic mesh fixation in laparoscopic extraperitoneal inguinal hernia repair. Ann Surg 2001;233:18–25.

27. Zieren J, Castenholz E, Jacobi C, Zieren HU, Muller JM. Is mesh fixation necessary in abdominal hernia repair? Results of an experimental study in the rat. Langenbecks Arch Surg 1999;382:71–5.

28. Lowham AS, Filipi CJ, Fitzgibbons RJJ, Stoppa R, Wantz GE, Felix EL, Grafton WB. Mechanisms of hernia recurrence after preperitoneal mesh repair: traditional and laparoscopic. Ann Surg 1997;225:422–31.

29. Tucker JG, Wilson R, Ramshaw BJ. Laparoscopic herniorrhaphy: technical concerns in prevention of complications and early recurrence. Am Surg 1995;61:36–9.

30. Felix E, Scott S, B. C, Geis P, Duncan TD, Sewell R, McKernan B. Causes of recurrence after laparoscopic hernioplasty: a multicenter study. Surg Endosc 1998;12:226–31.

31. Kraus M. Nerve injury during laparoscopic inguinal hernia repair. Surg Laparosc Endosc 1993;3:342–5.

32. Colborn G, Brick WG, Gadacz TR, Skandalakis J. Inguinal anatomy for laparoscopic herniorrhaphy. 2. Altered inguinal anatomy and variations. Surgical Rounds 1995;June:223–32.

33. Colborn G, Skandalakis J. Laparoscopic inguinal anatomy. Hernia 1998;2:179–91.

34. Khajanchee YS, Urbach DR, Swanstrom LL, Hansen PD. Outcomes of laparoscopic herniorrhaphy without fixation of mesh to the abdominal wall. Surg Endosc 2001;15:1102–7.

35. Ramshaw BJ, Shuler F, Jones H, Duncan TD, White J, Wilson R, Lucas GW, Mason EM. Laparoscopic Inguinal hernia repair. Lessons learned after 1224 consecutive cases. Surg Endosc 2001;15:50–4.

36. Ferzli GS, Frezza EE, Pecoraro AMJ, Ahern KD. Prospective randomized study of stapled versus unstapled mesh in a laparoscopic preperitoneal inguinal hernia repair. J Am Coll Surg 1999;188:461–5.

37. Smith AI, Royston CMS, Sedman PC. Stapled and nonstapled laparoscopic transabdominal preperitoneal (TAPP) Inguinal hernia repair. A prospective randomized trial. Surg Endosc 1999;13:804–6.

38. Hollinsky C, Hollinsky KH. Static Calcualtions for mesh fixation by intraabdominal pressure in laparoscopic extraperitoneal herniorrhaphy. Surg Laparosc Endosc 1999;9:106–9.

Addendum

No current discussion of controversies in laparoscopic inguinal hernia repair would be complete without addressing the recently published prospective randomized trial comparing laparoscopic inguinal hernia repair with open mesh repair [1]. This study, conducted at 14 Veterans Affairs Medical Centers, randomized nearly 2000 patients to undergo either laparoscopic hernia repair or the Lichtenstein open tension-free mesh repair for either primary or first-time recurrent inguinal hernias. The results of 24-month follow-up in just over 85% of the patients show that the overall recurrence rate was lower in the open group compared with the laparoscopic group (4.9% vs 10.1%). The intraoperative, immediate postoperative, and life threatening complication rate was also reported as lower in the open group. Reported benefits for the laparoscopic approach included less pain in the first 2 weeks, earlier resumption of vigorous activity, and a lower recurrence rate for repair of first-time recurrent hernias, especially when the repair was performed by an experienced surgeon (3.6% laparoscopic vs 17.4% open). The two types of repair were reported similar with respect to recurrence rate for primary hernias when the repair was performed by an experienced surgeon (5.1% laparoscopic vs 4.1% open). The incidence of chronic pain, long-term complications, and days to resumption of sexual activity was also similar between the two groups. Based on these results, the authors concluded that the open tension-free Lichtenstein hernia repair was superior to the laparoscopic mesh repair for primary inguinal hernias.

While seemingly condemning the laparoscopic approach for repair of primary inguinal hernias, this study actually demonstrates the benefits of laparoscopic inguinal hernia repair while underscoring the need for adequate training and experience in this technique. Less experienced surgeons had significantly more recurrences with the laparoscopic repair than with open repair (12.3% vs 2.5%), while no difference existed between experienced surgeons. The equivalent recurrence rate in the experienced group combined with the benefits of less pain and faster return to activity demonstrates the superiority of the laparoscopic repair when performed correctly.

With regards to complications, the majority of the reported life-threatening complications were likely anesthesia related (i.e., cardiac issues, anaphylactic drug reaction, and postoperative respiratory insufficiency). This highlights the need, as emphasized in this chapter, to carefully select patients who have an underlying state of health compatible with undergoing general anesthesia. The clinical significance of many of the other listed complications is also questionable such as claiming the presence of a peritoneal defect over the mesh at time of closure and presence of a seroma as complications. Complications in the „other" category were 3–5 times more likely in the laparoscopic group, yet we don't know what these other complications were. Knowing the etiology of these complications would be helpful in interpreting these data. In all, the typical hernia complications after hernia repair such as neuralgia, wound infection, or injury to cord structures or vessels are comparable between the two approaches.

This study supports our contention that surgeons committed to the comprehensive treatment of groin hernias should acquire skills in the laparoscopic technique through properly mentored training, and maintain these skills by applying this technique to carefully selected patients with primary inguinal hernias. This will allow surgeons to more successfully apply the laparoscopic approach to recurrent and bilateral inguinal hernias where even more patient benefit is realized.

1. Neumayer L, Giobbie-Hurger A, Jonasson O, et al. Open mesh versus laparoscopic mesh repair of inguinal hernia. N Engl J Med 2004;350:1819–27.

Commentary

ABE FINGERHUT

The three controversies in the chapter by Ritter and Smith include: (1) the role of the laparoscopic approach to inguinal hernia repair, (2) the question of which laparoscopic technique is best, and (3) the question whether the mesh should be fixed or not.

"Where does laparoscopy fit best" is indeed central to the debate. Is going through a previous incision a real problem? Finding a clear anatomical plane, leading to recognition of the essential anatomic landmarks and repair all the defects are as essential as uncertain. Lesions to the vessels and/or cord are the real dangers, and these structures are vulnerable in any approach. As mesh repairs increase (20% of revisional hernia repairs are previous mesh repairs) [1], avoiding previous surgical fields in the case of recurrence means using the traditional, anterior, transcutaneous, approach if the original technique was laparoscopic, or the transperitoneal approach if the original technique was pre-peritoneal.

That the young manual laborer will benefit most from the laparoscopic repair might be true: however, this has never been shown formally. Moreover, it has been stated that those patients with higher income [2] and without workers compensation [3] (Felix) return to work earlier. Is this the case of „the young manual laborer"?

What is the rationale behind saying that „the common benefits of avoiding previous surgical fields and the ability to address all types of groin hernia has lead to the laparoscopic approach being readily accepted for the repair ... of bilateral hernia". The authors' recommendations seemed to be based on one small (n=43 patients) randomized trial (Sarli), which favored the laparoscopic approach for patient comfort and return to work. While admittedly up to 50% of patients have unsuspected (asymptomatic) bilateral hernias, no one knows their natural history and no other controlled trial has yet shown any benefit in the simultaneous repair over the sequential repair [4]. Rather than stating that bilateral repair will save these patients a second operation (in Sarli's study, both sides can be treated in the same session, without any difference in time), the true question remains without an answer: "is it necessary to operate on asymptomatic hernia?"

As concerns the statement that "*Acquisition* and *maintenance* of experience and skills through ... laparoscopic herniorrhaphy for ... primary hernias ... will allow the surgeon to ... tackle more difficult recurrent and bilateral cases", I cannot agree that patients be considered the training or maintenance grounds, especially for a technique that has at the best modest or marginal benefits and does have some well recognized drawbacks [5].

As for the choice between the TAPP and TEP techniques, it is somewhat paradoxical to see that, in the opinion of the authors, the major indication for the TEP repair, which definitely has advantages over the TAPP repair, is to "avoid adherences", while this is supposed to be the advantage of the transperitoneal laparoscopic route. Where are the true arguments?

Last, as concerns the question of whether to fix or not, the authors "believe" that fixation is necessary. Of note, there was no difference in the recurrence rates of the two controlled trials mentioned (Smith and Ferzli). Additionally, the numbers of patients in these trials were *not* that small (502 patients in the study with TAPP, 92 in that with TEP). While no β error was calculated in the first (Smith), surgeons had previously performed more than 200 repairs before entering the trial. In the second, the authors stated that they did the necessary calculation, but do not provide the numbers: the conclusion was that mesh fixation can be avoided without compromising on results and with a savings of US$ 120 per patient (Ferzli). Swanstrom has shown the same. "Short" follow-up is not particular to these two studies (although a median of 16 and 8 months, respectively, are nothing to be ashamed of).

May I add a word of caution to the all too frequent comment that this or that (usually adverse) outcome might be due to the "learning curve", the case for at least five reports cited herein [References 10, 11, 18, 22, 24 above]. While the learning curve was not stated for every study, it is not known with certainty that recurrence(s) or complication(s) occurred early in the series of McCormack or Ramshaw. In those authored by Champault and Beets, the classical 50 laparoscopic repair cutoff value was stated. As regards the study by Felix, 1115 laparoscopic were performed in a "specialized hernia repair" center. Two of the TAPP complications occurred within 12 months (~150 patients). Lastly, in the study reported by Ramshaw (600 patients), four of the enterotomies and the two cystotomies were due to difficulties in dissection, and, excepting one balloon injury to the bladder, were not directly related to the laparoscopic technique. Every surgeon has a learning curve. It is not because the experience of one surgeon improves over time that the *overall* learning curve (that of the overall population of surgeons) changes. The recurrence rate per year after mesh repair is a straight upwards line, if patients are followed correctly [6–8]. The recently published multicenter trial of 2164 patients by Neumayer et al. [9] adds another dimension to the notion: the learning curve for laparoscopic repair may be as high as 250 cases. Recurrence was more frequent in the laparoscopic arm. Life-threatening complications occurred more often in the laparoscopic group, confirming earlier reports [6].

Just to play with numbers, let us say that the "learning curve" for laparoscopic hernia repair is between 30 and 50 procedures [10]. About 14% of all hernia repairs in the USA are laparoscopic, that is to say approximately 115,000 repairs for the year 2003 [5]. If we consider that 500 (this is probably a low estimate) "new" surgeons embark on this operation every year, then they will repair about 13% to 20% of these hernias on their "learning curve" (11.8% of hernia repairs by residents, $n=6444$, are done laparoscopically [11]). This leads to acknowledge: (1) why the recurrence rate of laparoscopic repair, like any other type of repair, will not decrease for the overall population of surgeons, although the rate for one individual surgeon or team will, and (2) if the new surgeon does not meet the minimum number (to be determined) necessary "to maintain his or her skills" for the more difficult recurrent or bilateral repairs, then the time (in the reduced working hours) invested in becoming "good" at the technique might be better spent elsewhere.

What would these numbers be if the learning curve were really 250 [9]?

References

1. Schumperlick V, Klinge U. Prosthetic implants for hernia repair. Br J Surg 2003;90: 1457–8.
2. Voyles CR. Tension-free mesh plug hernioplasty. Op Tech Gen Surg 1999;1:197–202.
3. Salcedo-Wasicek MD, Thirlby RC. Postoperative course after herniorrhaphy: a case-controlled comparison of patients receiving worker's compensation vs patients with commercial insurance. Arch Surg 1995;130:29–32.

4. Fischer S, Cassivi S, Paul A, Troidl H. Evidence-based medicine and special aspects in bilateral inguinal hernia repair. Hernia 1999;3:89–95.
5. Rutkow IM,. Demographic and socioeconomic aspects of hernia repair in the United States in 2003. Surg Clin North Am 2003;83:1045–51.
6. EU Hernia Trialists Collaboration. Repair of groin hernia with synthetic mesh: meta-analysis of randomized controlled trials. Ann Surg 2002;235:322–32.
7. Flum DR, Horvath K, Koepsell T. Have outcomes of incisional hernia repair improved with time? Ann Surg 2003;237:129–35.
8. Memon MA, Cooper NJ, Memon B, Memon MI, Abrams KR. Meta-analysis of randomized clinical trials comparing open and laparoscopic inguinal hernia repair. Br J Surg: 90;1479–92.
9. Neumeyer L, Giobbie-Hurder A, Jonasson O, Fitzgibbons R, Dunlop D, Gibbs D, Reda D, Henderson W. Open mesh versus laparoscopic mesh repair of inguinal hernia. N Engl J Med 2004;350:1819–27.
10. Davies CJ, Arregui ME. Laparoscopic repair for groin hernias. Surg Clin North Am 2003;83:1141–61.
11. Lo P, Ahmed N, Chung RS. Which laparoscopic operations are the fastest growing in residency programs? Surg Endosc 2001;15:S145.

Thyroid and Parathyroid Surgery

Kaare J. Weber, William B. Inabnet III

▶ **Key Controversy**

Choice of surgical approach
- Endoscopic approach
  - Cervical
  - Transaxillary
  - Anterior chest
- Video-assisted approach
- Mini-open or focused approach
  - Preoperative localization: ultrasound, sestamibi scintigraphy
  - Intraoperative localization: radio-guided probe

32.1
Introduction

Surgery of the thyroid and parathyroid is traditionally performed through a transverse cervical incision with very low morbidity and virtually no mortality. However, with the increasing acceptance of minimally invasive surgery, surgeons are now applying these techniques to the cervical region. Several minimally invasive approaches to the neck have evolved over the recent years. Gagner reported the first endoscopic parathyroidectomy in 1996 [1]. Huscher and colleagues followed with the description of complete endoscopic thyroidectomy [2]. With the endoscopic approach, several approaches to the thyroid and parathyroid glands have evolved, including the cervical approach, the transaxillary approach, and the breast or anterior chest wall approach, as well as video-assisted surgery [3–9]. In addition, advances in techniques have allowed surgeons to operate on both the thyroid and parathyroid glands through a mini-open or focused approach [10, 11]. In this chapter, each of these approaches will be described paying attention to their inherent advantages and disadvantages.

Of all of these techniques, the focused approach to parathyroidectomy seems to be the most commonly used approach by endocrine surgeons. Surgery of the parathyroid glands has seen a rapid change over the last several years with unilateral neck exploration for primary hyperparathyroidism now the standard approach at most centers. First described in 1982, the focused approach relies on preoperative localization, as well as intraoperative monitoring of parathyroid hormone (PTH) [12, 13]. The controversies that now exist include choice of preoperative localization along with the use of intraoperative PTH assay with and without radioguidance.

32.2
Discussion

32.2.1
Endoscopic Thyroidectomy and Parathyroidectomy

Endoscopic surgery for the thyroid and parathyroid glands can be approached through a variety of methods. Totally endoscopic approaches to parathyroidectomy and thyroidectomy were first reported in the late 1990s [1, 2], and since then several groups have reported their experience with the endoscopic approach [4, 5, 7, 9, 11, 13, 14].

32.2.1.1
Cervical Approach

The cervical approach utilizes small incisions in the neck. The technique for both thyroidectomy and parathyroidectomy requires general anesthesia and uses carbon dioxide to create a working space in the subplatysmal plane. Our approach to both thyroidectomy and parathyroidectomy utilizes three or four ports. Access is first gained through an incision along the anterior border of the sternocleidomastoid muscle in a superior location. Sharp dissection is used to identify the carotid artery. The space medial to the carotid artery but lateral to the strap muscles is developed using blunt dissection with either conventional instruments or insertion of a sponge to dissect the perithyroidal tissue plane. For both techniques, the strap muscles are retracted anteromedially to visualize the thyroid [3, 4].

During endoscopic thyroidectomy, the superior poles vessels are identified, isolated and divided with ultrasonic energy by working directly through the small incision. A purse-string suture is placed in the subcutaneous tissue and a 10-mm trocar is inserted. A working space is created with insufflation of carbon dioxide to a pressure of 10 mmHg. The tip of a 5-mm 0°-scope is first used to bluntly dissect the subplatysmal space and then switched to a 5-mm 30°-scope. A 5-mm trocar is then inserted at the sternal notch and two additional 3-mm trocars are placed at the midline and mid-portion of the sternocleidomastoid. After identifying and preserving the recurrent laryngeal nerve, the inferior thyroid artery is identified and ligated. The superior and inferior parathyroid glands are mobilized and preserved. The thyroid is next mobilized from the trachea, and the isthmus divided with the ultrasonic scalpel. The specimen is placed in a retrieval sac and removed through the initial 10-mm trocar site [3].

For parathyroidectomy, an endoscopic approach can be performed on the basis of pre-operative imaging and intra-operative PTH monitoring. The thyroid is retracted medially to dissect the posterolateral aspect of the gland in order to identify the parathyroid gland as well as the recurrent laryngeal nerve. The scope can be moved to as needed to various ports in order to facilitate the dissection of both the superior and inferior lobes as well as left and right lobes of the thyroid if required. After the abnormal gland is identified, care must be taken not the damage the capsule for risk of spillage and recurrence. After the vascular pedicle has been dissected, it can be ligated between clips or with an endoloop. The specimen is then removed in a retrieval sac fastened from the thumb of a rubber glove. Unless there is inappropriate reduction of intraoperative PTH levels, no attempt is made to identify the remaining parathyroid glands in order to preserve tissue planes [4].

The cervical endoscopic approach allows for bilateral neck exploration if warranted in addition to easy conversion to an open approach if required. Endoscopic magnification, as well as use of bipolar coagulation or ultrasonic energy can help prevent injury to the recurrent laryngeal nerve.

Initial reports from various institutions have demonstrated the safety and efficacy of the cervical approach [4, 14]. Over 5 years, 56 patients underwent attempted endoscopic parathyroidectomy. Six patients were converted to conventional surgery either due to large gland size or inability to locate the gland within a reasonable amount of time. Mean operative time for single gland removal was 121 min. Multiple gland excision took longer with an average of 270 min. While the operative times can be prolonged, they decrease with experience. There were no major complications including nerve injury. The excellent optics with high magnification and resolution likely contributes to the clear identification and preservation of the recurrent laryngeal nerve. Minor complications included hypercarbia as a result of prolonged carbon dioxide insufflation. Patients were discharged home after an average stay of 1.2 days. All patients have remained normocalcemic and asymptomatic with follow-up ranging anywhere from 1 month to 2 years [4].

32.2.1.2
Transaxillary Approach

Additional endoscopic methods to thyroidectomy and parathyroidectomy have been reported by several groups, including the transaxillary approach [15, 16]. This technique also requires general anesthesia and the use carbon dioxide to create a working space. Insufflation pressures are lower than the supraclavicular approach, thus reducing the risk for hypercarbia, respiratory acidosis, subcutaneous emphysema, and air embolism. A major advantage to this approach is the avoidance of a cervical incision by utilizing the axilla for placement of trocars. However, the view achieved by the axillary approach is limited, requiring division of the strap muscles for exposure, as well as only a unilateral exploration. Supporters of this technique believe that the axillary approach allows for a lateral view equivalent to open surgery facilitating identification of the nerve and parathyroid glands. The remote location of the incision does require a larger working space resulting in a greater technical challenge and subsequent increased operative times.

Ikeda and colleagues recently reported a retrospective study of 40 patients comparing endoscopic thyroidectomy by the axillary approach with conventional open surgery. None of the endoscopic procedures required conversion but operative time was significantly longer in the endoscopic group (168 vs 82 min). In addition, none of the patients developed hypercapnia. There were reports of subcutaneous emphysema of the neck and anterior chest that resolved in the postoperative period. There were no occurrences of recurrent laryngeal nerve or parathyroid injury in either group. Four patients in the endoscopic group complained of severe chest pain on the first postoperative day. One patient in the endoscopic group complained of slight hypesthesia while 13 patients in the open group complained of hypesthesia or paresthesia. None of the patients in the endoscopic group complained of dysphagia, while six patients in the open group complained of discomfort when swallowing. All patients undergoing the endoscopic axillary thyroidectomy were satisfied with the cosmetic result while 15 patients in the open group expressed dissatisfaction with the cosmetic results [15].

Experience with endoscopic parathyroidectomy via the axillary approach has been limited. Seven patients have been reported to undergo endoscopic axillary parathyroidectomy. Mean operative time was again prolonged (171 min). One patient had to be converted to open due to the presence of a thymic parathyroid adenoma. No recurrent nerve injuries occurred and cosmesis was excellent. Some patients did complain of discomfort in the anterior chest, which resolved after 3 months [16].

32.2.1.3
Anterior Chest Approach

The anterior chest approach to endoscopic thyroidectomy or parathyroidectomy utilizes port access at the nipple areolar complex or various positions below the clavicle depending on the surgeon, thus avoiding a cervical incision [14, 17, 18]. Similar to the axillary approach, this technique requires general anesthesia, low pressure carbon dioxide insufflation, as well as a flexible laparoscope. In addition, the strap muscles must be divided for adequate exposure. However, unlike the axillary approach, the anterior chest approach allows for bilateral neck exploration.

Several groups have demonstrated that the anterior chest approach to thyroidectomy is feasible and safe [17, 18, 19]. As with the other endoscopic approaches, operative time remains increased. In addition, hospital stay can also be prolonged as a result of routine use of drains in the postoperative period. Similar to the axillary approach, severe chest pain has been reported post-operatively. Conversion has also been reported as a result of excessive bleeding. A significant disadvantage of both the axillary and anterior chest approach is the lack of immediate access to bleeding either intraoperatively or postoperatively.

Preliminary results in five patients undergoing endoscopic parathyroidectomy by the anterior chest approach demonstrated that this procedure could be performed safely. Mean operative time was again prolonged (236 min). Hospital stay was 6 days. There was no evidence of recurrent laryngeal nerve injury. All patients had normal serum calcium and parathyroid hormone levels at follow-up. Cosmesis was excellent [7].

32.2.2
Video-assisted Thyroidectomy and Parathyroidectomy

Significant experience has been gained utilizing the minimally invasive video-assisted thyroidectomy (MIVAT) and parathyroidectomy (MIVAP) by Miccoli and colleagues [8, 9]. Using this technique, patients can undergo either regional anesthesia or general anesthesia. For MIVAP, preoperative localization with ultrasound or sestamibi scan is required. For both techniques, a 15-mm skin incision is made approximately at the level of the sternal notch. After the cervical midline is opened, the operative space is maintained with narrow retractors. Dissection is carried out with small instruments under endoscopic vision with a 30°, 5-mm scope.

Since describing MIVAT in 1998, Miccoli and colleagues have published a large multi-institutional experience demonstrating the feasibility of this technique [20]. A total of 336 patients underwent MIVAT at four separate institutions. The mean operative times for lobectomy and total thyroidectomy were 69 and 87 min, respectively. The mean length of stay was 1.9 days. Complication rates did not differ from standard thyroidectomy with seven transient and one definitive recurrent nerve palsies. In addition, there were nine transient and two definitive cases of hypoparathyroidism. Fifteen patients were converted to open procedures [20].

Results from a published series of 137 patients undergoing MIVAP demonstrate that outcome and operative time were the same as in traditional surgery with better cosmetic result and less painful course. Mean operative time was 56.1 min. Conversion to open was required in ten patients due to either incorrect preoperative localization, the presence of a second adenoma, carcinoma, or intrathyroidal adenoma. One patient experienced a recurrent laryngeal nerve palsy. Transient hypoparathyroidism occurred in six cases [21].

32.2.3
Mini-open or Focused Approach

Mini-open or focused approach is another non-endoscopic option available to endocrine surgeons. The procedure can be performed under either general or regional anesthesia. Advantages of regional anesthesia have been demonstrated by Lo Gerfo and colleagues with conventional thyroidectomy. These include decreased postoperative pain, easier reoperation for postoperative bleeding, and shorter operative time and hospital stay [22].

The minimally invasive open approach to thyroidectomy allows the surgeon to offer the advantages of regional anesthesia to the patient undergoing minimally invasive, non-endoscopic surgery. The technique utilizes a small 2- to 3-cm transverse skin incision approximately 3–4 cm above the sternal notch, slightly higher than a conventional incision. Subplatysmal flaps are created to 2 cm above the thyroid cartilage superiorly and to the level of the sternal notch inferiorly. The cervical fascia is then incised along the midline exposing the strap muscles which are elevated off the thyroid capsule. The higher skin incision allows for exposure of the superior poles vessels, which are taken first in order to deliver the gland through the incision. The recurrent nerve is then identified as it enters the larynx. While providing better exposure, the incision also provides excellent cosmetic results. At any time during the procedure, the incision can be extended for further exposure if required [23].

In a series of 89 patients by Ferzli and coworkers, thyroidectomy was attempted through a 2.5-cm incision. Most (63%) of the thyroidectomies were able to be completed with a 4-cm incision, 28% of patients had an incision length under 3 cm, and eight patients had an incision extending beyond 4 cm. Patients requiring larger incisions had thyroid glands measuring 7 cm or greater. This technique can be completed in approximately an hour (mean 76 min) similar to the conventional technique. Most patients were discharged home less than 23 h after surgery. Complications included cardiac arrhythmia requiring additional observation post-operatively. Transient hypocalcemia was reported in one patient. There were no recurrent laryngeal nerve injuries or palsies [23].

Mini-open or focused approach to parathyroidectomy is a unilateral exploration of the neck for a single adenoma localized preoperatively by ultrasound and/or technetium-99m sestamibi scan. The focused approach can be performed under general anesthesia or cervical block. Adequate removal of the diseased gland is confirmed with intraoperative PTH monitoring. Some surgeons rely on a gamma probe to guide the dissection in patients who have received technetium-99m sestamibi preoperatively [11, 13].

For unilateral neck exploration, a 2-cm incision is made in a natural skin cease based on preoperative localization studies or over the area of maximal radioactivity if a gamma probe is used. The sternocleidomastoid muscle is retracted laterally and the underlying strap muscles are separated. The thyroid lobe is mobilized and retracted anteromedially. Attempt is made to identify the recurrent laryngeal nerve particularly if the gland is in a deep location. Once the adenoma is identified, the vascular pedicle is dissected and ligated with small clips. Intraoperative PTH levels are drawn prior to the incision, after isolation and 5, 10, and 20 min after excision. A 50% reduction in the PTH level from the highest pre-excision value is considered adequate resection of all hypersecreting parathyroid tissue [11, 13].

Results have been excellent. Udelsman and colleagues have recently reported the outcome of 656 patients undergoing exploration for primary hyperparathyroidism [13]. A minimally invasive or focused approach was used in 255 patients. Patients underwent preoperative localization with sestamibi scans imaged with SPECT (single photon emission computed tomography). A positive scan was obtained in 96% of patients undergoing a focused approach. Anesthesia with cervical block was successful in 89% of patients with 29 requiring conversion to general anesthesia. Intraoperative PTH monitoring demonstrated a greater than 50% decreased from baseline in 97% of patients after excision of the adenoma. Mean operative time for the focused approach was 50% less than the traditional approach with mean operative time of 1.3 h. There were no deaths and the complication rate for minimally invasive parathyroidectomy was 1.2% compared with 3% for the conventional approach. The cure rate, defined as maintenance of eucalcemia 6 months after surgery, was 97%. Lastly, there was a seven-fold reduction in length of hospital stay as well as a 50% reduction in total hospital charges in the minimally invasive group [13].

32.2.3.1
Preoperative Localization

Because of the improvement in preoperative localization studies, surgeons can reliably explore the neck in a unilateral, focused approach. A variety of studies are available to localized abnormal parathyroid glands. Ultrasound and sestamibi scintigraphy are the first line tests for preoperative localization.

High-resolution ultrasonography has a sensitivity of 70–80% [24]. It is inexpensive and simple. It provides important anatomic information including the size and depth of the parathyroid adenoma and its relationship to surrounding structures. Ultrasound can also provide important information about the thyroid gland. However, the disadvantage of this technique is that sensitivity is directly related to the user. In addition, it is limited by acoustic shadows, which can result in blind spots.

Dual phase sestamibi scanning is a very reliable examination for preoperative localization with sensitivities ranging from 80 to 90% [24, 25]. Compared with ultrasound, sestamibi scanning has the advantage of evaluating ectopic parathyroid glands in the mediastinum as well as the tracheoesophageal groove. Disadvantages of this technique are the relative cost compared with ultrasound, as well as the requirement of radioisotope administration.

Some recommend the combined use of sestamibi scanning and high-resolution ultrasonography. The sensitivity of preoperative localization can be increased to well over 90% when the two modalities are utilized together [26].

32.2.3.2
Intraoperative Localization

Intraoperative localization with the gamma probe is an additional method surgeons can utilize to help localize parathyroid glands.

We recently examined our initial experience with intraoperative radioguidance during targeted parathyroidectomy. Sixty patients selected for radioguidance had a solitary adenoma visualized on technetium-99m sestamibi scintigraphy. A gamma probe was used to guide the dissection. We found that in almost 50% of patients, the probe provided confusing or inaccurate information. However, in the six patients with of persistent or recurrent hyperparathyroidism, the gamma probe aided in the localization of the abnormal gland by allowing optimal placement of the incision and by guiding the dissection in the re-operative neck. As a result, we believe that radioguidance may be more beneficial in persistent or recurrent hyperparathyroidism and in the reoperative neck where the dissection may be difficult [27].

32.3
Summary (Table 32.1)

— Over the last several years, a variety of minimally invasive techniques have evolved to approach the thyroid and parathyroid glands. They include totally endoscopic approaches, video-assisted approaches as well as mini-open or focused approaches.
— There have been no randomized, prospective studies comparing these techniques with the conventional open approach; however, many centers have demonstrated their feasibility and safety. Each have their inherent advantages and disadvantages and are summarized in Table 32.1.
— The obvious advantage of the endoscopic approaches is cosmesis, especially with the extra-cervical approaches where there are no visible neck scars. However, there are some inherent disadvantages to this approach including the potential complications from carbon dioxide insufflation, as well as significant post-operative pain from the extensive dissection with axillary or anterior chest approach.
— A significant disadvantage of both the axillary and anterior chest/breast approach is the lack of immediate access to bleeding either intra-operatively or postoperatively.
— The approach of choice for thyroidectomy will ultimately depend on the experience and skill of the surgeon as well as the desires of the patient.
— The principles of focused parathyroidectomy include a unilateral neck exploration based on preoperative imaging, intraoperative assessment of the adequacy of resection (i.e., PTH monitoring), and preservation of tissue planes around the normal parathyroid glands. All of the minimally invasive approaches adhere to these principles including the open focused, video-assisted, and endoscopic approaches. Endocrine surgeons should be familiar with all the different techniques so that the operative approach can be individualized.

References

1. Gagner M. Endoscopic subtotal parathyroidectomy in patients with primary hyperparathyroidism. Br J Surg 1996;83:875.
2. Huscher CSG, Chiodini S, Napolitano C, Recher A. Endoscopic right thyroid lobectomy. Surg Endosc 1997;11:877.

Table 32.1. Comparison of advantages and disadvantages of various approaches to thyroid and parathyroid surgery

Approach	GETA	CO_2 insufflation	Special equipment	Operative time	Invasiveness	Bilateral neck exploration	Pain	Cosmesis
Supraclavicular	Yes	Yes	Mini-scope and instruments	Increased	Dissection limited to neck	Yes	Decreased	Excellent
Transaxillary	Yes	Yes	Flexible laparoscope	Increased	Extra-cervical dissection with division of strap muscles	No	Increased	No visibible cervical scar
Anterior chest	Yes	Yes	Flexible laparoscope	Increased	Extra-cervical dissection with division of strap muscles	Yes	Increased	No visible cervical scar but possible areolar/ nipple deformity
Video-assisted	No	No	Traditional instruments	Equivalent	Dissection limited to neck	Yes	Decreased	Excellent
Mini-open/ focused	No	No	Traditional instruments	Decreased	Dissection limited to neck	No	Decreased	Excellent

3. Inabnet WB, Addis MD. Endoscopic thyroidectomy with CO_2 insufflation. Op Tech Otolaryngol Head Neck Surg 2002;13:242–3.
4. Gagner M, Rubino F. Endoscopic parathyroidectomy. In: Gagner M, Inabnet WB, eds. Minimally invasive endocrine surgery. Philadelphia: Lippincott, Williams & Wilkins; 2002.
5. Ikeda Y, Takami H, Sasaki Y, Kan S, Niimi, M. Endoscopic neck surgery by the axillary approach. J Am Coll Surg 2000;191:336–40.
6. Takami H, Ikeda Y. Minimally invasive thyroidectomy. Aust N Z J Surg 2002;72:841–2.
7. Ikeda Y, Takami H, Niimi S, Kan S, Sasaki Y, Takayama J. Endoscopic total parathyroidectomy by the anterior chest approach for renal hyperparathyroidism. Surg Endosc 2002;16:320–2.
8. Miccoli P, Berti P, Raffailli M, Conte M, Materazzi G, Galleri D. Minimally invasive video-assisted thyroidectomy. Am J Surg 2001;181:567–70.
9. Miccoli P, Bendinelli C, Vignali E, Mazzeo S, Cecchini G, Pinchera A, Marcocci C. Endoscopic parathyroidectomy: report of an initial experience. Surgery 1998;124:1077–80.
10. Park CS, Chung WY, Chang HS. Minimally invasive open thyroidectomy. Surg Today 2001;31:665–9.
11. Inabnet WB, Fulla Y, Bonnichon P, Icard P, Chapuis Y. Unilateral neck exploration under local anesthesia: the approach of choice for asymptomatic primary hyperparathyroidism. Surgery 1999;126:1004–9.
12. Tibblin S, Bondeson AG, Ljungberg O. Unilateral parathyroidectomy in hyperparathyroidism due to a single adenoma. Ann Surg 1982;195:245–52.
13. Udelsman R. Six hundred fifty-six consecutive explorations for primary hyperparathyroid. Ann Surg 2002;235:665–70.
14. Yeung GHC. Endoscopic thyroid surgery today: a diversity of surgical strategies. Thyroid 2002;12:703–6.
15. Ikeda Y, Takami H, Sasaki Y, Takayama J, Niimi M, Kan S. Clinical benefits in endoscopic thyroidectomy by the axillary approach. J Am Coll Surg 2003;196:189–95.
16. Ikeda Y, Takami H, Niimi M, Kan S, Sasaki Y, Takayama J. Endoscopic thyroidectomy and parathyroidectomy by the axillary approach – a preliminary report. Surg Endosc 2002;16:92–5.
17. Ikeda Y, Takami H, Tajima G, Sasaki Y, Takayama J, Kurihara H, Niimi M. Total endoscopic thyroidectomy: axillary or anterior chest approach. Biomed Pharmacother 2002;56:72s-78s
18. Ohgami M, IshiiS, Arisawa Y, Ohmori T, Noga K, Furukawa T, Kitajima M. Scarless endoscopic thyroidectomy: breast approach for better cosmesis. Surg Laparosc Endosc Percutan Tech 2000;10:1–4.
19. Inabnet WB, Gagner M. Endoscopic thyroidectomy: supraclavicular approach. In: Gagner M, Inabnet WB, eds. Minimally invasive endocrine surgery. Philadelphia: Lippincott, Williams & Wilkins; 2002.
20. Miccoli P, Bellantone R, Mourad M, Walz M, Raffaelli M, Berti P. Minimally invasive video-assisted thyroidectomy: multiinstitutional experience. World J Surg 2002;20:972–5.
21. Miccoli P, Berti P, Massimo C, Raffaelli M, Materazzi G. Minimally invasive video-assisted parathyroidectomy: lesson learned from 137 cases. J Am Coll Surg 2000;191:613–8.

22. Lo Gerfo P. Local/regional anesthesia for thyroidectomy: evaluation as an outpatient procedure. Surgery 1998;124:975–9.
23. Ferzli GS, Sayad P, Abdo Z, Cacchione RN. Minimally invasive, nonendoscopic thyroid surgery. J Am Coll Surg 2001;192:665–8.
24. Chapuis Y, Fulla Y, Bonnichon P, Tarla E, Abboud B, Pitre J, Richard B. Values of ultrasonography, sestamibi scintigraphy, and intraoperative measurement of 1–84 PTH for unilateral neck exploration of primary hyperparathyroidism. World J Surg 1996;20:835–40.
25. Kim CK, Kim S, Krynyckyi BR, Machac J, Inabnet WB. The efficacy of sestamibi para-thyroid scintigraphy for directing surgical approaches based on modified interpreta-tion criteria. Clin Nucl Med 2002;27:246–8.
26. Lumachi F, Zucchetta P, Marzola MC, Boccagni P, Angelini F, Bui F, D'Amico DF, Favia G. Advantages of combined technetium-99m sestamibi scintigraphy and high-reso-lution ultrasonography in parathyroid localization: comparative study in 91 patients with primary hyperparathyroidism. Eur J Endocrinol 2000;143:755–60.
27. Inabnet WB, Kin CK, Haber RS, Lopchinsky RA. Radioguidance is not necessary dur-ing parathyroidectomy. Arch Surg 2002;137:967–70.

Commentary

GÖRAN ÅKERSTRÖM

In 1982, Tibblin et al. [1] reported the first series of *unilateral parathyroid operation*. Without preoperative localization, however, most surgeons con-sidered a limited procedure inappropriate, and therefore a majority of pa-tients with hyperparathyroidism (HPT) was until recently subjected to con-ventional, bilateral cervical exploration. After pioneering evaluation of possi-bilities to apply minimally invasive procedures also for neck surgery, Gagner in 1996 reported the first endoscopic parathyroidectomy. With improvement in preoperative imaging of parathyroid glands, with sestamibi scintigraphy (MIBI), and due also to intense Internet marketing, the interest for minimally invasive parathyroid operations has thereafter markedly increased.

Endocrine surgeons in general have most easily adopted a unilateral *mini-open, focused approach* (MIP) with minimal incision over a preoperatively localized gland [2–4]. This operation has previously often been used in reop-erative parathyroid surgery. With appropriate selection of patients and using the quick intraoperative parathyroid hormone assay (IOPTH) to confirm ab-sence of additional pathological glands, the focused approach has with lim-ited follow-up had cure rates almost comparable with those of conventional open surgery. The MIP procedure can shorten operative time and hospital stay, and may in combination with regional anesthesia be performed ambula-tory with reduced hospital charges. Gamma probe radioguidance has been claimed to improve intraoperative localization of diseased glands, but has been abandoned at many centers because of imprecise results. This method may, as emphasized by the authors, be more important in reoperative parathyroid surgery.

Minimal video-assisted parathyroidectomy (MIVAP) may provide similar decrease in operative time and improved patient comfort [5]. It is said that this procedure can be adopted without a long learning curve by any experienced parathyroid surgeon. The proportion of patients eligible for MIVAP has increased with training to presently more than 70%. Preoperative localization with both MIBI and high-resolution ultrasonography (US) has improved the recruitment and success rate [5, 6].

Henry and colleagues have reported another method of *video-assisted parathyroidectomy with lateral approach*, which has also been considered attractive to learn for the endocrine surgeon [7]. Part of this operation is performed openly, with direct access via the incision for a trocar at the anterior border of the sternocleidoid muscle, and after endoscopic dissection the adenoma is delivered with open technique. Absence of dissection in the subplatysmal space minimizes the risk for subcutaneous emphysema. Possibly related to different stage of method development, somewhat lower proportion of patients (43%) has been considered eligible for this operation than for the MIVAP procedure. The conversion rate has also been slightly higher (16%, compared with 8% for MIVAP), reflecting that this method may require a somewhat longer learning period. The Henry method may be very efficient for glands behind the thyroid lobe or in the upper posterior mediastinum, whereas the MIVAP procedure may be preferred for glands at the lower thyroid pole or below it, and a combination of these methods can be recommended [5].

The *totally endoscopic method for parathyroidectomy* has been excellent in expert hands, but more difficult to learn for the endocrine surgeon without the extensive endoscopic expertise. The appropriate dissection plane may indeed be difficult to identify, and these operations are generally associated with longer operative times, and have a minimal but potential risk for subcutaneous emphysema.

The minimally invasive parathyroid operations are generally considered inappropriate for patients with multiglandular parathyroid disease (MGD) occurring in 10–15% of HPT patients, and are avoided also in familial and multiple endocrine neoplasia-associated HPT. The selection of patients is crucially dependent on high quality preoperative localization, which may be more equivocal in patients with only modest elevation of serum calcium who may have higher incidence of MGD. IOPTH can during operation strongly support the presence of single gland disease, but may not always show an appropriate 50% fall if baseline values are within the normal range [5]. Unfortunately, IOPTH may be misleading in patients with MGD, where it is most required [8]. The outcome of a minimally invasive operation therefore remains to some extent uncertain without follow-up, which for evaluation of real long-term results requires several years.

With open surgery 28% of thyroid operations, were reported possible to perform via an incision smaller than 3 cm, and may qualify as *minimally invasive open thyroid surgery* [9]. 63% needed an incision of 4 cm or larger, obviously dependent on the size of the lesion to remove. Exploration via a 4-cm or larger incision may not imply or require special minimally invasive techniques, as this is a common incision length in thyroid surgery. Placing the incision higher in the neck can make access easier, but may cause a more visible scar. In this context symmetry is crucial, and sometimes more important than incision length. Early ligature of superior pole vessels may facilitate delivery of the thyroid, and is common routine in thyroid surgery.

Minimally invasive video-assisted thyroidectomy (MIVAT) can be made with a 1.5-cm incision for thyroid nodules not exceeding 3 cm, with benign pathology and absence of thyroiditis or thyreotoxicosis. Total thyroidectomy has also been accomplished for nonaggressive papillary carcinoma.

Cervical endoscopic thyroidectomy has further advantage of causing almost no visible scar, but is generally more time consuming, and requires considerable longer learning period for an endocrine surgeon. *The transaxillary and chest approaches for endoscopic thyroidectomy* leave no visible scars in the neck, but are invasive, time-consuming procedures, performed by experts only. They also provide inefficient control of operative bleeding, and are unlikely to be commonly adopted by endocrine surgeons. Experience with these methods for parathyroidectomy is limited.

The authors of this chapter have succinctly described the new methods for neck surgery. It may be further emphasized that the results of the minimally invasive procedures have to be balanced against our present, generally extraordinary results of open neck surgery [10]. The scar after conventional neck incision is rarely annoying, and often not visible in commonly treated elderly patients, where it can often be concealed in a skin crease. An experienced endocrine surgeon can swiftly perform a conventional open procedure with minimal tissue trauma. Little additional time is often needed for the bilateral extension, which this far probably still remains as the safest procedure with superior long-term outcome in HPT. Nevertheless, the minimally invasive and endoscopic procedures represent important development and investment for the future, as they may in the long run provide improved image of anatomic details. It should, however, be crucial to select the new procedures for the appropriate patients, and maintain methods of conventional neck surgery as important basis for training. It has to be recognized that the minimally invasive, and especially the endoscopic operations, tend to be more difficult and require longer training period to be safely performed

References

1. Tibblin S, Bondeson AG, Ljungberg O. Unilateral parathyroidectomy in hyperparathyroidism due to single adenoma. Ann Surg 1982;195:245–52.
2. Udelsman R. Six hundred fifty-six consecutive explorations for primary hyperparathyroidism. Ann Surg 2002;235:665–70.
3. Monchik JM, Barellini L, Langer P, Kahya A. Minimally invasive parathyroid surgery in 103 patients with local/regional anesthesia, without exclusion criteria. Surgery 2002;131:502–8.
4. Sosa JA, Powe NR, Levine MA, Bowman HM, Zeiger MA, Udelsman R. Cost implications of different surgical strategies for primary hyperparathyroidism. Surgery 1998;124:1028.
5. Berti P, Materazzi G. Picone A, Miccoli P. Limits and drawbacks of video-assisted parathyroidectomy. Br J Surg 2003;90:743–7.
6. Arici C, Cheah K, Ituarte PHG, Morita E, Lynch TC, Siperstein AE et al. Can localization studies be used to direct focused parathyroid operations? Surgery 2001;129:720–9.
7. Henry J-F, Iacobone M, Mirallie E, Deveze A, Pili S. Indications and results of video-assisted parathyroidectomy by a lateral approach in patients with primary hyperparathyroidism. Surgery 2001;130:999–1004.
8. Proye CA, Goropoulos A, Franz C, Carnaille B, Vix M, Quievreux JL, Couplet-Lebon G, Racadot A. Usefulness and limits of quick intraoperative measurements of intact (1–84) parathyroid hormone in the surgical management of hyperparathyroidism: sequential measurements in patients with multiglandular parathyroid disease. Surgery 1991;110:1035–42.
9. Ferzli GS, Sayad P, Abdo Z, Cacchione RN. Minimally invasive, nonendoscopic thyroid surgery. J Am Coll Surg 2001;192:665–8.
10. van Heerden JA, Grant CS. Surgical treatment of primary hyperparathyroidism: an institutional perspective. World J Surg 1991;15:688–92.

Subject Index